Total Well-being

Editors

ALISON J. BRAINARD
LYNDSAY M. HOY

ANESTHESIOLOGY CLINICS

www.anesthesiology.theclinics.com

Consulting Editor
LEE A. FLEISHER

June 2022 • Volume 40 • Number 2

ELSEVIER

1600 John F. Kennedy Boulevard • Suite 1800 • Philadelphia, Pennsylvania, 19103-2899

http://www.theclinics.com

ANESTHESIOLOGY CLINICS Volume 40, Number 2
June 2022 ISSN 1932-2275, ISBN-13: 978-0-323-98781-3

Editor: Joanna Collett
Developmental Editor: Arlene Campos

Anesthesiology Clinics (ISSN 1932-2275) is published quarterly by Elsevier Inc., 360 Park Avenue South, New York, NY 10010-1710. Months of issue are March, June, September, and December. Periodicals postage paid at New York, NY and at additional mailing offices. Subscription prices are $100.00 per year (US student/resident), $375.00 per year (US individuals), $464.00 per year (Canadian individuals), $986.00 per year (US institutions), $1016.00 per year (Canadian institutions), $100.00 per year (Canadian student/resident), $225.00 per year (foreign student/resident), $498.00 per year (foreign individuals), and $1016.00 per year (foreign institutions). To receive student and resident rate, orders must be accompanied by name of affiliated institution, date of term, and the *signature* of program/residency coordinator on institutions letterhead. Orders will be billed at individual rate until proof of status is received. Foreign air speed delivery is included in all *Clinics'* subscription prices. All prices are subject to change without notice. POSTMASTER: Send address changes to *Anesthesiology Clinics,* Elsevier Health Sciences Division, Subscription Customer Service, 3251 Riverport Lane, Maryland Heights, MO 63043. Customer Service (orders, claims, online, change of address): Elsevier Health Sciences Division, Subscription Customer Service, 3251 Riverport Lane, Maryland Heights, MO 63043. **Tel:1-800-654-2452 (U.S. and Canada); 314-447-8871 (outside U.S. and Canada). Fax: 314-447-8029. E-mail: journalscustomerservice-usa@elsevier.com (for print support); journalsonlinesupport-usa@elsevier.com (for online support).**

Reprints. For copies of 100 or more of articles in this publication, please contact the Commercial Reprints Department, Elsevier Inc., 360 Park Avenue South, New York, NY 10010-1710. Tel.: 212-633-3874; Fax: 212-633-3820; E-mail: reprints@elsevier.com.

Anesthesiology Clinics, is also published in Spanish by McGraw-Hill Inter-americana Editores S. A., P.O. Box 5-237, 06500 Mexico D. F., Mexico.

Anesthesiology Clinics, is covered in *MEDLINE/PubMed (Index Medicus), Current Contents/Clinical Medicine, Excerpta Medica, ISI/BIOMED*, and *Chemical Abstracts*.

Contributors

CONSULTING EDITOR

LEE A. FLEISHER, MD, FACC, FAHA
Robert D. Dripps Professor and Chair of Anesthesiology and Critical Care, Professor of Medicine, Perelman School of Medicine, University of Pennsylvania, Philadelphia, Pennsylvania

EDITORS

ALISON J. BRAINARD, MD
Associate Professor of Anesthesiology, Co-Director of Well-being, Medical Director, Cherry Creek North Ambulatory Surgical Center, Department of Anesthesiology, University of Colorado, Aurora, Colorado

LYNDSAY M. HOY, MD
Assistant Professor, Department of Anesthesiology and Critical Care, University of Pennsylvania, Philadelphia, Pennsylvania

AUTHORS

DANIEL ABRAHAM, MD
Assistant Professor, Department of Anesthesiology and Critical Care, Perelman School of Medicine at the University of Pennsylvania, Philadelphia, Pennsylvania

ANOUSHKA M. AFONSO, MD, FASA
Assistant Professor, Department of Anesthesiology and Critical Care, Memorial Sloan Kettering Cancer Center, New York, New York

KAMNA S. BALHARA, MD, MA, FACEP
Assistant Professor of Emergency Medicine, Emergency Medicine Residency Program, Assistant Director, Health Humanities at Hopkins EM, Co-Director, Johns Hopkins School of Medicine, Johns Hopkins Department of Emergency Medicine, Baltimore, Maryland

OLIVER BAWMANN, MD
Resident Physician, Internal Medicine-Pediatrics Department, University of Colorado School of Medicine, Aurora, Colorado

LAURA K. BERENSTAIN, MD, FASA, ACC
Adjunct Professor of Clinical Anesthesiology, Cincinnati Children's Hospital Medical Center, Cincinnati, Ohio

ALAN ROBERT BIELSKY, MD
Associate Professor, University of Colorado School of Medicine. Director of Pain Service, Children's Hospital Colorado, Colorado

NATALIE J. BODMER, MD
Adult Cardiothoracic Anesthesiology Fellow, Department of Anesthesiology, Perioperative and Pain Medicine, Stanford University School of Medicine, Stanford, California

KENNETH B. BROWN, Jr., MD
Department of Anesthesiology, The University of North Carolina at Chapel Hill, Chapel Hill, North Carolina

STEPHANIE I. BYERLY, MD
Professor, Department of Anesthesiology and Pain Management, University of Texas Southwestern, Dallas, Texas

THOMAS J. CARUSO, MD, MEd
Clinical Professor, Department of Anesthesiology, Perioperative and Pain Medicine, Stanford University School of Medicine, Stanford, California

JOYCE M. CHANG, MD
Assistant Professor, Department of Anesthesia and Perioperative Care, University of California, San Francisco, San Francisco, California

FEI CHEN, PhD, MEd
Department of Anesthesiology, The University of North Carolina at Chapel Hill, Chapel Hill, North Carolina

MALISSA CLARK, PhD
Industrial and Organizational Psychology, Associate Professor, Department of Psychology, University of Georgia, Athens, Georgia

SHEELA PAI COLE, MD, FASE, FASA
Clinical Professor, Department of Anesthesiology, Perioperative and Pain Medicine, Stanford University, Stanford, California

ARIANNA COOK, MD, MPH
Department of Anesthesiology, The University of North Carolina at Chapel Hill, Chapel Hill, North Carolina

CHRISTOPHER COWART, MD
Assistant Professor, Department of Anesthesiology and Perioperative Medicine, Penn State College of Medicine, Hershey, Pennsylvania

ELIZABETH W. DUGGAN, MD, MA
Industrial and Organizational Psychology, Associate Professor, Department of Anesthesiology and Perioperative Medicine, The University of Alabama at Birmingham, Birmingham, Alabama

MICHAEL R. EHMANN, MD, MPH, MS, FACEP
Assistant Professor of Emergency Medicine, Emergency Medicine Residency Program, Associate Director, Health Humanities at Hopkins EM, Faculty, Johns Hopkins School of Medicine, Johns Hopkins Department of Emergency Medicine, Baltimore, Maryland

CAROLYN BERGER FOLEY, MD
Assistant Professor, Department of Anesthesiology, University of Colorado School of Medicine, Children's Hospital Colorado, Colorado

ANNERY G. GARCIA-MARCINKIEWICZ, MD, MSCE
Assistant Professor of Anesthesiology and Critical Care Medicine, The Children's Hospital of Philadelphia, Department of Anesthesiology and Critical Care, Philadelphia, Pennsylvania

MICHAEL A. GROPPER, MD, PhD
Professor and Chair, Department of Anesthesia and Perioperative Care, University of California, San Francisco, San Francisco, California

KUSH GUPTA, BS
Medical Student, Stanford University School of Medicine, Stanford, California

NATHAN IRVIN, MD, MSHPR, FACEP
Assistant Professor of Emergency Medicine, Health Humanities at Hopkins EM, Co-Director, Johns Hopkins School of Medicine, Johns Hopkins Department of Emergency Medicine, Baltimore, Maryland; Center Faculty for the Center for Mental Health and Addiction Policy Research at Johns Hopkins Bloomberg School of Public Health

HUNG-MO LIN, ScD
Professor, Department of Population Health Science and Policy, Icahn School of Medicine at Mount Sinai, New York, New York

LAUREN LISANN-GOLDMAN, MD
Cardiothoracic Anesthesiology Fellow, Department of Anesthesiology, Montefiore Medical Center, New York, New York

STEVEN R. LOWENSTEIN, MD, MPH
Professor of Emergency Medicine and Medicine, Associate Dean of Faculty Affairs, University of Colorado School of Medicine, Aurora, Colorado

BRYAN MAHONEY, MD
Associate Professor, Department of Anesthesiology, Perioperative and Pain Medicine, Mount Sinai Morningside and West Hospitals, New York, New York

ELIZABETH B. MALINZAK, MD
Assistant Professor, Department of Anesthesiology, Duke University, Durham, North Carolina

REBECCA D. MARGOLIS, DO, FAOCA
Assistant Professor, Department of Anesthesiology Critical Care Medicine, Children's Hospital Los Angeles, University of Southern California Keck School of Medicine, Los Angeles, California

SCOTT D. MARKOWITZ, MD
Vice Chair for Professional Development and Diversity, Professor of Anesthesiology, Equity, and Inclusion, Department of Anesthesiology, Washington University School of Medicine, St Louis, Missouri

SUSAN M. MARTINELLI, MD, FASA
Department of Anesthesiology, The University of North Carolina at Chapel Hill, Chapel Hill, North Carolina

MADELYN MENDLEN
Medical Student, University of Colorado School of Medicine, Aurora, Colorado

DORRE NICHOLAU, MD, PhD
Professor, Department of Anesthesia and Perioperative Care, University of California, San Francisco, San Francisco, California

BARBARA ORLANDO, MD, PhD
Associate Professor, Department of Anesthesiology, McGovern Medical School, The University of Texas Health Science Center at Houston, Memorial Hermann Hospital, Houston, Texas

TRAVIS REECE-NGUYEN, MD, MPH, FAAP
Clinical Assistant Professor, Department of Anesthesiology, Perioperative, and Pain Medicine, Division of Pediatric Anesthesiology, Stanford Medicine, Stanford, California

KELSEY M. REPINE, MD
Resident Physician, Anesthesiology Department, University of Colorado School of Medicine, Aurora, Colorado

LEELACH ROTHSCHILD, MD
Associate Professor of Clinical Anesthesiology, University of Illinois Hospital and Health Sciences System, Chicago, Illinois

AUDREY SHAFER, MD
Professor, Anesthesiology, Perioperative and Pain Medicine, Stanford University School of Medicine, Veterans Affairs Palo Alto Health Care System, Anesthesia, Palo Alto, California

SHAHLA SIDDIQUI, MD, DABA, MSc, FCCM
Assistant Professor, Department of Anesthesia, Critical Care and Pain Medicine, Beth Israel Deaconess Medical Center, Harvard Medical School, Boston, Massachusetts

JINA L. SINSKEY, MD, FASA
Associate Professor, Department of Anesthesia and Perioperative Care, University of California, San Francisco, San Francisco, California

SARAH S. TITLER, MD
Clinical Associate Professor, Department of Anesthesia, Division of Pediatric Anesthesia, Department of Pediatrics, University of Iowa, Iowa City, Iowa

ALBERT H. TSAI, MD
Clinical Assistant Professor, Department of Anesthesiology, Perioperative and Pain Medicine, Stanford University School of Medicine, Stanford, California

AMY E. VINSON, MD, FAAP
Assistant Professor of Anaesthesia, Department of Anesthesiology, Critical Care and Pain Medicine, Boston Children's Hospital, Harvard Medical School, Boston, Massachusetts

JO M. VOGELI, PhD
Assistant Professor, Health and Well-being Psychologist, Department of Anesthesiology Well-being Program, University of Colorado School of Medicine, Anschutz Medical Campus, Aurora, Colorado

CIERA WARD, MD
Christus Mother Frances Hospital, Anesthesia, Tyler, Texas

Contents

The collective threat to physician well-being is a complex issue with no clear solution. Even before the coronavirus disease 2019 pandemic, physicians suffered from widespread burnout and moral injury, with negative consequences for patient care, physician health, and the health care system. Initial clinician well-being efforts leaned heavily on individual-focused interventions. However, workplace culture and environment are key factors that affect burnout, and therefore clinician well-being efforts require both individual-focused and systems-level interventions. A sustainable culture of support in medicine is necessary to foster physician well-being.

Women represent approximately one-third of all anesthesiologists in the United States. Before the COVID-19 pandemic, research regarding gender bias in anesthesiology defined the scope of the problem. Unfortunately, the pandemic exposed and expanded the imbalances associated with gender, placing women anesthesiologists as both primary caregivers in the home and on the frontlines of health care. These systemic inequities exacerbated burnout in women anesthesiologists. Several initiatives that can improve well-being and the work culture for all anesthesiologists, including women, will also be discussed.

There are several work-related barriers to breastfeeding among physician mothers including: lack of appropriate place for breastmilk expression, unpredictable and inflexible schedules, and lack of time to breastfeed or express milk. In a survey of physician mothers, those who were in surgical and procedural subspecialties, including anesthesiology, reported a lack of lactation facilities in close proximity to the operating room as a barrier to breastfeeding. Unlike other physicians and clinicians in different health care environments, anesthesiology is unique in that there is often no built-in time for breaks or a predictable end time to the operating room schedule. A break system is typically established, within an institution, for meal break relief for trainees, Certified Registered Nurse Anesthetist, and Anesthesia Assistants. This system for breaks may not be sufficient to accommodate the frequency or length required for lactation sessions. In addition, these break systems do not typically provide relief for supervising anesthesiologists for meals or lactation sessions. A study of physician mothers across specialties identified anesthesiologists as significantly more likely than women of other medical specialties to self-report maternal discrimination. The study defined maternal discrimination as discrimination based on pregnancy, maternity leave, or breastfeeding. As a workforce and specialty, we must support our breastfeeding anesthesiologists and facilitate lactation needs on return to the workplace.

Increasing attention is being paid to both anesthesiologist well-being and commitments to diversity, equity, and inclusion. Sexual minorities (ie, members of the lesbian, gay, bisexual, transgender, queer/questioning, intersex, and asexual [LGBTQIA] communities) face many challenges in society and the workplace, including mental health conditions, discrimination, and increased risk for burnout. In this review, we outline the current state of mental health conditions and burnout in sexual minority individuals, discrimination and harassment faced both in society and the workplace, and steps that workplaces can take to become more inclusive and welcoming.

Addressing resident wellness is an important topic given the high risk for burnout and depression in resident physicians compared with the general U.S. population. This article provides an overview of various approaches to help conceptualize and intervene on resident wellness, based on the 9-strategies framework to improve wellness laid out by Shanafelt and colleagues. This article outlines the most relevant literature in each strategy followed by the authors' experience within their anesthesiology residency program.

Resident physician burnout and well-being are increasingly important and salient topics in medical training. Unfortunately, limited research exists regarding the efficacy of various burnout and wellness interventions for resident physicians. Better characterization of the causes of burnout and the components of well-being must necessarily precede implementation and evaluation of interventions. The authors advocate for an increased role for technology in implementing and studying wellness programming for resident physicians. In addition, they describe an intervention under development at the University of Colorado School of Medicine that uses a "Gratitude Journal" smartphone app to support trainee wellness.

Racism represents a public health crisis, adversely impacting patient outcomes and health care workplace inclusivity. Dismantling racism requires transforming both racist systems and individual and collective consciousness. Focusing on antiracism in health professions education through the transdisciplinary lens of the health humanities can spur self-reflection, critical thinking, and collaboration among health professions educators and trainees to create more equitable structures of care. This article describes how the health humanities provide a powerful framework for antiracist health professions education. The authors conclude with a snapshot of an existing humanities-based antiracist curriculum, with suggestions to facilitate implementation in other settings.

Mentorships play a critical role in the development of physician careers and should be tailored within a structured, evidence-based mentoring program to ensure mutual benefit and avoidance of pitfalls. We offer a narrative review of the current literature and commentary on mentoring at the medical student, GME trainee, and early career faculty levels within anesthesiology, and propose a framework on which an effective mentoring program can be implemented.

Early-career physicians face a broad range of challenges unique to their phase of life and career. Beginning in residency, anesthesiologists encounter stressors unique to their work environment, which, when coupled with their personal life demands, places significant burden and creates potential for burnout. In this article, the authors review the literature to explore the contributors of burnout in early-career anesthesiologists, evaluate the relationship between compassionate care and empathic distress, and propose strategies to prevent and treat burnout in this specific subset of anesthesiologists.

This article explores an often-untouched subject in anesthesiology residency: relationships. The authors examine the importance of fostering all types of relationships (eg, personal, professional, self) and the impact of the training process on relationships and total well-being. Common issues in relationships during anesthesiology residency are shared through real-life anecdotes from physicians who are currently in or have completed their residencies. Psychological principles including optimism bias, cognitive dissonance, social comparison, and self-efficacy are explored as contributing to dysfunction in relationships. Strategies are offered for each psychological domain as a resource for faculty and program leadership to improve the residency experience in anesthesiology.

> The practice of anesthesiology requires both clinical skills and the ability to navigate complex social situations. Leadership skills such as emotional intelligence, adaptability, conflict management, and negotiation are crucial for success but infrequently taught. Coaching is a thought-provoking process that enhances self-awareness and inspires the maximization of personal and professional potential. It has been used in the business world for personal and professional development for decades, and evidence now exists that coaching also provides benefits for physicians in both professional development and well-being.

> When describing health care provider wellness, diet and nutrition are typically not addressed. This, in combination with the lack of decent food and diet resources typically available to the typically busy health care provider, exposes a significant gap in the road to advancing clinician wellness. This article aims to describe the relationship between nutrition and well-being, and potential barriers to optimal nutrition encountered by health care providers in the workplace. Readily available and practical strategies to improve physician diet and nutrition include: mindful eating practices, home meal preparation, food journaling, and mobile applications. From an organizational level, once physicians are making more informed food choices it is the hospital's responsibility to make nutritional options available in the workplace.

> Poetry and medicine are related in multiple ways, including historical interests in healing, defined broadly, through words. More contemporary scholarship explores how poems, which include insights into the human condition, can enlarge our understanding of health, illness, mortality, and health care, including issues of diversity. Anesthesiology and poetry have particular affinities due to their structures, timeframes, and rhythms. Patients, physicians, and health care workers can benefit in terms of well-being by access to reading, reflecting on, and writing poetry.

> Burnout among critical care personnel has increased due to the additional psychological and physical demands of caring for critically ill patients with limited resources. Factors that increase the risk of burnout include compassion fatigue, lack of control over the work environment, difficult interpersonal relationships, and constant exposure to end-of-life issues. Organizational commitment to physician wellbeing depends on improving workplace efficiency, recognizing stressors in the critical care environment, and providing resources to help manage staffing shortages. Community building, training in communication, and team-building strategies are important steps in building collaboration and camaraderie in the workplace.

ANESTHESIOLOGY CLINICS

SERIES OF RELATED INTEREST

Critical Care Clinics

THE CLINICS ARE AVAILABLE ONLINE!
Access your subscription at:
www.theclinics.com

Foreword

Ensuring Well-Being in a Postpandemic World: Ensuring our Specialty Maintains its Resilience

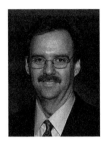

Lee A. Fleisher, MD, FACC, FAHA
Consulting Editor

Clinician well-being and burnout has been the subject of numerous academic studies and media attention as a cause of individuals leaving the field and medical errors. The COVID-19 pandemic has only exacerbated the issues with the stressors of taking care of ill individuals and the loneliness from continuously wearing masks. In this issue of *Anesthesiology Clinics*, the editors have assembled a series of articles with a focus on the unique challenges in specific populations. They also have numerous articles on strategies to enhance well-being.

We were fortunate to identify two leaders to edit this issue. Alison Brainard, MD is an Associate Professor at the University of Colorado in the Department of Anesthesiology. She is a member of the Occupational Health and the Physician Well-Being Committees within the American Society of Anesthesiologists (ASA). She is the co-director of well-being for the Department of Anesthesiology at the University of Colorado and is a founding member for the hospital's Faculty Engagement and Well-Being Committee. Alison has been leading the resident well-being curriculum for the last 6 years and has multiple publications on the topics of well-being and curricular design. Dr Brainard has spoken around the country on the topics of resiliency, second victim, peer support, and burnout. Lyndsay M. Hoy, MD, is an Assistant Professor in the Department of Anesthesiology and Critical Care at the Perelman School of Medicine at the University of Pennsylvania. She is currently a member of the ASA's Committee on Physician Well-Being, the department wellness champion for the Perelman School of Medicine Faculty Wellness Committee and the Penn GME Wellness Committee, co-lead for Penn Women in Anesthesiology, faculty co-director of Rx/Museum, and a board member of The LAM Foundation. She is a Harvard Macy fellow and recently completed the Stanford Physician Well-being Director course

Anesthesiology Clin 40 (2022) xiii–xiv
https://doi.org/10.1016/j.anclin.2022.02.001
1932-2275/22/© 2022 Published by Elsevier Inc.

and the Empowering Women Physicians coaching program. Together they have assembled a stellar group of authors.

Lee A. Fleisher, MD, FACC, FAHA
3400 Spruce Street, Dulles 680
Philadelphia, PA 19104, USA

E-mail address:
Lee.Fleisher@uphs.upenn.edu

Preface

Total Well-Being in Anesthesiology: Looking Beyond COVID-19

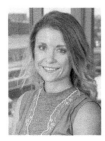 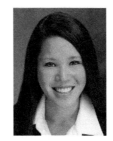

Alison J. Brainard, MD   Lyndsay M. Hoy, MD
Editors

It is admittedly impossible to predict where we will be in the COVID-19 pandemic by the time our readers receive this issue—hopefully, somewhere better, and not at the height of yet another surge or amid preparations for one. Indeed, it seems uncertainty has endured as the only reliable theme throughout these unsettling times. Likewise, physician well-being has emerged as a pandemic in its own right, as the ways in which we care for one another and ourselves—as individuals, medical professionals, and a society—have been upended. One thing has become abundantly clear: the adage of putting on your own oxygen mask before caring for others resonates now, perhaps more than ever.

Caring for the critically ill during a global pandemic, particularly when basic safety needs of frontline clinicians are compromised and science is met with skepticism, has wrought extraordinary personal and professional moral fatigue and injury. The suicide of emergency medicine physician Lorna Breen, MD, tragically epitomized the untold suffering and grief experienced by so many in health care. The long-term sequela in anesthesiology remains to be seen, and we have reason to worry—in a specialty already vulnerable to loneliness, feelings of despair, burnout, and isolation now exacerbated by the pandemic are pressing considerations for trainees, faculty, health care systems, and professional organizations alike. It is prescient to look beyond the pandemic and ask ourselves as a collective: what do anesthesiologists need to be well and stay well?

We are at a critical juncture in anesthesiology, one that has illuminated the interconnectedness of physician burnout, organizational accountability, institutional culture, systemic inequity, structural racism, gender bias, underrepresentation, social justice, psychological and physical workplace safety, peer support, patient safety, compassion

Anesthesiology Clin 40 (2022) xv–xvi
https://doi.org/10.1016/j.anclin.2022.01.015
1932-2275/22/© 2022 Published by Elsevier Inc.

fatigue, domestic caregiving responsibilities, and job security, among others. In urgently recognizing—and embracing—physician well-being as durational, we have the opportunity to disrupt, remodel, and invest in sustained wellness efforts while engendering compassion for ourselves and one another. We must intentionally and diligently assess the ongoing toll of the pandemic on anesthesiologists' well-being and continue to do so. We must all be stewards of wellness in anesthesiology by upholding a culture of care and making space for the conversations foregrounded in this issue and within our workplaces.

This inaugural well-being issue of *Anesthesiology Clinics* is an intentional effort to collate different institutions and organizations' wellness experiences, authored by peers and trainees both within our field and beyond. We hope this diverse compilation of perspectives yields insights to broaden our understanding of how to operationalize well-being in relevant clinical and educational contexts. From systems-based and individual interventions to "bottom-up" initiatives and curricula, the articles presented here thoughtfully advocate that timely action is essential if we want to attract and retain diverse, bright individuals within our field and to continue doing the work of caring for others.

We wish to thank Dr. Lee Fleisher for entrusting us with this timely and incredibly urgent issue. To Joanna Collett and Arlene Campos, we could not have done this without your patience and guidance. To our many authors, we are beyond grateful for your generosity of spirit, professionalism, and collegiality. We recognize that we approached you at a challenging moment and greatly appreciate your shared wisdom and lived experiences. We see this issue as a joint effort and collective embodiment of the ethos we hope will permeate and impact wellness and well-being efforts in anesthesiology across programs and institutions.

Alison J. Brainard, MD
Department of Anesthesiology, University of Colorado, 12401 East 17th Avenue, 7th Floor, Aurora, CO 80045, USA

Lyndsay M. Hoy, MD
Department of Anesthesiology and Critical Care, University of Pennsylvania, 3400 Spruce Street, 6 Dulles, Philadelphia, PA 19104, USA

E-mail addresses:
Alison.Brainard@cuanschutz.edu (A.J. Brainard)
Lyndsay.Hoy@pennmedicine.upenn.edu (L.M. Hoy)

The Wicked Problem of Physician Well-Being

Jina L. Sinskey, MD[a],*, Rebecca D. Margolis, DO[b,1], Amy E. Vinson, MD[c,2]

KEYWORDS

- Physician well-being • Wellness • Burnout • Professionalism

KEY POINTS

- The collective threat to physician well-being is a complex issue that is difficult to solve.
- The COVID-19 pandemic has exposed existing problems within the health care system, resulting in widespread clinician burnout and moral injury.
- Clinician burnout has negative consequences for patient care, physician health, and the health care system.
- Clinician well-being efforts require both individual-focused and systems-level interventions.
- A sustainable culture of support in medicine is necessary to foster physician well-being.

INTRODUCTION

The collective threat to physician well-being is a complex issue with no clear solution emerging despite nearly a decade's worth of efforts dedicated to battling physician burnout. Even before the coronavirus disease 2019 (COVID-19) pandemic, physicians were struggling under a health care system where they felt micromanaged and demoralized due to a combination of increasing clerical burden and physician performance metrics that eroded the meaning, autonomy, and purpose in their work.[1] The COVID-19 pandemic has widened and exposed these cracks and worsened the situation by hurtling physicians into a collective crisis of moral injury. Health care professionals were already being pushed to the breaking point, with 59% of practicing anesthesiologists in the United States at high risk for burnout at the dawn of the pandemic.[2] It is hard to fathom that the situation has improved since.

[a] Department of Anesthesia and Perioperative Care, University of California, San Francisco, CA, USA; [b] Department of Anesthesiology Critical Care Medicine, Children's Hospital Los Angeles, University of Southern California Keck School of Medicine, Los Angeles, CA, USA; [c] Department of Anesthesiology, Critical Care and Pain Medicine, Boston Children's Hospital & Harvard Medical School, Boston, MA, USA
[1] Present address: 839 North Frederic Street, Burbank, CA 91505.
[2] Present address: 300 Longwood Avenue, Bader 3, Boston, MA 02115
* Corresponding author. 550 16th Street, San Francisco, CA 94158.
E-mail address: Jina.Sinskey@ucsf.edu
Twitter: @JinaSinskeyMD (J.L.S.); @RebeccaMargolis (R.D.M.); @imswimming3 (A.E.V.)

Anesthesiology Clin 40 (2022) 213–223
https://doi.org/10.1016/j.anclin.2022.01.001
1932-2275/22/

The issue of physician well-being is a "wicked problem" in medicine. The term "wicked problem" was coined in the 1970s and refers to social or cultural problems that are ill-defined and inherently unsolvable (**Table 1**).[3] Unlike an arithmetical problem, a "wicked problem" does not have a clear-cut solution. Attempts at solutions tend to reveal new aspects of the problem, often changing the nature of the problem itself. For example, in the early months of the COVID-19 pandemic, masking and social distancing were the predominant solutions to flatten the curve, while a vaccine was being developed. Once the vaccine was created, it seemed as if the COVID-19 problem would be solved. However, issues of vaccine hesitancy, widespread misinformation, emerging variants, and inequitable global vaccine distribution then became the "new" problems.

The main characteristic of a "wicked problem" is that it is impossible to define. The word "well-being" itself is ambiguous because (1) it has no clear definition, (2) it is often used interchangeably with the word "wellness," and (3) its meaning has markedly transformed over time. Initial efforts to promote "wellness" in the workplace focused on the individual with institutions encouraging clinicians to maintain a healthy lifestyle and improve resilience. Over time, the definition of "well-being" evolved to encompass the effects of organizational and systemic factors that support a culture and environment where clinicians can thrive.[4] Yet, many physician well-being initiatives continue to fixate on the individual, reinforcing the idea that clinicians are solely responsible for their own burnout. When taking a step back to remember that "burnout" is by definition an occupational phenomenon,[5] it becomes unacceptable to place the onus on the

Table 1
Ten characteristics of "wicked problems" and implications for solving problems

Characteristics of "Wicked Problems"	Implications for Solving "Wicked Problems"
No clear definition of the problem	Requires a systems approach
No stopping rule	Unclear when the problem is solved because there is always the possibility of a better solution
Solutions are not right or wrong, they are better or worse	No clear consensus as to which solution will solve the problem
No immediate or ultimate test for a solution	Any solution creates waves of consequences over an extended period
"One shot" operation: each implemented solution has far-reaching consequences	No opportunity to learn by trial-and-error due to high stakes
Infinite number of potential solutions	It is a matter of judgment which solutions should be pursued and implemented
Every "wicked problem" is essentially unique	Effective solutions in one context cannot be directly transferred to another context
Every "wicked problem" is a symptom of an underlying, deeper issue	Solving a "wicked problem" often reveals a deeper problem that is more difficult to solve
No single explanation to the problem	The choice of explanation determines the way the problem is addressed
Problem solvers have no "right to be wrong"	Taking on "wicked problems" can be risky, and problem solvers must be fully responsible for their actions

Data from Rittel HWJ, Webber MM. Dilemmas in a general theory of planning. Policy Sci 1973;4(2):155–169.

individual. In this context, well-being efforts can ironically be turned into a weapon to blame and shame clinicians for a purported lack of personal optimization, potentially and paradoxically worsening clinician burnout.

Another characteristic of a "wicked problem" is that every attempt at a solution comes with high stakes because each implemented solution leaves "traces" that cannot be undone.[3] Every time physicians are asked to attend a mandatory well-being lecture during their free time or fill out a well-being survey without clear follow-up or accountable change, they lose confidence that the time and energy spent participating in such efforts translate into tangible improvements to their workplace and well-being. Over time, this can rightfully lead to further dissatisfaction, demoralization, and disengagement in the health care workforce.

Clinician burnout is a pressing issue with negative consequences for patient care, physician health, and the health care system.[6] The COVID-19 pandemic blew open the existing cracks in the health care system and continues to take an immeasurable toll on the physical, mental, and emotional health of health care professionals. A once highly motivated, engaged workforce of health care workers is now threadbare from moral injury, watching a nation divided and science repudiated. We are beginning to see an impending crisis of health care staffing shortages, and if for no other reason than the continued solvency of the overall health care system, we must reevaluate our approach to clinician well-being and course-correct before it is too late. If history is any teacher, we should expect reverberations in the health care workforce far exceeding those experienced following prior epidemics (eg, the 2003 SARS-CoV-1 outbreak in Canada), which were substantial.[7] Here we discuss the evolution of well-being efforts in medicine and how we can move forward to build a sustainable culture of physician well-being.

A Brief History of "Wellness" in Medicine

"In no relationship is the physician more often derelict than in his duty to himself."[8] This statement, uttered by Sir William Osler, considered by many to be the father of modern medical education, underscores a truth about our profession that has not changed considerably over the past century. Physicians enter medicine with a laudable intention to help others—to bestow kindness to their fellow man via the highly trained and executed stewardship of their gifts. To this day, physicians in training dutifully recite the Hippocratic Oath at white coat ceremonies where they solemnly vow to place patients' needs above their own. But who teaches them how to sustain this? Who lets them in on the secret that there are limits? Who prevents them from spiraling down the rabbit hole of competitive self-effacement and performative self-sacrifice? Certainly not the modern health care infrastructure that relies heavily on this mindset to ask a workforce already stretched thin to "do more with less."

There has always been dysfunction and unwellness in medicine. Storied physicians, including Osler himself, were plagued by depression, suicidality, and substance use disorders.[9,10] This burden of substance use disorder and suicide has declared itself and continues within our own ranks of anesthesiologists today.[11–13] The work of helping the sick has always and ever will be difficult, but the fulfillment of a worthy practice held a promise that has continually brought bright, diligent people to the medical professions.

It was not until 2012 that a sharp focus on physician well-being emerged. Shanafelt and colleagues[14] published the first large-scale study of burnout in the US physician population, revealing that nearly half of US physicians were at "high risk for burnout." Burnout, an occupational phenomenon, had been studied widely in a range of human service industries, but never in medicine on a large scale. This, understandably, caught the public's attention, and a flurry of lay press attention ensued with public now doubting the fitness of their physician workforce. At this point, with public scrutiny mounting, it was no longer a problem that could be ignored. For those already enmeshed in the work of physician support and well-being, this was a welcome change and justification for their ongoing work. But the focus was not as crisp as one would hope—the angle of attack was on physicians—something was wrong with doctors, so how do we fix them?

Over the coming years, hundreds of papers were published, focusing primarily on individual interventions to improve well-being, from meditation and mindfulness to nutrition, sleep, and physical fitness. Occasionally a pilot study would be published showing modest improvements in some metric of well-being, but this was rarely followed by larger randomized controlled trials. Throughout this time, a disdain for all things "wellness" was growing in the medical community—it was justified, as we will discuss in the next section.

Then in 2018, many forces began coming together, shifting focus from the individual to the systems and policies ultimately crafting the culture of medicine. Two national organizations in particular, the Accreditation Council for Graduate Medical Education (ACGME) and the National Academy of Medicine (NAM), have highlighted the importance of using a systems approach to address clinician well-being. In 2017, the ACGME revised its Common Program Requirements to emphasize the importance of positive learning and working environments for trainee well-being.[15] In 2019, the NAM issued a report titled "Taking Action Against Clinician Burnout: A Systems Approach to Professional Well-Being," which introduced 6 goals to enhance clinician well-being (**Table 2**).[4] National organizations, armed with datasets demonstrating the return on investment for well-being initiatives and the profound downstream effects of physician burnout on patient safety and quality of care, joined together to call for systemic change[16] and began focusing on pragmatic solutions. This seismic shift in approach was punctuated by an editorial by Thomas Schwenk,[17] where he stated that "Physicians in 2018 are the proverbial 'canary in the coal mine.' While the canary may be sick, it is the mine that is toxic. Caring for the sick canary is compassionate, but likely futile until there is more fresh air in the mine."

Fast forward 3 years, and we are grappling not only with a global pandemic but also a reckoning of systemic racism and societal unrest. We are living in "unprecedented times" and with that comes new approaches and perspectives. Owing to the collective, slow-moving trauma experienced by the health care community during the COVID-19 pandemic, we are now more openly discussing the topics of mental health, well-being, and injustice that were previously stigmatized into silence.

Well-Being 1.0: Where We Failed

Given the history of well-being in medicine, it is not surprising that the first iteration of clinician well-being efforts leaned heavily on individual interventions such as mindfulness classes, yoga, and resilience training. One reason is that the primary objective of initial well-being efforts was to address burnout, and at the time there was a tendency to think of burnout as an individual problem. However, burnout stems from chronic workplace stress that has not been successfully managed.[18] As workplace culture and environment affect burnout, individual-focused interventions alone cannot sufficiently address the issue, thus the inclusion of systems-level interventions is necessary.

Despite repeated calls for a systems approach to physician well-being, health care organizations have continued to predominantly allocate their attention and resources to individual-focused interventions. Physicians already exhibit high levels of resilience[6]

Table 2
National Academy of Medicine goals for eliminating clinician burnout and enhancing professional well-being

Goal	Description
Create positive work environments	Transform health care work systems by creating positive work environments that prevent and reduce burnout, foster professional well-being, and support quality care
Create positive learning environments	Transform health professions education and training to optimize learning environments that prevent and reduce burnout and foster professional well-being
Reduce administrative burden	Prevent and reduce the negative consequences on clinicians' professional well-being that result from laws, regulations, policies, and standards promulgated by health care policy and regulatory and standards-setting entities, including government agencies (federal, state, and local), professional organizations, and accreditors
Enable technology solutions	Optimize the use of health information technologies to support clinicians in providing high-quality patient care
Provide support to clinicians and learners	Reduce the stigma and eliminate the barriers associated with obtaining the support and services needed to prevent and alleviate burnout symptoms, facilitate recovery from burnout, and foster professional well-being among learners and practicing clinicians
Invest in research	Provide dedicated funding for research on clinician professional well-being

Data from National Academy of Medicine, National Academies of Sciences E and Medicine. Taking action against clinician burnout: a systems approach to professional well-being. The National Academies Press; 2019. https://doi.org/10.17226/25521.

and they are being tested time and time again during the COVID-19 pandemic. Individual-focused interventions without organizational efforts to improve the work environment will inevitably breed resentment and resistance due to incongruence between the organizational leadership's words ("we value your well-being") and actions ("we are not fully invested in your well-being").

Another reason for the predominance of individual-focused interventions is that they are nimbler and take less time to implement than systems-level interventions. The urgency and widespread negative consequences of physician burnout prompted health care institutions to act swiftly. This focus on immediate action, although well-intentioned, can hurt physician well-being efforts by promoting quick fixes rather than long-term solutions. In medical school, many of us learned the adage *ubi pus, ibi evacua* or "where there is pus, evacuate it." Even though it is faster and easier to put a bandage on the abscess instead of draining the pus, this will not make the abscess go away and in fact, will make things much worse. Superficial well-being initiatives that do not address core issues related to well-being conversely worsen burnout and precipitate a loss of trust in leadership and the organization.

The "quick fix" mindset to reduce burnout also led to rushed efforts to define and measure clinician burnout. It is impossible to solve a problem without having a thorough understanding of the problem itself. The Maslach Burnout Inventory (MBI) evaluates 3 key dimensions of emotional exhaustion, depersonalization, and a diminished sense of personal accomplishment.[5] Although the original goal of the MBI was to study which factors are associated with each of the 3 dimensions of burnout, numerous organizations have modified or misused the MBI to measure burnout as a single score to provide an individual diagnosis or organizational metric.[19] As mentioned earlier, with "wicked problems," the choice of explanation determines the way the problem is addressed. Thus, oversimplification of the concept of burnout inevitably leads to well-being interventions that are woefully inadequate or misdirected.

Well-being is much more than avoiding burnout. Well-being is the experience of positive perceptions and the presence of positive environments that enables individuals to thrive and achieve their full potential.[4] In medicine, positive perceptions and environments are driven by pragmatic solutions that improve physicians' daily clinical practice as opposed to initiatives that do little more than check off an arbitrary well-being box. Well-being permeates the entire work experience, and well-being efforts must begin with addressing physicians' basic physical and mental health needs, followed by patient and physician safety needs, before focusing on higher-order needs such as respect, appreciation, and connection.[20] Burnout is a symptom, not the underlying problem. A well-being strategy that fixates solely on decreasing burnout lacks dimension and represents a lost opportunity to build engagement; it also embodies a reactive, instead of proactive, approach to well-being.

As is the case with many issues in medicine, preventing burnout is more effective than treating established burnout. A population health approach has been proposed to address physician well-being through the promotion of professional fulfillment, prevention of burnout, and selective mitigation strategies for physicians at elevated risk for burnout.[21] Preemptive actions to promote physician engagement and protect against burnout help clinicians, patients, and health care organizations avoid many of the negative consequences of burnout, ultimately benefiting the entire health care system.

Eventually, we must drain the abscess. Every "wicked problem" is a symptom of an underlying, deeper problem. Physician burnout is a symptom of an unhealthy culture in medicine and health care industry that pushes physicians ever more toward moral injury.[1]

Well-Being 2.0: Shifting Focus to a Sustainable Culture

Moving the needle on improving well-being in medicine necessitates a cultural overhaul of the medical system, understanding that the well-being of health care providers is essential for a safe, efficient, and effective healthcare system. "Checking the well-being box" without changing the system is as useful as rearranging deck chairs on the Titanic. Where is the hope? Where do we go from here? As thought leaders and well-being pragmatists, we believe there is a way to lower the temperature on the boiling pot in which we are swimming and shift toward a more sustainable culture. Physician well-being experts have known the secret for years: the answer is not group yoga or mandatory resilience training; the answer is the hard work of culture change.

Stop the glorification of excessive self-sacrifice

We are part of a culture that has traditionally upheld perfection and unrealistic self-sacrifice. We expect overworked physicians who are barely clinging to the lowest level of Maslow's hierarchy of needs[20] to provide the highest level of complex, error-free care. Physicians perpetuate this mentality through the rituals of medical training. We give a pleased nod to a "tough" intern who arrives limping in pain or "help" a struggling colleague by placing an intravenous catheter for rehydration so they can finish a call shift. In medicine, we have created a culture where personal boundaries are discouraged and perceived as a lack of dedication to the profession. We create an artificial choice between a successful professional life and a fulfilling personal life, when in fact they should coexist. The archaic model of medical practice, where the male physician worked long hours and was supported by a full-time, unpaid wife at home, is now a rare reality. Although today's diverse workforce has evolved to increasingly resemble the society it serves, the demands on physicians continue to be based on this antiquated model.

How do we enact limits on the Hippocratic Oath? The 2017 Revised Declaration of Geneva contains the words: "I WILL ATTEND TO my own health, well-being, and abilities in order to provide care of the highest standard."[22] We must recognize, as a profession, that serving our own needs ultimately serves our patients, as demonstrated by the overused but accurate adage: "We must put on our own oxygen masks first." We must normalize physicians expressing the need to care for their own mental or physical health and those of their loved ones.

Litigation: stop blaming and shaming doctors
The litigious nature of the American health care system leaves little room for vulnerability. "First do no harm" often feels a distant second to patient satisfaction scores or online reviews. Physicians involved in a lawsuit are at increased risk for stress, personal consequences, and burnout.[23,24] Increased litigation against doctors has not been shown to improve patient safety or quality of care; more likely, it is contributing to the exodus from medicine, ultimately decreasing patient safety through limited access to care.[25,26] Clinicians may practice defensive medicine to avoid malpractice claims, which can lead to moral injury and damage the physician-patient relationship.[27] Well-designed and implemented liability reform is necessary to recapture the goal of upholding patient safety while minimizing the personal and professional trauma on doctors.

Normalize peer and mental health support
The lack of psychological safety in medicine is largely due to the lack of systems-level responses to events such as litigation, unanticipated bad outcomes, and critical events, leaving isolated clinicians to suffer in silence. Proactive, not reactive, robust support mechanisms must be established to respond to clinicians involved in these highly stressful events. These include peer support programs that can respond to clinicians in real time, provision of relief from clinical duties when appropriate, connection to professional mental health support, and longitudinal legal and risk management support. In other fields, such as law enforcement, there is mandatory time off after a critical event. However, in medicine, we are expected to proceed with the next case despite evidence that this is not in patients' or providers' best interests.[28] This mindset is built on the hubris and arrogance that physicians are somehow impenetrable. We are not have the capacity to care for those who are suffering without emotional repercussions nor should we desire this trait. We must normalize time off after critical events and provide a systems-level recognition of the emotional labor of medicine.

During the COVID-19 pandemic, state licensing requirements were temporarily suspended to mobilize physicians to states in dire need of providers. Yet predating the pandemic, many of these states enacted barriers to medical licensure if physicians had a history of seeking treatment for depression or anxiety or took an antidepressant medication, as 13.8% of Americans do.[29] To normalize physician self-care, state licensing organizations must give mental health parity with physical health. Nearly 40% of physicians report reluctance to seek care for mental health issues due to concerns about repercussions to their medical licensure.[30] We recognize the need for regulatory agencies to ensure the safety of future patients, but it should not come at the expense of a healthy physician workforce.

Stop the strip mining

Health care systems strive for efficiency. Although a desirable goal, it is not sustainable without a foundation of clinician well-being. The reimbursement structure of medicine in the United States is flawed and motivates health care institutions to prioritize short-term gains over sustainability. Clinicians are pressured to do more with fewer resources[31]; this production pressure can lead to moral injury when clinicians feel that patient care is compromised. This "carrot and stick" model devalues physicians' compassion and expertise, reducing them to a cog in the wheel. Harnessing physicians' intrinsic motivators, such as delivering high-level patient care and contributing to a shared purpose, is a more effective strategy to engage physicians.[32] Clinicians are a valuable and finite resource and must be recognized as such. It is insufficient for health care institutions to focus solely on recruitment; they must adopt long-term strategies focused on retention by investing in and supporting employees.

Empower physicians to be the architects of their own environment

Physicians are well aware of clinical and environmental stressors that threaten well-being, yet often feel disempowered to voice concerns and suggest improvements.[33] This renders a disservice to patients, clinicians, and health care organizations because physicians provide unique insight and potential solutions to burnout. Health care institutions must invest in physician leadership to empower individuals with the skills and resources to enact necessary change in their clinical practice and work environment.

Furthermore, physician leaders' time must be respected as a finite resource. Physicians are often asked to take on leadership roles without additional pay or protected nonclinical time.[34] This lack of adequate resources is a set up for failure. Leadership roles without protected time or compensation can lead to burnout due to exhaustion, feelings of incompetence, and a lack of achievement and productivity. In addition, physician leaders may experience resentment if the institution devalues their time and efforts.

Another way for health care institutions to invest in physician leaders is to offer physician leadership training. Medicine traditionally emphasizes intellectual rigor as the key to becoming a successful physician.[35] However, a physician cannot lead and effect change through academic excellence alone. An effective physician leader must, as David Chestnut posits, possess the attributes of "humility, servant leadership, self-awareness, kindness, altruism, attention to personal well-being, responsibility and concern for patient safety, lifelong learning, self-regulation, and honesty and integrity."[36] Although most physicians are responsible for leading patient care teams in the clinical setting,[37] health care organizations rarely invest in developing physicians as leaders.[33] Early leadership training for physicians represents an opportunity to improve the clinical work environment for all care team members and achieve better patient outcomes. Although some graduate medical education programs provide leadership training, it is not currently a widespread practice in medicine and health care systems.[38]

SUMMARY

"Do the best you can until you know better. Then when you know better, do better."

– Maya Angelou

Efforts to study and address physician well-being are relatively new, and our understanding of physician well-being continues to evolve. Early well-being initiatives focused predominantly on the individual because burnout was initially framed as an individual problem, but there is ample evidence that systems, policies, and organizations profoundly affect well-being. Therefore, both individual-focused and systems-level interventions are necessary. Rapid deployment of low-cost, one-off solutions are insufficient to adequately and holistically address physician well-being. We are in a crisis of burnout due to widespread moral injury and a longstanding culture of medicine that forces clinicians to "do more with less" and robs them of the meaning and purpose in their work.[31] The COVID-19 pandemic has exacerbated preexisting moral injury for many physicians, and the stakes are higher now than ever. We cannot afford to let this vicious cycle continue. If we want to make real progress to address physician well-being, we can no longer focus solely on extinguishing the immediate fires of physician burnout. We must take the long and difficult path to heal our professional culture and develop a sustainable culture of support in medicine.

FINANCIAL DISCLOSURE

The authors have nothing to disclose.

CONFLICTS OF INTEREST

J. L. Sinskey is the Vice Chair of the American Society of Anesthesiologists' Committee on Physician Well-being. R. D. Margolis is the cofounder of the Society for Pediatric Anesthesia's Special Interest Group for Physician Well-Being. A. E. Vinson is the Chair of the American Society of Anesthesiologists' Committee on Physician Well-being.

REFERENCES

1. Shanafelt TD, Schein E, Minor LB, et al. Healing the professional culture of medicine. Mayo Clin Proc 2019;94(8):1556–66.
2. Afonso AM, Cadwell JB, Staffa SJ, et al. Burnout rate and risk factors among anesthesiologists in the United States. Anesthesiology 2021;134(5):683–96.
3. Rittel HWJ, Webber MM. Dilemmas in a general theory of planning. Policy Sci 1973;4(2):155–69.
4. National Academies of Sciences, Engineering, and Medicine. Taking Action Against Clinician Burnout: A Systems Approach to Professional Well-Being. Washington, DC: The National Academies Press; 2019.
5. Maslach C, Jackson SE, Leiter MP. Maslach burnout inventory: manual. Mind Garden; 2018.
6. West CP, Dyrbye LN, Shanafelt TD. Physician burnout: contributors, consequences and solutions. J Intern Med 2018;283(6):516–29.
7. Rankin J. Godzilla in the corridor: the Ontario SARS crisis in historical perspective. Intensive Crit Care Nurs 2006;22(3):130–7.
8. Osler W, Silverman ME, Murray TJ, et al, American College of Physicians: American Society of Internal Medicine. The quotable osler.; 2008.
9. Morris SD, Morris AJ, Rockoff MA. Freeman allen: boston's pioneering physician anesthetist. Anesth Analg 2014;119(5):1186–93.
10. Schonwald G, Skipper GE, Smith DE, et al. Anesthesiologists and substance use disorders. Anesth Analg 2014;119(5):1007–10.
11. Warner DO, Berge K, Sun H, et al. Substance use disorder among anesthesiology residents, 1975-2009. JAMA 2013;310(21):2289–96.

12. Warner DO, Berge K, Sun H, et al. Substance use disorder in physicians after completion of training in anesthesiology in the United States from 1977 to 2013. Anesthesiology 2020;133(2):342–9.

13. Schernhammer ES, Colditz GA. Suicide rates among physicians: a quantitative and gender assessment (meta-analysis). Am J Psychiatry 2004;161(12): 2295–302.

14. Shanafelt TD, Boone S, Tan L, et al. Burnout and satisfaction with work-life balance among US physicians relative to the general US population. Arch Intern Med 2012;172(18):1377–85.

15. Accreditation Council for Graduate Medical Education. Improving physician well-being, restoring meaning in medicine. Accessed. https://www.acgme.org/what-we-do/initiatives/physician-well-being/. [Accessed 13 August 2021]. Available at.

16. Thomas LR, Ripp JA, West CP. Charter on physician well-being. JAMA 2018; 319(15):1541–2.

17. Schwenk TL. Physician well-being and the regenerative power of caring. JAMA 2018;319(15):1543–4.

18. Burnout an "occupational phenomenon": International classification of diseases. Accessed. https://www.who.int/news/item/28-05-2019-burn-out-an-occupational-phenomenon-international-classification-of-diseases. [Accessed 4 August 2021]. Available at.

19. Maslach C, Leiter MP. How to Measure Burnout Accurately and Ethically. Harv Business Rev 2021. Accessed. https://hbr.org/2021/03/how-to-measure-burnout-accurately-and-ethically. [Accessed 13 August 2021]. Available at.

20. Shapiro DE, Duquette C, Abbott LM, et al. Beyond burnout: a physician wellness hierarchy designed to prioritize interventions at the systems level. Am J Med 2019;132(5):556–63.

21. Trockel M, Corcoran D, Minor LB, et al. Advancing physician well-being: a population health framework. Mayo Clin Proc 2020;95(11):2350–5.

22. Parsa-Parsi RW. The revised declaration of geneva: a modern-day physician's pledge. JAMA 2017;318(20):1971–2.

23. Balch CM, Shanafelt T. Combating stress and burnout in surgical practice: a review. Thorac Surg Clin 2011;21(3):417–30.

24. Jones JW, Barge BN, Steffy BD, et al. Stress and medical malpractice: organizational risk assessment and intervention. J Appl Psychol 1988;73(4):727–35.

25. Mello MM, Frakes MD, Blumenkranz E, et al. Malpractice liability and health care quality: a review. JAMA 2020;323(4):352–66.

26. Forster HP, Schwartz J, DeRenzo E. Reducing legal risk by practicing patient-centered medicine. Arch Intern Med 2002;162(11):1217–9.

27. Kass JS, Rose RV. Medical malpractice reform: historical approaches, alternative models, and communication and resolution programs. AMA J Ethics 2016;18(3): 299–310.

28. Gazoni FM, Amato PE, Malik ZM, et al. The impact of perioperative catastrophes on anesthesiologists: results of a national survey. Anesth Analg 2012;114(3): 596–603.

29. Brody DJ, Gu Q. Antidepressant use among adults: United States, 2015-2018. NCHS Data Brief 2020;(377):1–8.

30. Dyrbye LN, West CP, Sinsky CA, et al. Medical licensure questions and physician reluctance to seek care for mental health conditions. Mayo Clin Proc 2017;92(10): 1486–93.

31. Shanafelt T, Trockel M, Ripp J, et al. Building a program on well-being: key design considerations to meet the unique needs of each organization. Acad Med 2019; 94(2):156–61.
32. Lubarsky DA, French MT, Gitlow HS, et al. Why money alone can't (Always) "Nudge" physicians: the role of behavioral economics in the design of physician incentives. Anesthesiology 2019;130(1):154–70.
33. Shanafelt T, Trockel M, Rodriguez A, et al. Wellness-centered leadership: equipping health care leaders to cultivate physician well-being and professional fulfillment. Acad Med 2020. https://doi.org/10.1097/ACM.0000000000003907.
34. Griesbach S, Theobald M, Kolman K, et al. Joint guidelines for protected nonclinical time for faculty in family medicine residency programs. Fam Med 2021;53(6): 443–52.
35. Emanuel EJ, Gudbranson E. Does medicine overemphasize IQ? JAMA 2018; 319(7):651–2.
36. Chestnut DH. On the road to professionalism. Anesthesiology 2017;126(5):780–6.
37. Blumenthal DM, Bernard K, Bohnen J, et al. Addressing the leadership gap in medicine: residents' need for systematic leadership development training. Acad Med 2012;87(4):513–22.
38. Thornton KC, Sinskey JL, Boscardin CK, et al. Design and implementation of an innovative, longitudinal wellness curriculum in an anesthesiology residency program. A A Pract 2021;15(2):e01387.

Burnout from Gender Inequity in a Pandemic

Elizabeth B. Malinzak, MD[a],*, Stephanie I. Byerly, MD[b]

KEYWORDS

- Women anesthesiologists • Gender equity • Well-being • Burnout
- COVID-19 pandemic

KEY POINTS

- Before the start of the COVID-19 pandemic in 2020, it was known that women anesthesiologists faced unique challenges related to their gender, including but not limited to, harassment, compensation inequity, decreased rates of promotion, less representation in leadership, and inequitable distribution of domestic duties.
- During the pandemic, enhanced clinical duties, domestic responsibilities, and stress made it easier to see the flawed narrative of work–life balance in medicine. Inflexible scheduling, undervalued caregiving responsibilities outside of work, and loss of academic and leadership productivity caused many women physicians to reduce their work hours, transition to part-time, or consider leaving medicine.
- Women physicians, and in particular anesthesiologists, have a higher rate of burnout and mental health issues than their male counterparts, which was exacerbated during the pandemic and continues to be an issue as the pandemic evolves and overwhelms health care systems and health care workers.
- Unless systemic change is enacted to shift work culture and institutional norms regarding gender, work, and caregiving, we will see long-lasting and possibly permanent effects on the well-being of women anesthesiologists.

INTRODUCTION

The percentage of women physicians in anesthesiology ranks in the lower third among all medical specialties. Women are 33% of anesthesiology residents, 25% of the overall anesthesiology workforce, and 37% of the academic anesthesiology workforce.[1–3] These numbers have remained relatively consistent since 2006.[3]

There is no appropriate stereotype for a woman anesthesiologist. Each is at a different point in their professional careers and personal lives, and each makes

[a] Department of Anesthesiology, Duke University, DUMC 3094, 2301 Erwin Road, Durham, NC 27710, USA; [b] Department of Anesthesiology and Pain Management, University of Texas Southwestern, 5323 Harry Hines Boulevard, Dallas, TX 75390, USA
* Corresponding author.
E-mail addresses: Elizabeth.malinzak@duke.edu (E.B.M.); Stephanie.Byerly@UTSouthwestern.edu (S.I.B.)
Twitter: @ebmalinzakmd (E.B.M.); @SByerlyMD (S.I.B.)

Anesthesiology Clin 40 (2022) 225–234
https://doi.org/10.1016/j.anclin.2021.12.001
1932-2275/22/© 2021 Elsevier Inc. All rights reserved.
anesthesiology.theclinics.com

decisions for themselves. This diversity of lived experiences highlights why broad assumptions about women anesthesiologists should be avoided. Unfortunately, in our culture and particularly in medicine, assumptions about women do exist. For example, there is an assumption that all women have a natural predilection for family life and children; this is applied to women without children as well. Additionally, the concept of intersectionality should be included, as many of the issues discussed here are often magnified for those who do not identify as cisgender and/or white.

We will briefly review the data regarding gender inequity in anesthesiology that were available before the COVID-19 pandemic in 2020. Next, we will discuss how the pandemic exposed the socially constructed norms, roles, and behaviors associated with gender that situates women anesthesiologists as both primary caregivers in the home and on the frontlines of health care. These systemic inequities continue to exacerbate burnout in women anesthesiologists. Finally, we will highlight initiatives that can improve well-being and the work culture for women anesthesiologists.

STATUS OF WOMEN ANESTHESIOLOGISTS PREPANDEMIC

Women anesthesiologists encounter unique challenges related to their gender that were well known before the beginning of the pandemic, including but not limited to harassment, compensation inequity, decreased rates of promotion, less representation in leadership, and inequitable distribution of domestic duties. Women anesthesiologists are more likely to perceive and experience gender-based discrimination, mistreatment, and sexual harassment than men in anesthesiology and report the highest rate of maternal discrimination among all medical specialties.[4–9] The most frequently identified sources of mistreatment include patients and nurses, followed by surgeons, and then other anesthesiologists.[5,6,10] Women anesthesiologists are paid less than their male counterparts for equitable work, with an annual pay gap of 8% (or approximately $32,000), and are overall more likely to have a lower salary range.[11] Over a 30-year career span and after investing in the same education and training, this translates to approximately 1 million dollars in lost earnings for women.

In academic medicine, women physicians are less likely to be promoted to associate, full professor, or department chair; there has been no narrowing of the gap over the last 35 years.[12] Contributing factors to promotion include publications, grants, speaking engagements, and awards. Women anesthesiologists have fewer publications as first or senior author in peer-reviewed anesthesiology journals and receive fewer career advancement awards.[13–18] Women anesthesiologists are less likely to receive invitations to speak at external departmental grand rounds.[19] At national anesthesiology meetings, all-men panels predominate, whereas women represent lower percentages of single or keynote speakers.[1,20,21] Between 1985 and 2020, only five women had delivered the prestigious Rovenstine lecture at the American Society of Anesthesiology (ASA) Annual Meeting.[1] Of the total Distinguished Service Awards given by all nine anesthesiology societies, women have been 12% of the recipients.[22]

Women anesthesiologists are a minority in anesthesiology leadership positions. To date, neither *Anesthesia & Analgesia* nor *Anesthesiology* has had a woman editor in chief.[2] There also has been little to no change in proportion of women editors for editorial boards of peer-reviewed anesthesiology journals over time.[2,23] The percentage of women chairs of academic anesthesiology departments has remained stagnant at 13% over the last 15 years.[24] The ASA has had five women presidents in 116 years; the first was Dr. Betty Stephenson in 1991.[17] Additionally, the proportion of women serving in the ASA House of Delegates continues to be well below the proportion of women in the anesthesiology workforce.[17] Notably, similar percentages of men and women anesthesiologists are eager to pursue leadership positions and identify similar barriers, including work–life conflict, lack of mentorship and sponsorship, and frustration with organizational support.[25]

At home, women physicians spend more time on domestic responsibilities, at an average of 8.5 more hours per week, regardless of marital or child status.[26,27] Additionally, women physicians, including those in dual-career relationships, are more likely to be the primary caregiver for children or elderly and are less likely to have a stay-at-home partner.[27]

THE PROGRESSION OF GENDER INEQUITY DURING THE COVID-19 PANDEMIC

The COVID-19 pandemic revealed the flawed narrative of work–life balance in medicine and the general culture of overwork.[28] It also threatened to regress the positive trends in gender equity and success in anesthesiology.

In the workplace, the pandemic brought forth significant workflow changes including increased administrative tasks, greater clinical responsibilities, and at times, the reduction of work hours.[29] Surge planning, new clinical protocols, and staffing challenges are a few of the many new administrative challenges.[30] As compared with other medical colleagues who can provide a large percentage of their care through telemedicine, most anesthesiologists must be physically present to provide patient care.[31] There was a greater need for intensive care physicians and intubation teams; many anesthesiologists were dispatched to unfamiliar clinical settings, worked longer hours, and cared for critically ill patients.[29,32] Conversely, some anesthesiologists experienced decreased work hours because of widespread cancellation of elective surgical cases or increased caregiving roles at home.[29,33] With the cancellation of elective surgeries, many anesthesiologists, specifically those in private practice, were furloughed or on unpaid leaves of absences, creating financial hardship.[34] In a survey from the California Society of Anesthesiologists, women anesthesiologists reported furlough status or being given involuntary vacation more often than men.[35]

In the academic setting, many faculty reduced their participation in scholarly and research activities to ensure the increasing clinical workloads were met. Many women anesthesiologists used their nonclinical time to focus on domestic responsibilities and childcare, resulting in a 33% larger drop in research hours and academic productivity compared to men.[36–42] Additionally, because women in academic medicine are more likely to have education roles, the adaptation to remote learning may have superseded other scholarly endeavors needed for promotion or leadership.[43,44] The percentage of articles on which women were first authors dropped during the pandemic, further increasing the existing authorship gender gap.[33,45–48] This occurred in spite of the surge in COVID-19-related publications, many of which were published in high impact journals and accrued more citations than non-COVID research.[45] Finally, there was reduced time for women physicians to attend virtual conferences because of personal responsibilities and institutional cost-cutting measures, reducing networking abilities.[49] The aforementioned workforce and academic elements that emerged during the pandemic will likely cumulatively contribute to the enhancement of the gender gaps in compensation, promotion, and leadership roles that women anesthesiologists already face.[36–38,42,50]

On the domestic front, there was an uptick in household responsibilities and caregiving needs because of school and daycare closings, disruption of children's activities, and stay-at-home orders. As most U.S. households lack elderly family members to rely on as backup, these responsibilities fell disproportionately to women.[28,36–38,41,51–55] Since the onset of the pandemic, parents in the United States have almost doubled their time spent on household tasks and childcare, with mothers contributing an average of 15 more hours per week more than fathers.[51] When virtual school and work-from-home became prevalent, it created a double-edged sword. Certainly, this new paradigm had the potential to facilitate the management of work–family roles, although multitasking, interruptions, and extended workday availability also increased.[38] Mothers were 50% more likely to be interrupted when working from home compared to fathers working from home.[41] In summary, augmented childcare and home schooling obligations coupled with disproportionate household responsibilities had an outsized impact on women anesthesiologists who struggled to meet family needs while also fulfilling increasing demands of pandemic-related work responsibilities.[56] As a consequence, more women anesthesiologists, particularly junior faculty, reduced work hours, considered leaving medicine altogether, or transitioned to part-time, secondary to pandemic stressors.[28,36,41,51,53]

Many anesthesiologists reported a heightened sense of personal precarity and sacrifice at the onset of the pandemic.[28,51] Women health care workers performing tracheal intubation of patients with suspected or confirmed COVID-19 were at increased risk of subsequent COVID-19 diagnosis or symptoms requiring self-isolation or hospitalization. This was likely due to the gendered design of personal protective equipment (PPE) and the limited availability of appropriately sized PPE.[57] There was anxiety about one's duty as a physician and the risk of contracting COVID, exposing family, and even death.[51,52,56,58] There was also a fear of leaving children as orphans, an unprecedented ethical dilemma for all physician parents torn between a dedication to the profession when needed most and a desire to protect their families; women in particular did not wish to be perceived as uncommitted to their job.[58,59] Breastfeeding women and mothers faced additional uncertainty regarding where and when to pump at work due to the potential risk of infection and/or if they should self-isolate from their infants and children while working in a high-risk environment.[56,59,60]

THE EFFECTS OF COVID-19 ON WELLNESS AND BURNOUT IN WOMEN ANESTHESIOLOGISTS

It is not surprising then that women physicians have a higher rate of burnout and mental health issues than their male counterparts. It has been known for years that women physicians experience depression and suicidality at higher rates than male physicians. A study in 1999 suggested that the incidence of depression among women physicians might be as high as 19.5%[61] along with suicide completion rates as much as 130% higher rate compared to women in the general population.[62]

The Medscape National Physician Burnout and Suicide Report is an annual compilation of survey results of physicians from all specialties. The 2021 Report included 12,339 physicians surveyed from August 30 to November 5, 2020. Overall, the rate of burnout for women was 51% compared to 36% for men. Only 49% of all physicians reported feeling happy to very happy compared to 69% of participants evaluated before the pandemic. The survey also reported that 1% of physicians had attempted suicide and 13% had thoughts about suicide.[63] Additionally, there were several studies published with data collected before the pandemic, suggesting that anesthesiologists and critical care physicians specifically are at high risk for burnout.[64,65] A recent article in *Anesthesiology* reported the prevalence of burnout among anesthesiologists is higher than previously known, with 59.2% of survey participants being at high risk for burnout and 13.8% meeting the criteria for burnout syndrome.[66] Such trends are likely worsening with the ongoing pandemic as it continues to overwhelm health care systems and its workers.

A rapid scoping review by Sriharan and colleagues reported that women health care workers are at increased risk for stress, burnout, and depression amid the pandemic.[67] Another study of 442 health care workers revealed that being woman,

Table 1	
Suggestions for improvement of work culture and well-being for anesthesiologists	
Group	**Recommendations**
Recommendations from ASA Committee on Systemic Life Imbalances	• Nontraditional and/or flexible scheduling adds value to a department or practice by giving flexibility to its members and their needs, as well as the ability to accommodate the surges and ebbs in surgical scheduling. • As the definitions of "a family" and of contemporary caregiver roles are changing rapidly, leaders need to create cultures in which physicians feel safe sharing information about caregiving responsibilities and feel secure in the knowledge that this will be used to support more equitable working environments. It is helpful to provide childcare and family care resource options, financial support, and leave time for caregiving needs. • Accommodations should be made for the loss of academic productivity due to changes in clinical duties, loss of academic time, stagnation of progress in a promotion track, and increased caregiving demands. • General wellness initiatives should be deployed, including but not limited to, well-being education, peer support, substance use disorder prevention and treatment, suicide prevention training, and diversity, equity, and inclusion initiatives.
ASA Statement on Creating a Culture of Well-Being for Health Care Workers	• Advocate for a culture of openness, normalization, and destigmatizing of mental health care in physicians. • Physicians should be able to seek care through mental health resources without fear of impact on licensure and credentialing. • The path to access these resources be easily accessible to individuals and that confidentiality be maintained. • Standardize state medical licensure and local credentialing questions to promote parity between mental and physical health, thus removing a barrier to seeking appropriate mental health care.
Other examples and suggestions	• There should be zero tolerance for harassment and microaggressions, as well as easily accessible reporting structures and psychologically safe spaces to discuss vulnerabilities. • Departments and practices should be transparent about compensation and standardize how professional effort is calculated among education, research, and clinical care. • Organizational leadership opportunities should be widely publicized to ensure that women have strong representation in the nomination, interview, and selection processes. • Rethink the traditional conference to include virtual options and childcare support. • Aim for deliberate representation. Having women as a part of the leadership group that makes pivotal decisions is imperative.

Box 1
Maslow's hierarchy of need
Basics: Physical and mental health needs
Safety: Patient and health care worker safety
Respect: Professional behavior among all health care workers
Appreciation: Recognition for practicing good patient care
Heal patients and contribute: Self-actualization, purpose-driven life

young, single, having less work experience, and working on the frontlines were associated with higher rates of depression, anxiety, and stress.[68] Some experts believe that up to 80% of health care worker burnout is related to health care system operations and the culture of the organization. The well-being of health care workers is essential to any health care system. The COVID-19 pandemic will have long-lasting and permanent effects on all health care workers. Those on the frontlines, including anesthesiologists and critical care physicians, are facing physical and emotional exhaustion as variants emerge and resurge.

A CALL TO ACTION AND RECOMMENDATIONS

In March 2020, a group of anesthesiologists called for the ASA to investigate systemic life imbalances that the pandemic exacerbated for women anesthesiologists. These included issues such as scheduling flexibility, caregiving, academic productivity, and well-being. The Ad Hoc Committee on Systemic Life Imbalances was subsequently formed. In addition to authoring a series of documents with specific suggestions (available at https://www.asahq.org/standards-and-guidelines/resources-from-asa-committees), in June 2021, the Ad Hoc Committee supported the overall recommendations as shown in **Table 1**. The committee also collaborated with members of the ASA Committee on Physician Well-Being and put forth a Statement on Creating a Culture of Well-Being for Health Care Workers. The statement recommends an expert opinion and evidence-based system that meets the Physician Wellness Hierarchy of Needs derived from Maslow's Hierarchy of Need as described in **Box 1**.[69] The recommendations include a team-based organizational platform as opposed to a top–down structure for establishing a more just culture of support and enabling a two-way communication between health care workers and hospital leadership. **Table 1** outlines these specific suggestions and recommendations as well as examples of other opportunities for work culture improvement to better support women anesthesiologists.

SUMMARY

We are caregivers—all of us. We care for our patients, but we also must care for loved ones and ourselves, said simply. We need to shift institutional perspectives of gender, work–life balance, and caregiving. With an eye toward strengthening the career trajectories of women anesthesiologists, the pandemic is an opportunity to build a more equitable workforce—namely initiating sustained institutional and systemic efforts to address gender disparities and fostering a culture of support that normalizes and destigmatizes mental health care in physicians. New paradigms and thought processes are critical to ensure the well-being of health care workers and the retention of women physicians.

CLINICS CARE POINTS

- Women anesthesiologists face unique challenges related to their gender, including but not limited to, harassment, compensation inequity, decreased rates of promotion, less representation in leadership, and inequitable distribution of domestic duties.

- During the pandemic, enhanced clinical duties and increased domestic and caregiving responsibilities caused burnout and mental health issues to intensify for many women anesthesiologists, causing them to reduce their work hours, transition to part-time, or consider leaving medicine.

ACKNOWLEDGEMENT

Thank you to the editors for such amazing work in finalizing this article. It's even more beautiful than I remember! I appreciate your investment. Elizabeth Malinzak.

DISCLOSURE

The authors have nothing to disclose.

REFERENCES

1. Moeschler SM, Gali B, Goyal S, et al. Speaker Gender Representation at the American Society of Anesthesiology Annual Meeting: 2011-2016. Anesth Analg 2019;129(1):301–5.
2. Bissing MA, Lange EMS, Davila WF, et al. Status of Women in Academic Anesthesiology: A 10-Year Update. Anesth Analg 2019;128(1):137–43.
3. Gonzalez LS, Fahy BG, Lien CA. Gender distribution in United States anaesthesiology residency programme directors: trends and implications. Br J Anaesth 2020;124(3):e63–9.
4. Miller J, Katz D. Gender Differences in Perception of Workplace Experience Among Anesthesiology Residents. J Educ Perioper Med 2018;20(1):E618.
5. Shams T, El-Masry R. Cons and pros of female anesthesiologists: Academic versus nonacademic. J Anaesthesiol Clin Pharmacol 2015;31(1):86–91.
6. Zdravkovic M, Osinova D, Brull SJ, et al. Perceptions of gender equity in departmental leadership, research opportunities, and clinical work attitudes: an international survey of 11 781 anaesthesiologists. Br J Anaesth 2020; 124(3):e160–70.
7. Adesoye T, Mangurian C, Choo EK, et al. Perceived Discrimination Experienced by Physician Mothers and Desired Workplace Changes: A Cross-sectional Survey. JAMA Intern Med 2017;177(7):1033–6.
8. Kraus MB, Dexter F, Patel PV, et al. Motherhood and Anesthesiology: A Survey of the American Society of Anesthesiologists. Anesth Analg 2020;130(5): 1296–302.
9. Association of American Medical Colleges Faculty Roster. 2019. Available at: https://www.aamc.org/data-reports/faculty-institutions/interactive-data/2019-us-medical-school-faculty. Accessed August 31, 2021.
10. McKinley SK, Wang LJ, Gartland RM, et al. Yes, I'm the Doctor": One Department's Approach to Assessing and Addressing Gender-Based Discrimination in the Modern Medical Training Era. Acad Med 2019;94(11):1691–8.
11. Hertzberg LB, Miller TR, Byerly S, et al. Gender Differences in Compensation in Anesthesiology in the United States: Results of a National Survey of Anesthesiologists. Anesth Analg 2021;133(4):1009–18.

12. Richter KP, Clark L, Wick JA, et al. Women Physicians and Promotion in Academic Medicine. N Engl J Med 2020;383(22):2148–57.

13. Miller J, Chuba E, Deiner S, et al. Trends in Authorship in Anesthesiology Journals. Anesth Analg 2019;129(1):306–10.

14. Pagel PS, Freed JK, Lien CA. Gender Composition and Trends of Journal of Cardiothoracic and Vascular Anesthesia Editorial Board Membership: A 33-Year Analysis, 1987-2019. J Cardiothorac Vasc Anesth 2019;33(12):3229–34.

15. Galley HF, Colvin LA. Next on the agenda: gender. Br J Anaesth 2013;111(2):139–42.

16. Flexman AM, Parmar A, Lorello GR. Representation of female authors in the Canadian Journal of Anesthesia: a retrospective analysis of articles between 1954 and 2017. Can J Anaesth 2019;66(5):495–502.

17. Toledo P, Duce L, Adams J, et al. Diversity in the American Society of Anesthesiologists Leadership. Anesth Analg 2017;124(5):1611–6.

18. Mayes LM, Wong CA, Zimmer S, et al. Gender differences in career development awards in United States' anesthesiology and surgery departments, 2006-2016. BMC Anesthesiol 2018;18(1):95.

19. Sharpe EE, Moeschler SM, O'Brien EK, et al. Representation of Women Among Invited Speakers for Grand Rounds. J Womens Health (Larchmt) 2020;29(10):1268–72.

20. Shillcutt SK, Lorenzen KA. Whose Voices Are Heard? Speaker Gender Representation at the Society of Cardiovascular Anesthesiologists Annual Meeting. J Cardiothorac Vasc Anesth 2020;34(7):1805–9.

21. Lorello GR, Parmar A, Flexman AM. Representation of women amongst speakers at the Canadian Anesthesiologists' Society annual meeting: a retrospective analysis from 2007 to 2019. Can J Anaesth 2020;67(4):430–6.

22. Ellinas EH, Rebello E, Chandrabose RK, et al. Distinguished Service Awards in Anesthesiology Specialty Societies: Analysis of Gender Differences. Anesth Analg 2019;129(4):e130–4.

23. Lorello GR, Parmar A, Flexman AM. Representation of women on the editorial board of the Canadian Journal of Anesthesia: a retrospective analysis from 1954 to 2018. Can J Anaesth 2019;66(8):989–90.

24. Chandrabose RK, Pearson ACS. Organizing Women in Anesthesiology. Int Anesthesiol Clin 2018;56(3):21–43.

25. Matot I, De Hert S, Cohen B, et al. Women anaesthesiologists' attitudes and reported barriers to career advancement in anaesthesia: a survey of the European Society of Anaesthesiology. Br J Anaesth 2020;124(3):e171–7.

26. Jolly S, Griffith KA, DeCastro R, et al. Gender differences in time spent on parenting and domestic responsibilities by high-achieving young physician-researchers. Ann Intern Med 2014;160(5):344–53.

27. Ly DP, Jena AB. Sex Differences in Time Spent on Household Activities and Care of Children Among US Physicians, 2003-2016. Mayo Clin Proc 2018;93(10):1484–7.

28. Brubaker L. Women Physicians and the COVID-19 Pandemic. JAMA 2020;324(9):835–6.

29. Margolis RD, Strupp KM, Beacham AO, et al. The effects of COVID-19 on pediatric anesthesiologists: A survey of the members of the Society for Pediatric Anesthesia. Anesth Analg 2021;134(2):348–56.

30. Siegrist KK, Latham GJ, Huang J, et al. Anesthesia Professionals: Helping to Lead the COVID-19 Pandemic Response From Behind the Drape and Beyond. Semin Cardiothorac Vasc Anesth 2020;24(2):121–6.

31. Rubin R. COVID-19's Crushing Effects on Medical Practices, Some of Which Might Not Survive. JAMA 2020;324(4):321–3.

32. McCartney CJ, Mariano ER. COVID-19: bringing out the best in anesthesiologists and looking toward the future. Reg Anesth Pain Med 2020;45(8):586–8.
33. Andersen JP, Nielsen MW, Simone NL, et al. COVID-19 medical papers have fewer women first authors than expected. Elife 2020;9.
34. Anesthesia Practices See Major Financial Hit as Physician Anesthesiologists Pivot During COVID-19 to Treat Patients in Critical Care and ICUs, ASA Survey Highlights. 2020. Available at: https://www.asahq.org/about-asa/newsroom/news-releases/2020/05/anesthesia-practices-see-major-financial-hit-as-anesthesiologists-pivot-during-covid-19. Accessed September 2, 2021.
35. Hertzberg LB. COVD-19 Impact Survey. 2020. http://www.csahq.org/docs/default-source/practice-management-docs/covid-19-survey-economic-impact-v2-(1).pdf?sfvrsn=e8b5c146_2. Accessed August 30, 2021.
36. Jones Y, Durand V, Morton K, et al. Collateral Damage: How COVID-19 Is Adversely Impacting Women Physicians. J Hosp Med 2020;15(8):507–9.
37. Narayana S, Roy B, Merriam S, et al. Minding the Gap: Organizational Strategies to Promote Gender Equity in Academic Medicine During the COVID-19 Pandemic. J Gen Intern Med 2020;35(12):3681–4.
38. Jagsi R, Fuentes-Afflick E, Higginbotham E. Promoting Equity for Women in Medicine - Seizing a Disruptive Opportunity. N Engl J Med 2021;384(24):2265–7.
39. Yule AM, Ijadi-Maghsoodi R, Bagot KS, et al. Support for Early-Career Female Physician-Scientists as Part of the COVID-19 Recovery Plan. Acad Med 2021;96(5):e16–7.
40. Malisch JL, Harris BN, Sherrer SM, et al. Opinion: In the wake of COVID-19, academia needs new solutions to ensure gender equity. Proc Natl Acad Sci U S A 2020;117(27):15378–81.
41. National Academies of Sciences, Engineering, and Medicine; Policy and Global Affairs; Committee on Women in Science, Engineering, and Medicine; Committee on Investigating the Potential Impacts of COVID-19 on the Careers of Women in Academic Science, Engineering, and Medicine. In: Dahlberg ML, Higginbotham E, editors The Impact of COVID-19 on the Careers of Women in Academic Sciences, Engineering, and Medicine. Washington (DC): National Academies Press (US); 2021.
42. Garrido P, Adjei AA, Bajpai J, et al. Has COVID-19 had a greater impact on female than male oncologists? Results of the ESMO Women for Oncology (W4O) Survey. ESMO Open 2021;6(3):100131.
43. Mayer AP, Blair JE, Ko MG, et al. Gender distribution of U.S. medical school faculty by academic track type. Acad Med 2014;89(2):312–7.
44. Das D, Lall MD, Walker L, et al. The Multifaceted Impact of COVID-19 on the Female Academic Emergency Physician: A National Conversation. AEM Educ Train 2021;5(1):91–8.
45. Wehner MR, Li Y, Nead KT. Comparison of the Proportions of Female and Male Corresponding Authors in Preprint Research Repositories Before and During the COVID-19 Pandemic. JAMA Netw Open 2020;3(9):e2020335.
46. Williams WA 2nd, Li A, Goodman DM, et al. Impact of the Coronavirus Disease 2019 Pandemic on Authorship Gender in The Journal of Pediatrics: Disproportionate Productivity by International Male Researchers. J Pediatr 2021;231:50–4.
47. Nguyen AX, Trinh XV, Kurian J, et al. Impact of COVID-19 on longitudinal ophthalmology authorship gender trends. Graefes Arch Clin Exp Ophthalmol 2021;259(3):733–44.
48. Ipe TS, Goel R, Howes L, et al. The impact of COVID-19 on academic productivity by female physicians and researchers in transfusion medicine. Transfusion 2021;61(6):1690–3.

49. Matulevicius SA, Kho KA, Reisch J, et al. Academic Medicine Faculty Perceptions of Work-Life Balance Before and Since the COVID-19 Pandemic. JAMA Netw Open 2021;4(6):e2113539.

50. Woodhams C, Dacre J, Parnerkar I, et al. Pay gaps in medicine and the impact of COVID-19 on doctors' careers. Lancet 2021;397(10269):79–80.

51. Halley MC, Mathews KS, Diamond LC, et al. The Intersection of Work and Home Challenges Faced by Physician Mothers During the Coronavirus Disease 2019 Pandemic: A Mixed-Methods Analysis. J Womens Health (Larchmt) 2021;30(4):514–24.

52. Soares A, Thakker P, Deych E, et al. The Impact of COVID-19 on Dual-Physician Couples: A Disproportionate Burden on Women Physicians. J Womens Health (Larchmt) 2021;30(5):665–71.

53. Hardy SM, McGillen KL, Hausman BL. Dr Mom's Added Burden. J Am Coll Radiol 2021;18(1 Pt A):103–7.

54. Nishida S, Nagaishi K, Motoya M, et al. Dilemma of physician-mothers faced with an increased home burden and clinical duties in the hospital during the COVID-19 pandemic. PLoS One 2021;16(6):e0253646.

55. Hu X, Dill MJ. Changes in Physician Work Hours and Patterns During the COVID-19 Pandemic. JAMA Netw Open 2021;4(6):e2114386.

56. Sarma S, Usmani S. COVID-19 and Physician Mothers. Acad Med 2021;96(2):e12–3.

57. El-Boghdadly K, Wong DJN, Owen R, et al. Risks to healthcare workers following tracheal intubation of patients with COVID-19: a prospective international multi-centre cohort study. Anaesthesia 2020;75(11):1437–47.

58. Rosanel S, Fogel J. Moral Dilemma of a Physician and Mother in the Midst of the COVID-19 Pandemic. South Med J 2020;113(8):384–5.

59. Chowdhry SM. Trying To Do It All: Being a Physician-Mother during the COVID-19 Pandemic. J Palliat Med 2020;23(5):731–2.

60. Robinson M. A Mother's Gold. JAMA 2021;325(22):2253–4.

61. Frank E, Dingle AD. Self-reported depression and suicide attempts among U.S. women physicians. Am J Psychiatry 1999;156(12):1887–94.

62. Schernhammer ES, Colditz GA. Suicide rates among physicians: a quantitative and gender assessment (meta-analysis). Am J Psychiatry 2004;161(12):2295–302.

63. Kane L. Medscape national physician burnout & suicide report 2021. 2021. Available at: https://www.medscape.com/slideshow/2021-lifestyle-burnout-6013456. Accessed September 20, 2021.

64. Vargas M, Spinelli G, Buonanno P, et al. Burnout Among Anesthesiologists and Intensive Care Physicians: Results From an Italian National Survey. Inquiry 2020;57. 46958020919263.

65. Moss M, Good VS, Gozal D, et al. An Official Critical Care Societies Collaborative Statement: Burnout Syndrome in Critical Care Healthcare Professionals: A Call for Action. Crit Care Med 2016;44(7):1414–21.

66. Afonso AM, Cadwell JB, Staffa SJ, et al. Burnout Rate and Risk Factors among Anesthesiologists in the United States. Anesthesiology 2021;134(5):683–96.

67. Sriharan A, Ratnapalan S, Tricco AC, et al. Occupational Stress, Burnout, and Depression in Women in Healthcare During COVID-19 Pandemic: Rapid Scoping Review. Front Glob Women's Health 2020;1(20).

68. Elbay RY, Kurtulmus A, Arpacioglu S, et al. Depression, anxiety, stress levels of physicians and associated factors in Covid-19 pandemics. Psychiatry Res 2020;290:113130.

69. Maslow AH. A theory of human motivation. Psychol Rev 1943;50:370–96.

Lactation in Anesthesiology

Annery G. Garcia-Marcinkiewicz, MD, MSCE[a],*, Sarah S. Titler, MD[b,c]

KEYWORDS

- Lactation • Anesthesiology • Anesthesiologists • Breastfeeding

KEY POINTS

- Anesthesiologists face multiple barriers to lactation in the workplace
- Lactation provides many benefits to mother, infant, and employer
- Supporting breastfeeding anesthesiologists contributes to inclusion and supports diversity within our specialty

PERSONAL EXPERIENCE FROM AUTHOR AGM

Two lactation pump breast shields rested between my chest and my left elbow. With my right hand I typed patient notes and placed orders in the computer as quickly as I could. With my left hand, I held the service phone between my shoulder and left ear as I triaged a patient issue. The emergency airway pager was clipped on my scrub pants over my right hip, its high-pitched alarm threatening to go off at any moment. Sweat dripped down my back.

Deep breaths. I can do this …

Please Let Down Reflex, please let down any milk that my body is able to produce. My baby needs it, and I am running out of time …

Wish I could be more hydrated …

Beeeeeeep! "Airway emergency: ED trauma bay ETA: now!"

I immediately pull the pumps off my chest. My milk containers completely spill—I just lost all my baby's food. No time to cry. Scrub top back on and now I need to run and save that airway!

There has got to be a better way…

[a] The Children's Hospital of Philadelphia, Department of Anesthesiology and Critical Care Medicine, 34-01 Civic Center Boulevard, Philadelphia, PA 19104, USA; [b] Department of Anesthesia, Division of Pediatric Anesthesia, University of Iowa, 200 Hawkins Drive, Iowa City, IA 52242, USA; [c] Department of Pediatrics, University of Iowa, Iowa, USA
* Corresponding author.
E-mail address: garciamara@chop.edu

Anesthesiology Clin 40 (2022) 235–243
https://doi.org/10.1016/j.anclin.2022.01.014

PERSONAL EXPERIENCE FROM AUTHOR SST

Breastfeeding was always my plan, even long before I considered starting a family. "Breast is best," right? I experienced low breastmilk supply and tried everything to increase my supply. I perceived this lack of breast milk supply as a failing on my part as a mother. "My body was built for this, so why can't I do it?" I thought to myself while guzzling water, ingesting milk promoting supplements, pumping after breastfeeding, and feeling generally defeated. Before returning to work, I had established a breastmilk pumping routine at home. I thought, "If I just keep this up at work then I can at least provide some of my baby's nutrition." When I returned to work, I realized that finding time to pump breastmilk was extremely difficult, in part because I felt very vulnerable. As faculty, there was no one assigned to provide relief for lactation sessions—I had to fit them in when I could. As my milk supply consistently dwindled, I was not in a space emotionally whereby I felt I could advocate for my lactation needs. In hindsight, I believe my department would have been supportive but I did not want to inconvenience my colleagues or the board runner for lactation sessions. I felt guilty. Then, one day while trying to squeeze in a pumping session amid supervising two trainees, I was called back stat to my operating room for airway concerns. As I pulled my shirt down and ran back to the operating room, I remember thinking: "I waited until I was faculty to have kids because I thought it would be easier. Boy, was I wrong." On further reflection, I also wondered: "Why is this the expectation of anesthesiologists when we return from maternity leave? How can I keep up this clinical schedule and still provide food for my baby?"

We are two mothers of five young children, as well as full-time clinical anesthesiologists, educators, and researchers in busy academic practices. We are beyond proud of this and we both love what we do. Author AGM gave birth to her three children while a resident, fellow, and young attending, respectively. Author SST gave birth to both of her children as an attending. The journey to this point was not easy. We made the intentional choice to become a full-time academic anesthesiologists who provide patient care, teach trainees, and pursue clinical research. While each of these work-related commitments has brought professional fulfillment, we also encountered lactation barriers that many anesthesiologists and physicians regularly face. Although every lactation experience is different and wrought with unique challenges, we are primarily concerned with addressing, optimizing, and normalizing the return-to-work process for breastfeeding physician anesthesiologists, including how to provide day-to-day lactation support within the perioperative space.

Physician mother's breastfeeding initiation rates are higher than the general population of mothers in the United States.[1] However, many physician mothers do not breastfeed for as long as intended secondary to work-related barriers to breastfeeding.[2] These work-related barriers to breastfeeding include: lack of appropriate place for breastmilk expression, unpredictable and inflexible schedules, and lack of time to breastfeed or express milk. In fact, work-related barriers may have an outsized impact on physician mothers' breastfeeding behavior compared with her education or breastfeeding intentions, when considering the duration of lactation.[1] Interestingly, clinical breastfeeding advocacy and anticipatory guidance for patients is often rooted in the physician's own breastfeeding behavior.[3] Furthermore, physician mothers' breastfeeding continuation rates are lower compared with other high-risk groups for early breastfeeding cessation.[4] As physician mothers, we generally have characteristics associated with higher breastfeeding initiation and continuation rates, thus early cessation of breastfeeding is unexpected. We contend that breastfeeding anesthesiologists, in particular, are faced with unique work-related barriers to lactation throughout our training and careers that contribute to early cessation.

The American Academy of Pediatrics (AAP) recommends exclusive breastfeeding for the infant's first 6 months of life, with continued breastfeeding for at least the first year of life.[5] There are several benefits to breastfeeding for infants and mothers. Infants who are breastfed have reduced risks of severe lower respiratory infections, asthma, acute otitis media, atopic dermatitis, sudden infant death syndrome, gastrointestinal infections, necrotizing enterocolitis (in premature infants), and probable reductions in obesity and diabetes mellitus.[6,7] Mothers who breastfeed benefit from increased birth spacing and may derive protection against breast cancer, ovarian cancer, type II diabetes mellitus, and hypertension.[6-8] Mothers who have early cessation of breastfeeding or who do not breastfeed may have an associated increased risk of maternal postpartum depression.[6]

Several health care leaders have released statements promoting the benefits and importance of breastfeeding. Dr Ruth Petersen, Director of the Division of Nutrition, Physical, Activity, and Obesity (DNPAO) at the National Center for Chronic Disease Prevention and Health Promotion, stated, "Breastfeeding provides unmatched health benefits for babies and mothers. It is the gold standard for infant feeding and nutrition."[7] Former Surgeon General Dr. Jerome Adams also stated: "Given the importance of breastfeeding on the health of mothers and children, it is critical that we take action to support breastfeeding. Women who choose to breastfeed face numerous barriers. Only through the support of family, communities, clinicians, health care systems and employers will we be able to make breastfeeding the easy choice."[7] Public health breastfeeding advocacy makes a difference: the percentage of breastfeeding babies increased from 73% in 2004 to 84% in 2016.[7]

How Breastfeeding Works

Human milk production is a complex secretory process involving several control systems in the body. During pregnancy and the initial postpartum period, milk production is an endocrine-driven process and later transitions to an autocrine process (ie, local control of milk synthesis). Essentially, the amount of milk produced depends on the amount of milk removed from the breast.[9,10] Ideally, infants would latch immediately and feed as often as necessary. These feeding cycles change in frequency and length based on infant age and maternal milk production, with newborns requiring the highest frequency of feedings on average needing to be fed every 2 hours and gradually decreasing in frequency with age. Lactation consultants advocate having the infant directly latch on, which provides the most ideal physiologic conditions allowing for a whole host of infant–mother cues that boost breastfeeding success, including skin to skin touch, smell, tactility, a quiet environment, and more.[11] Lactating women who are returning to work are encouraged to maintain the feeding cycles established at home. Many women attempt to create a reserve of breast milk by expressing milk between infant feedings. This expressed milk can then be frozen and stored to be used when the mother is not available for direct breastfeeding. Typically, these self-produced "milk banks" are consumed by the baby on the mother's return to work. Milk volume may decrease abruptly for some women on return to work, secondary to the stress of milk expression and the loss of physiologic cues associated with milk let-down (eg, skin to skin, baby cries, etc.). Lactation pumping schedules at work are critical to maintaining milk production; many women feel extreme pressure to bring home volumes of milk to maintain baby's intake at home. Simply maintaining breastmilk production is an enormous stressor on a new mother.

Lactation and Anesthesiology Challenges

A survey of physician mothers across specialties identified anesthesiologists as significantly more likely than women of other medical specialties to self-report maternal discrimination. Maternal discrimination was defined as discrimination based on pregnancy, maternity leave, or breastfeeding.[12,13] Particularly among physician mothers who are anesthesiologists, one study found that lacking adequate facilities or time to express breast milk was a reported concern.[14] In a survey of facilities whereby anesthesia is provided, 68% of respondent facilities reported no designated lactation space proximal to patient care areas.[15] Unlike clinicians in different health care environments, anesthesiology is unique in that once the patient is anesthetized there is often not a built-in mechanism for faculty relief from patient care for breastmilk pumping sessions. The case must either conclude or the anesthesiologist must be relieved for a breastmilk pumping session by a colleague. Unless carefully planned in advance, the operating room schedule does not have built-in time for a breastmilk pumping sessions for faculty anesthesiologists.[16] Remote anesthetizing locations are similar if not more challenging (eg, MRI suite) whereby lactation spaces also may not exist or are too distanced from patient care.[17] Although other clinicians may face similar barriers with lactation, anesthesiologists are unable to pump in between seeing clinic patients or plan pumping times (ie, "I will go during my lunch-break at 12:30"). Furthermore, in many practices, anesthesiologists supervise multiple operating rooms, with a typical model involving attending supervision of advanced practice providers (eg, nurse anesthetists, anesthesia assistants) and residents. The typical workflow in the perioperative space is very challenging for lactating anesthesiologists to find sufficient time for a breastpumping session, particularly when supervising more than one anesthetic.[18]

Access to Lactation Rooms

Many health care spaces have designated lactation rooms for employees. However, surgeons and physicians in procedural-based specialties report lack of proximity to lactation facilities as a significant barrier to breastfeeding.[2,4] In many hospitals, lactation rooms are far from the operating rooms, forcing lactating clinicians to choose between leaving the patient care area or pumping in a nondesignated location that lacks basic hygiene and/or the necessary equipment. Only 19.7% of physician survey respondents reported using designated lactation rooms for breastmilk pumping.[19] Most respondents reported using their office, call rooms, car, empty patient rooms, bathrooms, locker rooms, and closets for breastmilk expression.[19] The need for lactation spaces close to patient care areas was recognized by The American Accreditation Council for Graduate Medical Education (ACGME) in 2019. The ACGME now requires lactation spaces for Graduate Medical Education (GME) anesthesiology training programs. The lactation space should include "clean and private facilities for lactation that have refrigeration capability, with proximity for safe patient care" and "it would be helpful to have additional support within these locations that may assist the resident with the continued care of patients, such as a computer and a phone."[20] The ACGME further stated that providing the time for lactation sessions is as important as the lactation space.

Time

The operating room is a fast-paced, unpredictable environment, and the conventional expectation is that staffing breaks will take no more than 15 minutes. This break typically includes nutrition, hydration, and restroom use. However, a breastmilk pumping session is a multistep, time-intensive process that requires access to a lactation room, disinfecting and cleaning the surface, and supplies that will be used, attaching the breastmilk pump to self, expressing breastmilk with the use of the breastmilk pump (this step may take 20 to 40 minutes), removing the supplies when pumping is complete, cleaning and storing the pump supplies, storing and refrigerating the expressed breastmilk, using the restroom, and accessing hydration and nutrition (**Fig. 1**). We contend that the 15-minute break paradigm from clinical duties is insufficient time for an adequate breastmilk pumping session. The clinical rotation, case durations, and lactation session relief also need to be considered when creating the clinical assignments for lactating anesthesia clinicians.[16–18]

Lactation Room Facility

Fig. 2 demonstrates the components of an ideal lactation room.

1. Easily accessible, private, and near clinical duties
2. Functional, clean, with an interior lock, and outer-door in-use signage
3. Hospital grade pump available for use
4. Equipped with a wipeable chair, sink, hand sanitizer, soap, paper towels, additional pumping supplies, surface disinfectant wipes, and microwave to assist with sterilization of breast-pumping equipment
5. Refrigerator for breast milk storage
6. A computer and phone to respond to clinical needs

Case Study-the Anaphylaxis Crisis

Author AGM

My baby was 4- months old, and I had been working for about a month since the conclusion of my maternity leave. The conclusion of my maternity leave also brought with it the conclusion of my stored breast milk supply. My baby was at a point in which she needed the very milk that I was pumping for her next meal. This became unsustainable. I needed an alternative for her own safety and my own sanity. I could not be under so much pressure. We had planned on this happening, as had occurred with my 2 other children when I returned to work. We would start formula as a supplement to her diet. This had worked before as I was able to provide about 50:50 breastmilk: formula to my 2 other children for about a year.

Coming home after a very busy day at work, I longed to decompress, eat, drink some water, pump, and be with my children. About 5 minutes into my arrival and after

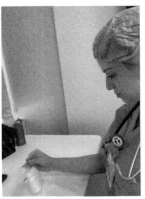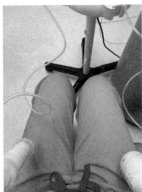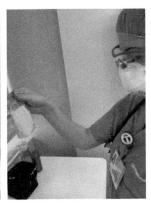

Fig. 1. Lactation at work.

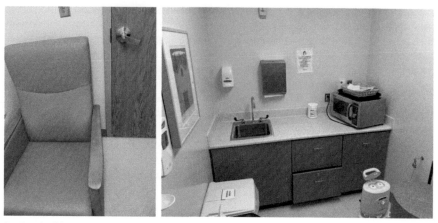

Fig. 2. Ideal lactation space in the workplace.

the second dose of ordinary infant formula, the provider caring for my baby calls for my immediate help. My baby developed a diffuse rash which quickly turned into hives. She became increasingly agitated and was struggling to breathe—she was in anaphylaxis. We quickly called emergency services who provided the necessary doses of epinephrine followed by a hospital admission, whereby we learned she developed anaphylaxis to cow's milk in infant formula (**Fig. 3**). Although cow's milk allergy is one of the most common food allergies in early life with a prevalence of 0.5% to

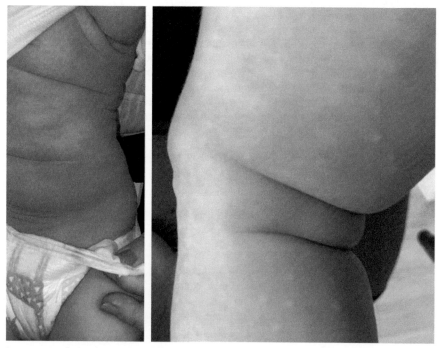

Fig. 3. Breastfed infant anaphylaxis to cow's milk formula.

3%, it rarely if ever presents as anaphylaxis.[13] But it did happen which emphasized the importance of continuing this child's access to breastmilk. Someone then told me that my lactation cycle was "impractical" and that I needed to "choose between motherhood or my career." I was at a crucial juncture: do I quit my job to safely nourish my child? I knew that with the ordinary demands of my clinical work I was unable to keep up with my baby's breastmilk needs.

Ultimately, I chose both. I spoke with advisors, colleagues, and supervisors. I described the circumstances and my strong desire to continue with my career. This was the right decision for me, and I received an incredible amount of support and understanding from my professional community. I told myself: I will never stop trying to do my best at both (**Fig. 4**).

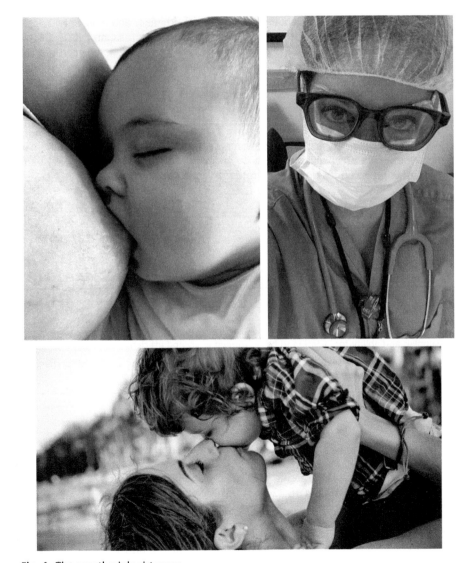

Fig. 4. The anesthesiologist mom.

Future Directions to Improve Lactation in Anesthesiology

As Dr. Jerome Adams stated: "We need to make breastfeeding the easy thing to do." The benefits of breastfeeding for mother and baby were described above. Breastfeeding has benefits beyond the mother and infant — it benefits the employer.[21] Supporting lactating women promotes wellness in the workplace by increasing workplace satisfaction, employee productivity and loyalty, and postpartum employee retention.[21] Making breastfeeding easier for anesthesiology clinicians is one of the most urgent and equitable ways to increase wellness and satisfaction in our workplace and specialty. To accomplish this, we should consider the following:

1. Increase the number of lactation spaces for anesthesiology clinicians and make these spaces more accessible from the operating room suite.
2. Improve the quality of these lactations spaces so that they can be equipped with the supplies and ability for lactation to be performed easily and efficiently.
3. Improve the system to allow for lactation sessions without pressuring the individual receiving or giving the break. For example, a lactating clinician should not feel guilty requesting a lactation session, just as there should be a colleague who is not overburdened with clinical care and is available to provide said lactation session relief.
4. Encourage supportive behavior, education, language, and small acts to change perspectives and workplace culture around breastfeeding.

Supporting lactating anesthesia clinicians is a practical way of maintaining gender diversity in our specialty, and one of the greatest forms of support for a fellow human being. Women are an invaluable presence in our field and the current system needs revision to improve conditions around returning to work after parental leave.

DISCLOSURE

The authors have nothing to disclose.

CLINICS CARE POINTS

- To make lactation easier and possible for anesthesiology clinicians, we need to increase the number of lactation spaces and make them more accessible from the operating room suite.
- The quality of lactation spaces needs to improve so that they can be equipped with the supplies and ability for lactation to be performed easily and efficiently.
- We must encourage supportive behavior, education, language, and small acts to change perspectives and workplace culture around breastfeeding.

REFERENCES

1. Sattari M, Levine D, Bertram A, et al. Breastfeeding intentions of female physicians. Breastfeed Med 2010;5(6):297–302.
2. Cantu RM, Gowen MS, Tang X, et al. Barriers to Breastfeeding in Female Physicians. Breastfeed Med 2018;13(5):341–5.
3. Sattari M, Levine D, Neal D, et al. Personal breastfeeding behavior of physician mothers is associated with their clinical breastfeeding advocacy. Breastfeed Med 2013;8(1):31–7.
4. Sattari M, Levine D, Serwint JR. Physician mothers: an unlikely high risk group-call for action. Breastfeed Med 2010;5(1):35–9.

5. Section on B. Breastfeeding and the use of human milk. Pediatrics 2012;129(3): e827–41.
6. Ip S, Chung M, Raman G, et al. Breastfeeding and maternal and infant health outcomes in developed countries. Evid Rep Technol Assess (Full Rep 2007;(153): 1–186.
7. Prevention CfDCa. Breastfeeding, why it Matters. Available at: https://www.cdc. gov/breastfeeding/about-breastfeeding/why-it-matters.html. Accessed 2021.
8. Victora CG, Bahl R, Barros AJ, et al. Breastfeeding in the 21st century: epidemiology, mechanisms, and lifelong effect. Lancet 2016;387(10017):475–90.
9. Kent JC. How breastfeeding works. J Midwifery Womens Health 2007;52(6): 564–70.
10. Kent JC, Prime DK, Garbin CP. Principles for maintaining or increasing breast milk production. J Obstet Gynecol Neonatal Nurs 2012;41(1):114–21.
11. KWaJ Riordan. Breastfeeding and human lactation. 5 edition. Jones and Bartlett Learning; 2015.
12. Adesoye T, Mangurian C, Choo EK, et al. Perceived Discrimination Experienced by Physician Mothers and Desired Workplace Changes: A Cross-sectional Survey. JAMA Intern Med 2017;177(7):1033–6.
13. Kraus MB, Thomson HM, Dexter F, et al. Pregnancy and Motherhood for Trainees in Anesthesiology: A Survey of the American Society of Anesthesiologists. J Educ Perioper Med 2021;23(1):E656.
14. Pearson ACS, Dodd SE, Kraus MB, et al. Pilot Survey of Female Anesthesiologists' Childbearing and Parental Leave Experiences. Anesth Analg 2019; 128(6):e109–12.
15. Titler SS, Dexter F. Low Prevalence of Designated Lactation Spaces at Hospitals and Ambulatory Surgery Centers in Iowa: An Educational Tool for Graduates' Job Selection. A A Pract 2021;15(11):e01544.
16. Titler S, Dexter F, Epstein RH. Percentages of Cases in Operating Rooms of Sufficient Duration to Accommodate a 30-Minute Breast Milk Pumping Session by Anesthesia Residents or Nurse Anesthetists. Cureus 2021;13(1):e12519.
17. Titler SS, Pearson ACS. Supporting Lactation Within an Academic Anesthesia Department: Obstacles and Opportunities. Anesth Analg 2020;131(4):1304–7.
18. Titler SS, Dexter F, Epstein RH. Suggested Work Guidelines, Based on Operating Room Data, for Departments with a Breast Milk Pumping Supervising Anesthesiologist. Breastfeed Med 2021;16(7):573–8.
19. Melnitchouk N, Scully RE, Davids JS. Barriers to Breastfeeding for US Physicians Who Are Mothers. JAMA Intern Med 2018;178(8):1130–2.
20. ACGME. ACGME Common Program Requirements (Residency). 2018. Available at: https://acgme.org/Portals/0/PFAssets/ProgramRequirements/CPRResidency2019. pdf. Accessed February 5 2020.
21. Committe USB. Federal Workplace Law: what are the benefits to employers. 2021. Available at: http://www.usbreastfeeding.org/p/cm/ld/fid=234. Accessed October 27 2021.

Burnout, Mental Health, and Workplace Discrimination in Lesbian, Gay, Bisexual, Transgender, Queer/Questioning, Intersex, and Asexual Anesthesiologists

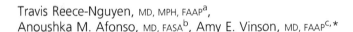

Travis Reece-Nguyen, MD, MPH, FAAP[a],
Anoushka M. Afonso, MD, FASA[b], Amy E. Vinson, MD, FAAP[c],*

KEYWORDS

- Burnout • Well-being • LGBTQIA • Mental health • Underrepresented in medicine

KEY POINTS

- Burnout is prevalent in anesthesiologists; in anesthesiologists, identifying as a sexual minority is an independent predictor of being at high risk for burnout.
- Those identifying as LGBTQIA are underrepresented in medicine and anesthesiology.
- LGBTQIA anesthesiologists face many legislative challenges at the local, state, and federal levels, which compounds issues of mental health and workplace discrimination and harassment.
- Given that not every state has legal protections in place, all nondiscrimination policies and diversity statements should include "sexual orientation" and "gender identity."

INTRODUCTION: BURNOUT AS AN OCCUPATIONAL HAZARD

Burnout as an occupational phenomenon entered the mainstream discourse in the mid-seventies with the work of psychologist Herbert Freudenberger, who described a cascade of behaviors, reactions and manifestations of work-related stress,

[a] Department of Anesthesiology, Perioperative, and Pain Medicine, Division of Pediatric Anesthesiology, Stanford Medicine, 453 Quarry Road, MC: 5663, Stanford, CA 94305, USA; [b] Department of Anesthesiology & Critical Care, Memorial Sloan Kettering Cancer Center, 1275 York Avenue, C-336, New York, NY 10065, USA; [c] Department of Anesthesiology, Critical Care and Pain Medicine, Boston Children's Hospital and Harvard Medical School, 300 Longwood Avenue, Bader 3, Boston, MA 02115, USA
* Corresponding author.
E-mail address: Amy.vinson@childrens.harvard.edu

Anesthesiology Clin 40 (2022) 245–255
https://doi.org/10.1016/j.anclin.2022.01.002
1932-2275/22/© 2022 Elsevier Inc. All rights reserved.

anesthesiology.theclinics.com

ultimately leading to a state of full burnout.[1] Shortly thereafter, in the interest of quantifying and further classifying the major symptoms, psychologist Christina Maslach and her colleagues developed the Maslach Burnout Inventory (MBI), a 22-item survey questionnaire that categorizes the symptoms of burnout into 3 dimensions: emotional exhaustion, depersonalization and a low sense of personal accomplishment.[2] Burnout was subsequently studied in many human service-related fields, particularly in occupations involving helping others and self-sacrifice. The concept of burnout was not widely applicable to physicians until 2012 when Tait Shanafelt and colleagues published a large study on burnout in U.S. physicians.[3] They demonstrated that nearly half of U.S. physicians were at high risk for burnout, defined as scoring high on either the emotional exhaustion or depersonalization subscales. Emotional exhaustion was the most prevalent domain followed by depersonalization and a low sense of personal accomplishment, in that order. Demographics included in this initial study included sex and age, but there were no reported differences in burnout rate between sexes and only slightly decreased risk with increasing age (odds ratio (OR): for each year older, 0.99).[3]

Since that time, interest in physician burnout has rapidly accelerated, with substantive efforts currently underway to ascertain the root causes of physician burnout and its impact on the lives of physicians and other clinicians, patient care, and ultimately, the health care system and society as a whole. Many national organizations have made clinician well-being a priority, including the National Academy of Medicine (NAM), who recently published a collaborative work product entitled, "Taking Action Against Clinician Burnout: A Systems Approach to Professional Well-being."[4] In this publication, the NAM collaborative outlines a rubric by which all health care stakeholders can work collaboratively to address imbalances in job demands and resources to align the workplace structures with the workforce values.

In discussions of physician burnout, it is important to recognize that burnout exists on a spectrum and can be measured several different ways with a variety of validated instruments, including the MBI. The predominant definition of "high risk for burnout" is understood to be reaching a threshold level of one or both dimensions of emotional exhaustion and/or depersonalization on the MBI, as described by Shanafelt and colleagues in 2012.[3] A more recent paper by Afonso and colleagues, on burnout in US attending anesthesiologists adds a new metric, "burnout syndrome," which they define as reaching threshold levels for all 3 domains of burnout simultaneously, to more fully appreciate the factors associated with more severe burnout.[5]

The recent paper by Afonso and colleagues studies burnout in attending anesthesiologists in the US with nearly 4000 survey responses. It demonstrated that 59% of respondents were at high risk for burnout and nearly 14% had burnout syndrome. More importantly, however, were the associations with demographic and practice factors revealed. Modest independent practice-related risk factors for high risk for burnout included longer work hours, staffing shortages, and not having a confidant at work. Demographic risk factors included lesbian, gay, bisexual, transgender, queer/questioning, intersex, and asexual (LGBTQIA) status, lack of support at home, and age less than 50 year old. Independent practice-related risk factors for burnout syndrome included staffing shortages and not having a confidant at work. Demographic risk factors included lack of support at home and age less than 50 year old. However, the most profound associations concerned the question: "How supported do you feel in your work-life?", whereby answers of little or no support carried an odds ratio of 6.7 (95% confidence interval (CI): 5.3%–8.5%) for being high risk for burnout and 10.0 (95% CI: 5.4%–18.3%) for burnout syndrome.[5]

THE SEXUAL MINORITY COMMUNITY IN ANESTHESIOLOGY

Sexual minorities face several well-documented challenges in medicine, including an increased rate of mental health conditions, discrimination in the workplace, and more recently, occupational burnout.[5] In this review, we will outline unique challenges faced by members of the LGBTQIA community in medicine as well as strategies for creating an inclusive, supportive, and welcoming environment for these professionals. To aid the reader less experienced in issues pertaining to sexual minorities, we have compiled definitions of key terms, as described by the Human Rights Campaign, a long-standing advocacy organization for sexual minorities.[6] (**Table 1**) We will use the terms "sexual minority" and LGBTQIA interchangeably and will use other terms (eg, LGB) when referencing studies and reports with a slightly more narrow focus.

Table 1
Definitions of key sexual minority terms

Term	Definition
Ally	"A term used to describe someone who is actively supportive of LGBTQ people. It encompasses straight and cisgender allies, as well as those within the LGBTQ community who support each other."
Asexual	"The lack of a sexual attraction or desire for other people."
Bisexual	"A person emotionally, romantically, or sexually attracted to more than one sex, gender, or gender identity though not necessarily simultaneously, in the same way or to the same degree. Sometimes used interchangeably with pansexual."
Cisgender	"A term used to describe a person whose gender identity aligns with those typically associated with the sex assigned to them at birth."
Coming Out	"The process in which a person first acknowledges, accepts and appreciates their sexual orientation or gender identity and begins to share that with others."
Gay	"A person who is emotionally, romantically, or sexually attracted to members of the same gender. Men, women, and nonbinary people may use this term to describe themselves."
Gender expression	"External appearance of one's gender identity, usually expressed through behavior, clothing, body characteristics or voice, and which may or may not conform to socially defined behaviors and characteristics typically associated with being either masculine or feminine."
Gender Identity	"One's innermost concept of self as male, female, a blend of both or neither—how individuals perceive themselves and what they call themselves. One's gender identity can be the same or different from their sex assigned at birth."
Homophobia	"The fear and hatred of or discomfort with people who are attracted to members of the same sex."
Intersex	"Intersex people are born with a variety of differences in their sex traits and reproductive anatomy. There is a wide variety of differences among intersex variations, including differences in genitalia, chromosomes, gonads, internal sex organs, hormone production, hormone response, and/or secondary sex traits."
Lesbian	"A woman who is emotionally, romantically or sexually attracted to other women. Women and nonbinary people may use this term to describe themselves."

(continued on next page)

Table 1 (continued)	
Term	**Definition**
Nonbinary	"An adjective describing a person who does not identify exclusively as a man or a woman. Nonbinary people may identify as being both a man and a woman, somewhere in between, or as falling completely outside these categories."
Outing	"Exposing someone's lesbian, gay, bisexual transgender or gender nonbinary identity to others without their permission. Outing someone can have serious repercussions on employment, economic stability, personal safety or religious or family situations."
Queer	"A term people often use to express a spectrum of identities and orientations that are counter to the mainstream. Queer is often used as a catch-all to include many people, including those who do not identify as exclusively straight and/or folks who have nonbinary or gender-expansive identities. This term was previously used as a slur, but has been reclaimed by many parts of the LGBTQ movement."
Questioning	"A term used to describe people who are in the process of exploring their sexual orientation or gender identity."
Sexual Orientation	"An inherent or immutable enduring emotional, romantic or sexual attraction to other people. Note: an individual's sexual orientation is independent of their gender identity."
Transgender	"An umbrella term for people whose gender identity and/or expression is different from cultural expectations based on the sex they were assigned at birth. Being transgender does not imply any specific sexual orientation."
Transitioning	"A series of processes that some transgender people may undergo to live more fully as their true gender. This typically includes social transition, such as changing name and pronouns, medical transition, which may include hormone therapy or gender-affirming surgeries, and legal transition, which may include changing legal name and sex on government identity documents. Transgender people may choose to undergo some, all or none of these processes."

Please visit the Human Rights Campaign website for additional information related to sexual minorities.

BURNOUT IN THE LESBIAN, GAY, BISEXUAL, TRANSGENDER, QUEER/QUESTIONING, INTERSEX, AND ASEXUAL COMMUNITY

Apart from the initial description of the MBI, whereby it was noted that respondents who identified as being part of a racial minority had similar rates of burnout to the entire studied cohort,[2] burnout studies have not typically focused on underrepresented communities in medicine, including the LBGTQIA community. Afonso and colleagues, demonstrated that identifying as underrepresented based on the LGBTQIA status inferred an increased risk of being "high risk for burnout" (odds ratio 2.21; 95% CI: 1.35%–3.63%; $P = .0002$).[5] Notably, only 2.7% of respondents in this study identified as underrepresented based on the LGBTQIA status, which is significantly less than the estimated 4.5% of the U.S. population who identify as members of the LGBT community.[7] While the LGBTQIA community is not classified as "underrepresented in medicine" by the Association of American Medical Colleges (AAMC),[8] and while the proportion of individuals in medicine identifying as LGBTQIA may be increasing,[9] these numbers certainly suggest an underrepresentation of LGBTQIA individuals within the anesthesiology community.

In another recent study of medical students, using the Oldenburg Burnout Inventory, 5.4% of respondents identified as a sexual minority (ie, specifically Lesbian, Gay, or Bisexual [LGB]). In addition to increased self-reported discriminatory experiences, those identifying as LGB had higher rates of burnout (adjusted relative risk (ARR): 1.63; 95 CI: 1.41%–1.89%), with those who experienced higher levels of mistreatment having a much higher risk of burnout (19.8%; 95% CI: 8.3%–31.4% in LGB students vs 2.3%; 95% CI: 0.2%–4.5%; $P < .001$ in heterosexual students).[10]

LEGISLATIVE HISTORY AND CURRENT CHALLENGES FOR THE LESBIAN, GAY, BISEXUAL, TRANSGENDER, QUEER/QUESTIONING, INTERSEX, AND ASEXUAL COMMUNITY

To better understand the context of professional burnout experienced by LGBTQIA anesthesiologists, we must recognize the compounding effects of external factors, particularly the legislative challenges faced by this community over the last several decades and the recent surge of anti-LGBTQIA bills across the country. According to the Human Rights Campaign, more than 250 anti-LGBTQIA bills have been introduced in state legislatures in 2021, 17 bills are already signed into law and 11 bills await governors' signatures. Indeed, 2021 has wrought the worst LGBTQIA legislative setbacks in recent history.[11]

According to the Movement Advancement Project (a nonprofit think tank established in 2006 to "help speed equality and opportunity for all"), in 2020 approximately 46% of LGBTQIA Americans live in states with positive LGBTQIA policy climates, whereas 45% live in states with negative policy climates.[12] It is, therefore, unsurprising that the minority stress experienced by LGBTQIA anesthesiologists will vary greatly by geography. Numerous studies[13–16] show the direct, negative impact that aggressive anti-LGBTQIA legislation has on sexual and gender minority Americans' mental health. Hatzenbuehler and colleagues investigated changes in mental health for LGB Americans during the antigay marriage campaigns of 2009 and discovered increased mood disorder (36.6%), generalized anxiety disorder (248.2%), alcohol use disorder (41.9%), and psychiatric comorbidity (36.3%) for those LGB Americans living in states which banned gay marriage, while there was no appreciable increase in those living in states without gay marriage bans. Significant state-by-state variability is seen in almost all LGBTQIA policy.[16]

The Movement Advancement Project notes that, as of 2020, only 20 states and Washington, D.C. explicitly prohibited discrimination of LGBTQ people in housing, public accommodations, and employment.[12] Unfortunately, the rise of discriminatory religious exemption claims, now legal in 13 states with at least 40 remaining bills under consideration in 2021, allows health care workers, adoption agencies, and some private companies to refuse service for LGBTQIA people based solely on their gender identity or sexual minority status. There are 13 states whereby it is illegal to discriminate against patients with LGBTQ in the health care system. Said simply, living in different states can profoundly impact an individual's ability to access discrimination-free, medically necessary care. We must acknowledge the repercussions of the recent deluge of antitransgender legislation across the country. In 2021 alone, there have been at least 35 bills seeking to prohibit transgender youth from accessing gender-affirming medical care, almost 70 bills that would prohibit transgender youth from playing sports on teams that align with their gender identity, and at least 15 "bathroom bills" that falsely claim sexual harassment to preclude trans-individuals from using their appropriate public bathrooms. Despite conversion therapy being categorized as torture by the United Nations Human Rights Council and the United Nations Committee Against Torture in 2015,[17] only 18 states and Washington, D.C. have legal bans prohibiting its practice. As anti-LGBTQIA bills are publicly debated and voted into law, LGBTQIA individuals are rendered vulnerable and stigmatized, potentially leading to worsened mental health.

Perhaps the most prominent contributor to LGBTQIA burnout in anesthesiology is the anxiety and fear surrounding workplace discrimination and harassment. The Federal Employment Non-Discrimination Act (ENDA), which would protect lesbian, gay, bisexual, and transgender Americans from employer discrimination (under Title VII of the Civil Rights Act of 1964), has been *proposed and defeated eleven times* from 1994 to 2013.[18,19] Interestingly, this legislation still afforded religious exemption, (including hospitals with religious affiliation), and allowed all employers the freedom to not offer LGBTQ spousal/partner benefits. After numerous failed attempts to pass ENDA, the Federal Equality Act, a new iteration of anti-LGBTQIA discrimination legislation, has been proposed in Congress four times since 2015. The highly anticipated Equality Act would amend the Civil Rights Act of 1964 to prohibit discrimination based on sexual orientation and gender identity in employment, education, public housing, and other federally funded programs. The Equality Act recently passed in the House in February 2021 but is expected to once again fail in the Senate, despite 76% of American support for LGBTQIA protections according to the Public Religion Research Institute.[20] In June 2020, the United States Supreme Court determined that sexual orientation and gender identity were considered tenets of sexual discrimination, and employers who fire someone for being gay or transgender violate Title VII of the Civil Rights Act of 1964 (*Bostock v Clayton* (2020)).[21] Although a considerable victory, this ruling does not cover areas of discrimination outside of employment. Notably, *Castro v. Yale University* (Feb 2021)[22] determined that attending physicians in academic medical centers can file lawsuits for sex-based discrimination under both Title VII and Title IX.

MENTAL HEALTH CHALLENGES FOR THE LESBIAN, GAY, BISEXUAL, TRANSGENDER, QUEER/QUESTIONING, INTERSEX, AND ASEXUAL COMMUNITY

The LGBTQIA community suffers from poorer mental health compared with nonsexual minority individuals.[23] This review will focus specifically on the mental health of those in the medical community who identify as a sexual minority.

In one study of 4673 medical students who self-reported their sexual orientation, 5% identified as a sexual minority. Those identifying as a sexual minority had higher rates of depressive symptoms (ARR: 1.59; 95% CI: 1.24%–2.04%) and anxiety symptoms (ARR: 1.64; 95% CI: 1.08%–2.49%). They were also more likely to report harassment and isolation compared with their cisgender heterosexual peers.[24] Additionally, Wang and colleagues, reported data from 2890 third-year medical residents, adjusting for depression and anxiety before residency, and showed that the 10% who identified as a sexual minority reported significantly higher levels of depression and anxiety than their sexual majority peers. They reported a lower sense of belonging during the second year of residency, a time that was also associated with higher depression and anxiety.[25] Another cross-sectional study of U.S. medical trainees evaluated whether medical student burnout differs by sexual orientation. Of the 26,123 analyzed responses from medical students, 5.4% identified as LGB (lesbian, gay, or bisexual) with an increased odds of burnout of 63%. This association persisted, though attenuated, after adjusting for mistreatment, which is also prevalent in the LGB community. Mistreatment is significantly higher in lesbian, gay or bisexual students with these students having an 8-fold higher predicted probability of burnout compared with heterosexual medical students.[10]

Beyond medical school, sexual minority physicians have increased rates of anxiety disorder and major depression. In 2020, Duba and colleagues reported data from 2003 young physicians determining if the prevalence of sexual orientation-based discrimination (SOBD) was associated with increased anxiety and depression in this population. SOBD was reported almost twice as frequently in participants with anxiety disorder and major depression.[26]

Further, a meta-analysis of 21,201 sexual minority individuals in the US, Canada, Europe, Australia, and New Zealand showed a higher lifetime prevalence of suicide attempts (11%, 95% CI: .08%–.15%), compared with heterosexual groups (4%, 95% CI: .03%–.05%).[27] Community-based surveys of sexual minority individuals suggest that up to 20% have attempted suicide, which is a much higher rate than the general U.S. population surveys. Sexual orientation was significantly associated with suicide attempts in adolescents and youths (OR = 2.26, 95% CI: 1.60%–3.20%). Gay or bisexual men were more likely to report suicide attempts compared with heterosexual men (OR = 2.21, 95% CI: 1.21%–4.04%).[28] These are alarming trends, particularly given the increased risk of suicide in the field of anesthesiology.[29]

Given the increased risk of poorer mental health in the LGBTQIA community, further work must be conducted for medical schools and workplaces to support safe and inclusive learning and working environments. Programs should emphasize and prioritize target-based interventions for sexual minority mental health, as the repercussions can be devastating for LGBTQIA individuals in the medical community.[24]

DISCRIMINATION IN THE WORKPLACE FOR MEMBERS OF THE LESBIAN, GAY, BISEXUAL, TRANSGENDER, QUEER/QUESTIONING, INTERSEX, AND ASEXUAL COMMUNITY

Prior data demonstrate that members of sexual minority communities are subject to more episodes of workplace discrimination in the form of harassment, stress, and ultimately burnout.[30,31] In one examination of 326 sexual minority employees, coping tactics such as "concealment-focused identity management strategy" (ie, "avoidance" or "closeting") were explored as well as positive behaviors of "disclosure-focused identity management strategy."[30] The authors found that those with higher levels of disclosure had higher job satisfaction, but only if low discrimination was also present in the workplace.[30] In another study of LGBT employees in higher education, heterosexist and gender harassment occurred in a concordant fashion. Those with the lowest perceived institutional support reported the most harassment and the severity of harassment was associated with occupational burnout and job dissatisfaction.[31]

In another assessment of workplace mistreatment, using data from the 2016 and 2017 AAMC Graduation Questionnaire, responses from 1463 (5.3% of the entire cohort) LGB graduating medical students were analyzed. The AAMC found that far more LGB students reported sexual orientation-based discrimination and multiple episodes of mistreatment than their heterosexual counterparts (23.1% vs 1.0%, $P < .001$ and 16.4% vs 3.6%, $P < .001$ respectively). Even more concerning were the increased rates of reporting public humiliation, unwanted sexual advances, offensive comments or name-calling, and receiving lower grades or evaluations due to sexual orientation.[10]

Actionable steps toward improving the inclusivity of our workplaces and increasing support of LGBTQIA clinicians:

A 2013 Williams Institute report demonstrated that LGBT-supportive policies and workplace climates are linked to greater job commitment, improved workplace relationships, increased job satisfaction, and improved health outcomes among LGBTQ employees.[32] There are currently no objective rating systems to measure support for LGBTQIA clinicians in anesthesiology departments across the country. The workplace climate is improved for all minoritized individuals when departments provide education about diversity and how to avoid discrimination, structural racism, microaggressions, and implicit bias.[33] Ultimately, departments should avoid performative allyship and provide tangible and meaningful support for LGBTQIA employees. The Gay and Lesbian Medical Association (GLMA) published a concise list of recommendations that can be used by departments to help improve the experiences of LGBT clinicians.[34]

- All nondiscrimination policies and diversity statements should include "sexual orientation" and "gender identity," as not all states have legal protections in place.
- Health benefit coverage must treat same-sex spouses and domestic partners equally and include transgender care.
- Departments should require comprehensive transgender health education for all staff and trainees, actively support transgender and gender-diverse clinicians by ensuring correct names/pronouns are used, guarantee single-stall bathroom availability, and support clinicians against any form of discrimination from patients and/or colleagues.
- Departments should intentionally increase LGBTQIA medical student/resident recruitment as well as the quality of LGBTQIA health care education in medical school. Although the AAMC definition of Under-Represented in Medicine) (URM) does not include LGBTQIA applicants, it is important to acknowledge that LGBTQIA applicants are, indeed, underrepresented and should be considered as such in the admissions process.
- Departments should create a psychologically safe space during recruitment interviews that include required implicit bias training of all interviewers. Displaying pronouns and pride memorabilia, coupled with allowing applicants to self-identify as LGBTQIA on official paperwork will send a clear message of support for LGBTQIA clinicians in your department.
- Equity in academic promotion practices, efforts to mitigate the minority tax, and sponsorship/mentorship for career advancement may improve LGBTQIA staff retention. Often, LGBTQIA clinicians are heavily involved in diversity, equity, and inclusion (DEI) efforts within their departments though this work is rarely acknowledged for promotion and clinical commitment. Leadership must give LGBTQIA faculty/staff a voice; diversity alone does not equal inclusion.

SUMMARY

Members of the LGBTQIA community are a growing cohort in the medical and anesthesiology workforce. Our best current data suggest that they are underrepresented in medicine, but that their representation is increasing. Sparse data exist as to the presence of LGBTQIA individuals in medical leadership positions and is an area in need of further investigation. We know that LGBTQIA individuals face increased rates of mental health conditions, suicidality, workplace discrimination, and burnout. We also know that the impact of these negative forces is greatly reduced, if not eliminated entirely, by working in a supportive environment free of harassment. As we move forward in medicine toward a greater commitment to diversity, equity, and inclusion, the LGBTQIA community should not be left behind. Efforts for inclusivity and welcoming of these professionals must be intentional, with an emphasis on junior colleagues in medical school, residency, and fellowship, who are more vulnerable to the impact of workplace discrimination, nearer to their own "coming out" struggles and often lacking in significant familial support. If we are to create a welcoming caregiving environment for patients with LGBTQIA and families, we must do the same for our own. Surely such efforts will lead to a more fulfilled, engaged, and welcoming workforce.

DISCLOSURE

The authors have nothing to disclose.

REFERENCES

1. Freudenberger HJ. Staff Burn-Out. J Soc Issues 1974;30(1):159–65.
2. Maslach C, Jackson SE. The measurement of experienced burnout. J Organ Behav 1981;2(2):99–113.
3. Shanafelt TD, Boone S, Tan L, et al. Burnout and Satisfaction With Work-Life Balance Among US Physicians Relative to the General US Population. Arch Intern Med 2012;172(18):1377–9.
4. Well-Being NA of S Engineering, and Medicine; National Academy of Medicine; Committee on Systems Approaches to Improve Patient Care by Supporting Clinician. Taking Action Against Clinician Burnout: A Systems Approach to Professional Well-Being. Washington, DC: The National Academies Press; 2019.
5. Afonso AM, Cadwell JB, Staffa SJ, et al. Burnout Rate and Risk Factors among Anesthesiologists in the United States. Anesthesiology 2021;134(5):683–96.
6. Campaign THR. Glossary of Terms [Internet]. Available at: https://www.hrc.org/resources/glossary-of-terms. Accessed November 1, 2021.
7. Conron KJ, Goldberg SK. Adult LGBT Population In The United States. 7AD. Available at: https://williamsinstitute.law.ucla.edu/wp-content/uploads/LGBT-Adult-US-Pop-Jul-2020.pdf. Accessed November 1, 2021.
8. Colleges A of AM. Underrepresented in Medicine Definition [Internet]. Available at: https://www.aamc.org/what-we-do/equity-diversity-inclusion/underrepresented-in-medicine. Accessed November 1, 2021.
9. Tanner L. U.S. medical schools boost LGBTQ students, doctor training. 2020. Available at: https://apnews.com/article/ky-state-wire-health-us-news-ap-top-news-medical-schools-985d50d0a7b1b593acd0dd791e8c3118. Accessed November 1, 2021.
10. Samuels EA, Boatright DH, Wong AH, et al. Association Between Sexual Orientation, Mistreatment, and Burnout Among US Medical Students. Jama Netw Open 2021;4(2):e2036136.
11. Ronan W. Officially Becomes Worst Year in Recent History for LGBTQ State Legislative Attacks as Unprecedented Number of States Enact Record-Shattering Number of Anti-LGBTQ Measures Into Law [Internet]. Available at: https://www.hrc.org/press-releases/2021-officially-becomes-worst-year-in-recent-history-for-lgbtq-state-legislative-attacks-as-unprecedented-number-of-states-enact-record-shattering-number-of-anti-lgbtq-measures-into-law. Accessed November 1, 2021.

12. Project MA. Mapping LGBTQ Equality: 2010 TO 2020. 2020. Available at: https://www.lgbtmap.org/2020-tally-report. Accessed November 1, 2021.
13. Hatzenbuehler ML, Keyes KM, Hasin DS. State-Level Policies and Psychiatric Morbidity In Lesbian, Gay, and Bisexual Populations. Am J Public Health 2011;99(12):2275–81.
14. Rostosky SS, Riggle EDB, Horne SG, et al. Marriage Amendments and Psychological Distress in Lesbian, Gay, and Bisexual (LGB) Adults. J Couns Psychol 2009;56(1):56–66.
15. Raifman J, Moscoe E, Austin SB, et al. Difference-in-Differences Analysis of the Association Between State Same-Sex Marriage Policies and Adolescent Suicide Attempts. Jama Pediatr 2017;171(4):350.
16. Hatzenbuehler ML, McLaughlin KA, Keyes KM, et al. The Impact of Institutional Discrimination on Psychiatric Disorders in Lesbian, Gay, and Bisexual Populations: A Prospective Study. Am J Public Health 2011;100(3):452–9.
17. UN Human Rights Council. Report of the Office of the United Nations High Commissioner for Human Rights, Discrimination and Violence against Individuals Based on Their Sexual Orientation and Gender Identity. vol 13. 2015:38. A/HRC/29/23
18. S.815 - Employment Non-Discrimination Act of 2013 [Internet]. Available at: https://www.congress.gov/bill/113th-congress/senate-bill/815. Accessed November 1, 2021.
19. H.R.5 - Equality Act [Internet]. Available at: https://www.congress.gov/bill/117th-congress/house-bill/5. Accessed November 1, 2021.
20. PRRI. Despite Partisan Rancor, Americans Broadly Support LGBTQ Rights [Internet]. 3AD. Available at: https://www.prri.org/research/despite-partisan-rancor-despite-partisan-rancor-americans-broadly-support-lgbtq-rights-broadly-support-lgbtq-rights/. Accessed November 1, 2021.
21. ScotusBlog. Bostock v. Clayton County, Georgia. Available at: https://www.scotusblog.com/case-files/cases/bostock-v-clayton-county-georgia/. Accessed November 1, 2021.
22. casetext. Castro v. Yale Univ. Available at: https://casetext.com/case/castro-v-yale-univ. 2AD [Accessed October 12 2021.
23. Russell ST, Fish JN. Mental Health in Lesbian, Gay, Bisexual, and Transgender (LGBT) Youth. Annu Rev Clin Psycho 2015;12(1):1–23.
24. Przedworski JM, Dovidio JF, Hardeman RR, et al. A Comparison of the Mental Health and Well-Being of Sexual Minority and Heterosexual First-Year Medical Students. Acad Med 2015;90(5):652–9.
25. Wang K, Burke SE, Przedworski JM, et al. A Comparison of Depression and Anxiety Symptoms Between Sexual Minority and Heterosexual Medical Residents: A Report from the Medical Trainee CHANGE Study. Lgbt Health 2020;7(6):332–9.
26. Duba A, Messiaen M, Boulangeat C, et al. Sexual-orientation based discrimination is associated with anxiety and depression in young physicians. A national study. J Affect Disord 2020;274:964–8.
27. Hottes TS, Bogaert L, Rhodes AE, et al. Lifetime Prevalence of Suicide Attempts Among Sexual Minority Adults by Study Sampling Strategies: A Systematic Review and Meta-Analysis. Am J Public Health 2016;106(5):e1–12.
28. Miranda-Mendizábal A, Castellví P, Parés-Badell O, et al. Sexual orientation and suicidal behaviour in adolescents and young adults: systematic review and meta-analysis. Br J Psychiat 2017;211(2):77–87.
29. Plunkett E, Costello A, Yentis SM, et al. Suicide in anaesthetists: a systematic review. Anaesthesia 2021;76(10):1392–403.

30. Velez BL, Moradi B, Brewster ME. Testing the Tenets of Minority Stress Theory in Workplace Contexts. J Couns Psychol 2013;60(4):532–42.
31. Rabelo VC, Cortina LM. Two Sides of the Same Coin: Gender Harassment and Heterosexist Harassment in LGBQ Work Lives. L Hum Behav 2014;38(4):378–91.
32. Badgett MVL, Durso LE, Kastanis A, et al. The Business Impact of LGBT-Supportive Workplace Policies [Internet]. 2013. Available at: https://williamsinstitute.law.ucla.edu/wp-content/uploads/Impact-LGBT-Support-Workplace-May-2013.pdf.
33. Ajayi AA, Rodriguez F, Perez V de J. Prioritizing Equity and Diversity in Academic Medicine Faculty Recruitment and Retention. Jama Heal Forum 2021;2(9): e212426.
34. Snowdon S. Recommendations for Enhancing the climate for LGBT students and employees in health professional schools: a GLMA white paper. Washington, DC: GLMA; 2013.

A Perspective on Wellness in Anesthesiology Residency Programs: A Multi-Strategy Approach

Kenneth B. Brown Jr, MD*, Arianna Cook, MD, MPH,
Fei Chen, PhD, MEd, Susan M. Martinelli, MD, FASA

KEYWORDS

- Resident wellness • Anesthesiology residency • Well-being • Burnout
- Graduate medical education

KEY POINTS

- Resident wellness is tied to program leadership, workplace community, professional development, work-life integration, and resiliency.
- Residency programs need a multilevel approach at the individual, departmental, and hospital levels to address resident well-being and decrease burnout rates.
- While a myriad of strategies for addressing burnout and improving well-being exist, implementing these approaches is often challenging given individual resident needs, lack of quality research, and implementation support.

INTRODUCTION

Physicians, particularly resident physicians, are at a higher risk for burnout and depression than the general U.S. population.[1] Given this concerning trend, medical organizations including the American Medical Association (AMA) and the Accreditation Council of Graduate Medical Education (ACGME) have focused efforts in combating physician burnout and improving well-being. In 2017, the ACGME revised the Common Program Requirements for accredited residency and fellowship programs to address well-being more comprehensively and emphasized the promotion of psychological, emotional, and physical well-being.[2]

Unfortunately, addressing resident wellness and burnout is challenging given its multiple contributing factors. Anesthesiology and surgical residents have a higher burnout prevalence compared with medicine and pediatric residents, suggesting that medical specialty can contribute to burnout risk.[3,4] Anesthesiology resident

Department of Anesthesiology, University of North Carolina at Chapel Hill, 101 Manning Drive, Chapel Hill, NC 27514, USA
* Corresponding author.
E-mail address: Kenneth_brown@med.unc.edu

Anesthesiology Clin 40 (2022) 257–274
https://doi.org/10.1016/j.anclin.2022.01.003   **anesthesiology.theclinics.com**
1932-2275/22/© 2022 Elsevier Inc. All rights reserved.

burnout rates were as high as 40% to 50% and depression rates between 10% and 22%.[3,5] Residents report that long work hours and sleep deficit contributed to poor working conditions.[6] Anesthesiology residents work an average of 64 to 70 hours per week and typically work overnight shifts as well as 24-h shifts.[6] They can have call shifts as frequent as every third night.[6] Working more than 50 hours per week has been associated with detrimental effects including sleep deprivation, decreased alertness, depression, and overall poor general physical health marked by weight gain, muscular pain, and cardiovascular decline.[7] One study showed that anesthesiology and intensive care residents accumulated 64.7 hours of sleep debt in a 2-month period.[8] Sleep debt has been associated with increased rates of depression and behavior problems as well as reduced quality of life, anxiety, and work performance.[7,8] Finally, high workload, work intensity, and poor workplace environment contribute to higher rates of burnout and exhaustion in anesthesiology residents.[6,9]

Resident well-being and burnout directly influence resident health and also negatively impact the quality of patient care and patient safety.[10] Residents have noted that their well-being directly affected their relationships with both patients and colleagues.[10] Burnout also negatively impacts professionalism; physicians who are burned out are three times more likely to have low patient satisfaction ratings.[11] Residents with burnout are twice as likely to be involved in patient safety incidents and provide suboptimal care.[11] A cross-sectional survey of 2773 anesthesiology residents showed that 33% of respondents with high burnout and depression risk self-reported multiple medication errors in the previous year compared with 0.7% of low-risk respondents.[11] Lower burnout rates are associated with improved decision-making and patient safety.[10] Residents with higher well-being are motivated to be more productive and can better perform their work duties.[10]

To improve well-being, residency programs must focus on addressing its multiple domains including professional development, relationships, physical health, and mental health.[12] However, this is a daunting task given the lack of overall quality research on resident wellness programs. Several program directors (PDs) indicated that a lack of support and resources for resident wellness initiatives often prevents them from implementing such programming.[12]

What follows is an overview of various approaches to conceptualize and intervene on resident wellness, based on the 9-organization strategy framework laid out by Shanafelt and colleagues.[13] We aim to provide a brief overview of the most relevant literature to each strategy, covering both general and anesthesiology-specific literature. Each section will conclude with our experience addressing these areas in our program. A summary of the strategies found in the literature is listed in **Table 1** and a summary of the specific strategies used at our program can be found in **Table 2**.

STRATEGY 1: ACKNOWLEDGE AND ASSESS THE PROBLEM
Overview

Understanding wellness and burnout in concrete terms, and closely monitoring these issues helps organizations respond to the ever-changing demands of the workplace on residents. Burnout and wellness can be difficult to measure and study. The Physician Well-Being Index is one example of a validated tool used to measure wellbeing.[14] The Maslach Burnout Inventory helps monitor the risk of burnout. Organization-level wellness assessments like the Mayo Well-Being Index aid in the direction of larger efforts at the departmental level.[13,15] Several metrics have been associated with wellness, such as overall time spent at work and the meaning that trainees find in their work. There are also efforts to highlight contributing factors that have been overlooked

Table 1
Example of specific interventions from the literature for each of the 9 strategies for improving wellness

Strategy	Intervention	Description	Reference
Strategy 1: Acknowledge and Assess the Problem	Validated tools such as PWBI and the MBI in wellness research	Questionnaires that Quantify well-being and burnout	[13,14]
	The Mayo WelL-being Index	Brief questionnaire that allows institution to track the well-being of employees, allowing them to target departments when wide-scale burnout occurs	[12]
Strategy 2: Harness the Power of Leadership	Effective communication between leaders and residents	Use specific instruction during complex clinical situations and two-way communication	[19]
	Leaders serving as role models	Residents learn their leadership skills from their superiors	[20]
Strategy 3: Develop and Implement Targeted Interventions	Development of a wellness committee	A comprehensive program encompassing mentorship, wellness education, and resident community	[23–25]
Strategy 4: Cultivate Community In the Workplace	Strengthen Peer Relationships	Participation in charity events, designated resident common work area, and planned out-of-hospital social events	[30]
	Strengthen Faculty-Resident Relationships	Planned nonmedical lectures such as financial wellness	[30]
Strategy 5: Use Rewards and Incentives Wisely	Formal Time-Banking Mechanisms	Stanford developed and studied a program to allow attendings to offer to cover shifts and bank that time for personal use later	[31]
Strategy 6: Align Values and Strengthen Culture	Patient Care	Patient census caps, transfer of nonclinical tasks to nonresident providers	[32]
	Intellectual Engagement	Protected didactic time	[32]
	Respect	"Doctor" badges mechanisms for addressing harassment	[32]
	Cultivation of Culture	Peer discussion groups, residency social events	[32]

(continued on next page)

Table 1
(continued)

Strategy	Intervention	Description	Reference
Strategy 7: Promote Flexibility and Work-life Integration	Part-time Residency	Approximate UK opportunities for 50% or 75% time residency programs	34
	Automated Block Scheduling	Using a computer algorithm to create block schedules for residents in a blinded, equitable way	40
	Alternate Shift Structures	Trialing casino-shifts in which shift changes ocurr at 0400 and 1200, following the pattern of the sun	41
	Family and Medical Leave	ABA policy for paid family leave	68
	Time-Banking	See Strategy 5 above	31
Strategy 8: Provide Resources to Promote Resilience and Self-Care	Mind fitness training	5-session course focusing on meditation training, self-awareness exercises, and discussions of difficult events	50
	Resilience curriculums	Workshops focusing on positivity, gratitude, and empathy training, time management skills, and coping with difficult events; mindfulness exercises, understanding grit, coping with positive and negative emotions	24,51
Strategy 9: Facilitate and Fund Organizational Science	Use of new, validated questionnaires for studies	2-question survey is available to more rapidly assess for burnout	62
	Use of biomarkers and physiologic data to quantify well-being and burnout	Use of physiologic parameters such as heartrate or biomarkers such as S 100B have been correlated to burnout	63,64

Legend: AMA–American Board of Anesthesiologygy, MBI–Maslach Burnout Inventory, PWBI–Physician Well-Being Index, UK–United Kingdom.

in the past, including the impact of work-life integration, sexism, and racism that trainees may face.[16–18] We should continue to strive to accurately describe factors contributing to well-being and burnout to more fully understand and address these issues.

Our program

In our residency program at the Department of Anesthesiology at the University of North Carolina, we have taken several approaches to define these issues and advance awareness within our department and for our residents. We have an active Wellness Committee that facilitates 2 to 3 Grand Rounds per year to continually foreground

Table 2
Examples of specific interventions from our program at the University of North Carolina for each of the 9 strategies for improving wellness

Strategy	Intervention	Description	Reference
Strategy 1: Acknowledge and Assess the Problem	Wellness Grand Rounds	2–3 Ground Round presentations on wellness topic to keep wellness at the forefront	
Strategy 2: Harness the Power of Leadership	Chair Involvement	Monthly conferences with residents, professionalism lectures intern year	
	Program Director Involvement	Monthly resident-program director meeting, bi-annual personal meetings, open-door policy	
	Other Faculty Involvement	Involvement in simulation, board preparation, morning lectures, Attendings provide daily resident feedback	
	Chief Residents' Involvement	Residents participate in chief resident selection	
Strategy 3: Develop and Implement Targeted Interventions	Pebble in the shoe	Addressing small-scale, actionable issues such as replacing broken keyboards in particular ORs	26
	Confession Sessions	Regular gatherings of interns and CA-1 residents under the guidance of a CA-3 resident to discuss difficult situations	29
	Anesthesia Family Day	Help support persons (family and friends) better understand the stresses of resident life, thus improving communication and increasing residents' personal support	67

(continued on next page)

Table 2
(continued)

Strategy	Intervention	Description	Reference
Strategy 4: Cultivate Community in the Workplace	Resident Community Building	Participation in multidisciplinary House Staff Council, annual funded class retreats, designated resident workroom, monthly out-of-hospital social events, significant other support groups, peer-to-peer mentorship	
	Resident-Faculty Community Building	Assigned faculty mentors	
Strategy 5: Use Rewards and Incentives Wisely	Earned Reading Days	Time after a set point in the afternoon is recorded and banked, when 10 h of time has been accumulated residents get a personal day at the discretion of the daily coordinators	
Strategy 6: Align Values and Strengthen Culture	Academic Medicine Rotation	5 wk program for UNC Anesthesia interns with class retreat, lectures covering leadership, fellowships, public health, and a quality improvement project with an assigned faculty mentor	22
	Confessions Sessions	See strategy 3 above	29
	Wellness Committee	Resident-led subcommittee that coordinates resident social activities, Confession Sessions, orientations for incoming CA-1s, donation drives, among other initiatives	
	Diversity, Equity and Inclusion Committee	Committee with representatives from the entire anesthesia department focusing on promoting diversity through monthly talks, monthly newsletters including information on relevant cultural events, among other initiatives	

Strategy	Initiative	Description	
Strategy 7: Promote Flexibility and Work-life Integration	Scheduling efforts	Scheduling chief resident takes into consideration holiday preference and vacation requests for block schedule creation, allowed the ability to request "no-call" days	
	Earned Reading Days	See above	
	Guaranteed postcall day for Home call	Guaranteed postcall day after home call	
Strategy 8: Provide Resources to Promote Resilience and Self-Care	Taking Care of Our Own	Mental health services for residents and faculty to address depression or help cope after an adverse event	62
	Kudos system	Anonymous form to provide Kudos for classmates or others in the department, released in a monthly email from the program director	
	Coffee and snacks in the resident library	Coffee and snacks help to boost resident morale	
Strategy 9: Facilitate and Fund Organizational Science	Departmental Wellness Research	We continue to research and aim to publish on our Family Day project, whereby we bring resident support people together to describe to them the field of anesthesia, the challenges of residency, and procedures we commonly perform. Our department has several on-going and future projects to further efforts in the field.	67

Legend: CA–clinical anesthesia, OR–operating room, UNC–University of North Carolina.

Table 3
An overview of wellness focused Grand Rounds that have recently been presented at the University of North Carolina Department of Anesthesiology

Grand Rounds Topic	Description
WELLBEING DURING THE PANDEMIC ANDCONTINUED RESILIENCE	Discuss how to evaluate individualized mental well-being and strategies to improve personal resilience
COGNITIVE, VOCAL, AND BREATHING TOOLS FOR EFFECTIVE & EMPATHETIC COMMUNICATION	Give physical and mental exercises to help mitigate burnout and build trust in the workplace
ADDICTION TO RECOVERY	Discuss the disease of addiction, understand how to recognize and intervene with an impaired colleague, and how to seek personal treatment
CONFLICT RESOLUTION	Provide training to professionally address conflicts in the workplace
COVID-19 & MAKING CULTURALLY RELEVANT DECISIONS	Focus on addressing COVID-19 related issues that have impacted individuals and more specifically individuals from diverse, underrepresented, or vulnerable groups
BIAS 101: A PRIMER ON IMPLICIT BIAS	Education on implicit biases and expanding training to address our personal biases
RELATIONSHIP-CENTERED PRACTICE AND DIFFICULT DISCUSSIONS	Provide tools to build strong relationships with patients for work fulfillment and to deal with difficult discussions with patients

departmental wellness (**Table 3**). These presentations range from guest speakers sharing personal accounts of burnout to our department's internal pain psychologists providing insight into the unique stressors of the COVID-19 pandemic and teaching coping mechanisms.

Furthermore, we have monthly resident meetings with the PDs to encourage open dialogue about tangible issues within the department and residency program. Setting intentional parameters to promote productive, solution-driven conversations have proven to be helpful. Finally, institution-wide interventions, including graduate medical education (GME) town halls for residents of all specialties, allow our broader community to collectively discuss the working atmosphere in our hospital. We recommend promoting similar strategies for training programs where no such analogs currently exist.

STRATEGY 2: HARNESS THE POWER OF LEADERSHIP
Overview

Leadership in the workplace is directly related to resident wellness. Resident supervisors include the department chair, PDs, daily supervising attendings, and chief residents. Residents regard positive resident–leadership interactions as beingimpactful on the overall workplace environment.[19,20] Lack of strong leadership and support for resident autonomy has been linked to burnout, specifically the depersonalization component.[19] In one study, residents rated specific instructions, especially during complex clinical situations, and two-way communication as important leadership skills.[20] Additionally, residents felt their leadership skills were primarily gained through direct observation of current leaders, suggesting the outsized impact of strong role modeling on a resident's future clinical success and leadership potential.[21]

Our program

Selecting effective leadership and maintaining strong relationships between residents and their supervisors can prove challenging. Our department chair engages with residents at the outset, teaching various professionalism topics during their intern Academic Medicine Rotation (described in detail under Strategy 6).[22] He also hosts monthly Chair's Conferences to prepare residents for oral boards. These interactions increase his face time and accessibility to residents. The PD holds monthly resident-PD meetings as discussed under Strategy 1, conducts bi-annual individual resident meetings, maintains an open-door policy for any resident in need, and connects residents with faculty mentors. Other faculty leaders are actively involved in resident training through simulation events, oral board practice, weekly morning lectures, and daily operating room pairings. At the end of each workday, attendings give in-person feedback to residents and complete an evaluation that ensures consistent, honest feedback to facilitate personal growth and allows the residents to provide feedback to the faculty. Residents also participate in the selection of chief residents and class representatives who serve on the Program Evaluation Committee to provide a resident voice in program decision making.

STRATEGY 3: DEVELOP AND IMPLEMENT TARGETED INTERVENTIONS
Overview

Although it can be challenging to initiate, implementing strategies targeted to improve resident well-being and decrease burnout is imperative. Specific interventions aiming for feasible outcomes may feel more manageable.[13] The Department of Anesthesiology at the University of Saskatchewan implemented a comprehensive wellness program involving the creation of a wellness committee, peer support groups, and regular wellness lectures focused on resilience and coping strategies, which cumulatively led to improved resident wellness.[23,24] The Department of Anesthesiology at the University of Colorado created and then evaluated a wellness program consisting of wellness lectures, quarterly wellness Grand Rounds, monthly peer mentorship meetings, quarterly wellness dinners, and group retreats.[25] This program similarly demonstrated positive impacts on resident well-being.

Our program

Our department has taken targeted approaches to improve well-being in our residency program. Initially, we developed a Departmental Wellness Committee with a faculty-led Resident Wellness Subcommittee. Over time, the Resident Wellness Subcommittee transitioned to a resident-led and resident-run committee. Our monthly resident-PD meetings serve as a focus group to identify specific areas of concern, allowing residents to address areas of concern both large and small. Another department-wide intervention we use is the "Pebble in the Shoe" program, developed by the AMA, in which easily resolvable logistical issues—fixing broken keyboards in particular operating rooms, adjusting the temperature of call rooms, among others—are solicited then quickly remedied.[26] Several studies point to the efficacy of Balint Groups, small collections of clinicians led by a trained facilitator to help the group unpack and process topics of concern, medical or otherwise, and can provide space for problem identification and problem solving.[27,28] Our program has used a similar approach called "Confession Sessions," first described by Karan and colleagues in which one class of residents meet with a more senior resident to discuss issues in a safe space.[29] This provides junior residents with experienced peer support and helps them to recognize that many experiences are shared.

Our program has developed and implemented an intervention that includes resident support persons (ie, family and friends). The CA-1 Family Anesthesia Day brings CA-1 residents and their support persons together to learn about wellness, burnout, substance abuse, and available local support resources.[30] The support persons also gain hands-on experience with simulated anesthesia procedures. The goal of this program is to help support persons better understand the stresses of resident life, thus improving communication and increasing residents' personal support outside of work.

STRATEGY 4: CULTIVATE COMMUNITY IN THE WORKPLACE
Overview

Cultivating a strong community of support for residents is important to their overall professional and personal success. Strong peer and faculty relationships have been noted to provide critical support to residents and to reduce burnout.[27,31] The Department of Emergency Medicine at the University of Alberta found that creating a resident wellness program led to stronger resident–resident and resident–faculty relationships.[32] These relationships were strengthened through charity events, the creation of a nonmedical library, financial wellness advice through a financial tips bulletin board, and out-of-work social events.[32] Intentionally fostering a community focused on resident wellness correlated with higher empathy and wellness scores and lower rates of anxiety and depression.[32]

Our program

At our institution, the residents' surrounding community is cultivated at multiple levels. The institution has a House Staff Council comprised of multidisciplinary residents who advocate for trainee well-being as well as create a collegial resident community. Our program also works to build community among residents through various social activities including annual class retreats and the designated resident workroom, which gives residents a place to relax and interact. The residents run the Resident Wellness Subcommittee which spearheaded initiatives such as monthly anesthesia events at local venues and a significant other support groups. The residents also created "anesthesia families," which are assigned groups composed of residents from each level of training (ie; intern, CA-1, CA-2, and CA-3) and encourage peer mentorship and support. To foster a faculty–resident community, each resident is assigned a faculty mentor who can provide support and career guidance throughout residency. During the COVID-19 pandemic, all institution or department-sponsored wellness events and meetings adhered to CDC guidelines.

STRATEGY 5: USE REWARDS AND INCENTIVES WISELY

The literature is sparse with regards to evaluating resident wellness through the lens of rewards and incentives. When this topic appears in the literature, it is primarily focused on attending physicians. As such, we highly encourage the medical community to intentionally explore the value of rewards and incentives with respect to resident well-being. For example, there is a paucity of literature addressing moonlighting in relation to well-being. Moonlighting is a common method for residents to gain access to additional financial resources and mitigate their financial strain. However, it may increase trainee workload and contribute to burnout. Our program has achieved a successful balance of providing supervised moonlighting opportunities on weekend days and weekday evenings; this approach has been well-received by residents who self-select for these extra shifts.

Additionally, Stanford Medicine implemented a faculty-level reward intervention. The intervention consists of 2 components: establishment of formal advising for career-life planning, and a program to quantify favors performed by one physician for another. The latter is predicated on paying it forward or time banking by helping colleagues. This strategy resulted in statistically significant improved wellness and perceived flexibility scores.[33] Anesthesiology is a demanding specialty wherein providers have little control over their schedules, particularly during residency. At our institution, we have a similar system in place that automatically logs noncall time spent in the operating room after 4:30 PM Once a resident has accumulated 10 overtime hours, the individual is eligible for an Earned Reading Day, to be assigned as scheduling permits. Time banking has been well received by our residents and has positively contributed to overall well-being.

STRATEGY 6: ALIGN VALUES AND STRENGTHEN THE CULTURE
Overview

Communities are predicated on mutual values and a culture of support among individuals within that community. Internal medicine chief residents at Brigham and Women's Hospital wrote that, in addition to fostering community, programs should strive to create a safe, respectful learning environment that is protective of trainees and their education.[34] Coupled with evidence on the negative impact of harassment (eg, sexual or otherwise) on well-being and burnout, promoting resident respect within a training program is vital.[35] Another perspective piece emphasized the importance of identifying residents as learners, rather than laborers; this approach promotes a shared culture of inquisitiveness, dedication, and self-improvement.[36] In summary, community is not something that will easily occur on its own. Rather, it requires intentional development through the promotion of a shared values system and a culture of respect throughout the hospital system.

Our program

Our program strives to create a positive, affirming culture by promoting respect for each other, intentionally enculturating every resident into the department, and emphasizing the role of the resident as a learner. We accomplish this through a variety of departmental initiatives, including our Diversity, Equity, and Inclusion Committee which holds monthly round table discussions and distributes monthly newsletters highlighting cultural and diversity events. Interns participate in an Academic Medicine Rotation, a leadership series headlined by lectures from our Chair introducing departmental-driven values and strategies. This course also allows our interns to develop a sense of camaraderie and a social support system among themselves. Finally, our department emphasizes the role of residents as learners. We are one of the few anesthesiology programs with a dedicated Education Specialist. We have clinical support from nurse anesthetists that allows our residents to participate in out-of-operating room electives that develop them as anesthesiology consultants. We also have a Citizenship Policy that, among other things, incentivizes participation in lectures and workshops by providing additional individual and class funding. These elements cumulatively create a dynamic environment with a clearly defined culture and set of values that guide our program.

STRATEGY 7: PROMOTE FLEXIBILITY AND WORK-LIFE INTEGRATION
Overview

Maintaining work-life balance can be challenging for physicians given the nature of their work. This may be especially true during residency given the difficult balancing act of working, learning, and maintaining a personal life. Finding and maintaining equilibrium is increasingly emphasized and has resulted in significant output in the literature, yet often with conflicting conclusions. A multidisciplinary survey assessing surgery, internal medicine, and anesthesiology residents showed no correlation between sleep or work hours and overall well-being and burnout.[37] Conversely, a systematic review indicated that time away from work and increased sleep is correlated with improved wellness.[38] Furthermore, there is disagreement regarding the correlation of ACGME duty hours on burnout, with some studies concluding there is no impact while others suggest a reduction in hours results in decreased burnout.[31,39,40]

Despite conflicting data, residents need to find balance to pursue interests outside of medicine and engage in basic self-care such as doctor and mental health appointments.[40] Many attempts to strike the proper balance between work and personal time have been instituted. For instance, the United Kingdom allows emergency medicine residents to work part-time, either 50% time or 75% time at the cost of atat extending their residency.[36] Other interventions aimed at improving work-life integration have targeted resident schedules. Automated scheduling tools are one example, using algorithms to create year-long block schedules for residents by incorporating preferred vacation time and elective requests to maximize the number of first choice placements.[41] This approach is associated with increased resident satisfaction.[41] Shift schedules, however, are more difficult to optimize. The implementation of casino-shifts for emergency medicine residents, which aim to have shift changes following the pattern of the sun and typically occur at 0400 and 1200, as opposed to standard 12-hour overnight call demonstrated no difference in overall wellness.[42] Schedule predictability has been shown to reduce burnout, though this is particularly difficult to implement in anesthesiology.[43]

Some authors have emphasized that work and life should be balanced and integrated, rather than striving to maximize life independent of work.[44] One way to do so may be through fostering community in the workplace, facilitating friendship and belonging even while at work. Much of what was discussed in Strategy 4, such as establishing physical spaces for the community and facilitating activities both in and out of the hospital may facilitate work-life integration. Finally, sick time and parental leave are important resident policies.[36] Wolpaw called for greater implementation of policies similar to the 2019 American Board of Anesthesiology (ABA) update that allows up to 2 months of family and medical leave before triggering extensions to residency.[45] One study surveying residents across 25 subspecialties found that residents truncated their maternity leave for fear of extending residency training.[46] The implementation of personal days has helped residents access personal medical care and improved overall flexibility to manage life events, independent of sick leave.[27,47]

Our program

We have attempted to implement several changes to promote flexibility and work-life integration. We adopted the ABA guidelines for medical and family leave. As mentioned above, we use Earned Reading Days to bank time for later use at the discretion of the daily coordinator. Residents also receive an automatic postcall day following Home call even if they are not called in overnight, which results in several weekdays off during the year to accommodate personal care appointments. The designated scheduling chief resident collects resident vacation week preferences and holiday preferences at the onset of the academic year. Yet, the unpredictability of operating room schedules remains a significant stressor for residents. Finally, transparency regarding rules and expectations for scheduling requests in addition to accommodating no-call days have proven beneficial.

STRATEGY 8: PROVIDE RESOURCES TO PROMOTE RESILIENCE AND SELF-CARE
Overview

Arguably one of the simplest ways to both promote resident well-being and address burnout is to focus interventions on the individual scale such as mindfulness training and improving capacity for empathy. Several studies suggest that the development of certain personal characteristics correlates with lower rates of burnout. "Grit," defined as the intrinsic drive to persist and achieve delayed gratification, has been linked to greater well-being in residency, and high baseline levels of resiliency are associated with lower rates of burnout.[48,49] Wellness didactic programs have been well received by residents, with one study showing a 69% participation rate and another demonstrating 60% of residents believed a course on stress-mitigation would be beneficial.[50,51]

Attempts have been made to determine the efficacy of interventions on personal resilience. One trial comparing surgical residents enrolled in a mindfulness training course against nonparticipants found the intervention group had a one-point decrease on a scale of 10 in stress scores at the end of the intervention.[52] Another study demonstrated that 6 workshops focusing on topics such as time management, empathy training, and resilience resulted in decreased burnout levels in obstetrics and gynecology residents, but only for those who attended more than 4 workshops.[53] A systematic review found mixed results, noting that improving coping skills seemed to increase well-being, though only 3 small-scale studies were assessed.[38] In contrast, several studies found no impact of resilience training on overall well-being or burnout rates.[27,54–57] Some sources suggest improving resident well-being and burnout depends primarily on addressing organizational and structural issues.[47,58–60] Finally, individualized approaches to improving resilience such as adequate access to mental health resources remain difficult to implement, with one survey indicating that 32.8% of resident respondents from across specialties at the Mayo Clinics endorsed a reluctance to seek mental health care.[61]

Albeit controversial, resiliency training likely has a place in multimodal wellness programming as there are minimal downsides even if the benefits remain unclear. Thus, we recommend that wellness programs incorporate this in some capacity. There likely needs to be a combination of individualized and systemic interventions at the departmental and hospital level to improve resident wellness.

Our program

Our institution offers a system-wide mental health program for physicians called Taking Care of Our Own, which has been highly utilized in our department.[62] This program provides confidential access to psychologists and psychiatrists who can assist in addressing depression, coping after adverse clinical events, and managing burnout. In addition, our department has a policy to provide support and relief from clinical duties for clinicians who experience an unanticipated adverse perioperative outcome. Another identified stressor for our residents is financial constraints, given residents' high debt burdens and limited training salaries. To address these concerns, our department created a faculty-led financial literacy program comprised of a financial lecture series, which has been welcomed by the residents.[63] Other well-received departmental programming and gestures include Grand Rounds presentations on mindfulness facilitated by departmental pain psychologists, free coffee pods and snacks in the resident library, and a kudos system to facilitate gratitude and community among residents.

STRATEGY 9: FACILITATE AND FUND ORGANIZATIONAL SCIENCE
Overview

Robust research efforts to deepen our collective understanding of burnout and wellness are essential. The use of validated well-being indices and scales (eg, Physician Well-Being Index, Maslach Burnout Inventory) are instrumental in studying wellness and burnout.[14,15] However, some of these tools can be burdensome due to their length. One study demonstrated that a two-question assessment showed similar accuracy for measuring burnout prevalence, potentially offering a method that may lead to higher compliance in execution.[64] Alternatively, some studies have turned to use unique approaches to quantify wellness and burnout.[64] For instance, studies have found correlations between burnout and physical attributes such as heart rate variability and the blood marker S100 B.[65,66] However, the scalability and ease of implementation of these approaches is limited.

Our program

Our institution uses the Mayo Wellbeing Index for all clinicians.[13] Aggregate data are provided to our department to track burnout and well-being over time. We also encourage active resident and faculty participation in scholarly work regarding wellness to contribute to the field and improve our program. For example, we are currently conducting a multi-institutional study assessing the impact of our annual CA-1 Family Day experience.[67] Encouraging the study of wellness and contributing to the growing dialogue will help our department and specialty.

SUMMARY

Statistically speaking, burnout is an issue that we all deal with in our residency programs. While a myriad of strategies for addressing burnout and improving well-being exist, implementation is often challenging. In addition, residents are a heterogenous group and have a multitude of lived experiences that contribute to a dynamic spectrum of burnout; interventions that some find helpful may not be welcomed by others. A comprehensive model such as Shanafelt's 9 strategies may be a useful roadmap to help faculty and trainees reflect on their individual program's wellness offerings and consider opportunities for improvement in managing burnout.[13] Some of the examples provided here may be easily adaptable for other training programs. Ultimately, there is a need for innovation in both organization-level and individual-level interventions. These interventions need to be evaluated and disseminated through the literature so others may benefit.

CLINICS CARE POINTS

- Programs can implement validated assessment methods such as the Physician Well-Being Index, the Mayo Well-Being Index, or the Maslach Burnout Inventory when assessing resident wellness
- To address wellness at the individual level, programs should consider resident preferences when designing schedules and offer easy access to mental health programs

- To address wellness at the departmental level, programs can consider incorporating wellness-focused grand rounds and developing a Wellness Committee with resident-run resident subcommittees
- To address wellness at the organizational level, hospital systems should attempt to foster a culture that respects residents as learners and they should develop a multidisciplinary resident council to facilitate resident communication with graduate medical education leadership

DISCLOSURE

The authors have nothing to disclose.

REFERENCES

1. Arnold J, Tango J, Walker I, et al. An evidence-based, longitudinal curriculum for resident physician wellness: the 2017 resident wellness consensus summit. West J Emerg Med 2018;19(2):337–41.
2. Improving physician well-Being, restoring the meaning in medicine. Accreditation Council for Graduate Medical Education. Available at: https://www.acgme.org/what-we-do/initiatives/physician-well-being/. Accessed September 29, 2021.
3. Rodrigues H, Cobucci R, Oliveira A, et al. Burnout syndrome among medical residents: a systematic review and meta-analysis. PLoS One 2018;13(11):e0206840.
4. Dyrbye LN, Burke SE, Hardeman RR, et al. Association of clinical specialty with symptoms of burnout and career choice regret among US resident physicians. JAMA 2018;320(11):1114–30.
5. Sun H, Warner DO, Macario A, et al. Repeated cross-sectional surveys of burnout, distress, and depression among anesthesiology residents and first-year graduates. Anesthesiology 2019;131(3):668–77.
6. Wong LR, Flynn-Evans E, Ruskin KJ. Fatigue risk management: the impact of anesthesiology residents' work schedules on job performance and a review of potential countermeasures. Anesth Analg 2018;126(4):1340–8.
7. Institute of Medicine (US). Committee on optimizing graduate medical trainee (resident) hours and work schedule to improve patient safety. impact of duty hours on resident well-being. In: Ulmer C, Wolman DM, Johns MME, editors. Resident duty hours: enhancing sleep, supervision, and safety. Washington (DC): National Academies Press (US); 2009. Available at. https://www.ncbi.nlm.nih.gov/books/NBK214939/.
8. Ehooman F, Wildenberg L, Manquat E, et al. Connected devices to evaluate sleep, physical activity and stress pattern of anaesthesiology and intensive care residents. Eur J Anaesthesiol 2020;37(7):616–8.
9. Danhakl V, Miltiades A, Ing C, et al. Observational study evaluating obstetric anesthesiologist residents' well-being, anxiety and stress in a North American academic program. Int J Obstet Anesth 2019;38:75–82.
10. Ratanawongsa N, Wright SM, Carrese JA. Well-being in residency: effects on relationships with patients, interactions with colleagues, performance, and motivation. Patient Education Couns 2008;72(2):194–200.
11. de Oliveira GS Jr, Chang R, Fitzgerald PC, et al. The prevalence of burnout and depression and their association with adherence to safety and practice standards: a survey of United States anesthesiology trainees. Anesth Analg 2013;117(1):182–93.

12. Tran EM, Scott IU, Clark MA, et al. Assessing and promoting the wellness of United States ophthalmology residents: a survey of program directors. J Surg Educ 2018;75(1):95–103.

13. Shanafelt TD, Noseworthy JH. Executive leadership and physician well-being: nine organizational strategies to promote engagement and reduce burnout. Mayo Clin Proc 2017;92(1):129–46.

14. Dyrbye LN, Satele D, Sloan J, et al. Utility of a brief screening tool to identify physicians in distress. J Gen Intern Med 2013;28(3):421–7.

15. Maslach C, Jackson SE, Leiter MP. Maslach burnout inventory. 3rd edition. In: Zalaquett CP, Wood RJ, editors. Evaluating stress: a book of resources. Palo Alto (California): Scarecrow Education; 1997. p. 191–218.

16. Perina DG, Marco CA, Smith-Coggins R, et al. Well-being among emergency medicine resident physicians: results from the ABEM longitudinal study of emergency medicine residents. J Emerg Med 2018;55(1):101–109 e102.

17. AlSayari RA. Using single-item survey to study the prevalence of burnout among medical residents-influence of gender and seniority. Saudi J Kidney Dis Transpl 2019;30(3):581–6.

18. Ban KA, Chung JW, Matulewicz RS, et al. Gender-based differences in surgical residents' perceptions of patient safety, continuity of care, and well-being: an analysis from the flexibility in duty hour requirements for surgical trainees (FIRST) trial. J Am Coll Surg 2017;224(2):126–136 e122.

19. Yrondi A, Fournier C, Fourcade O, et al. Burnout compared between anaesthesiology and psychiatry residents in France: an observational study. Eur J Anaesthesiol 2017;34(7):480–2.

20. van der Wal MA, Schonrock-Adema J, Scheele F, et al. Supervisor leadership in relation to resident job satisfaction. BMC Med Educ 2016;16:194.

21. van der Wal MA, Scheele F, Schonrock-Adema J, et al. Leadership in the clinical workplace: what residents report to observe and supervisors report to display: an exploratory questionnaire study. BMC Med Education 2015;15:195.

22. Martinelli SM, McGraw KA, Kalbaugh CA, et al. A novel core competencies-based academic medicine curriculum: description and preliminary results. J Educ Perioper Med 2014;16(10):E076.

23. Chakravarti A, Raazi M, O'Brien J, et al. Anesthesiology resident wellness program at the university of Saskatchewan: concept and development. Can J Anaesth 2017;64(2):185–98.

24. Chakravarti A, Raazi M, O'Brien J, et al. Anesthesiology resident wellness program at the university of Saskatchewan: curriculum content and delivery. Can J Anaesth 2017;64(2):199–210.

25. Janosy NR, Beacham A, Vogeli J, et al. Well-being curriculum for anesthesiology residents: development, processes, and preliminary outcomes. Paediatr Anaesth 2021;31(1):103–11.

26. AMA Launches STEPS Forward to Address Physician Burnout. J Miss State Med Assoc 2016;57(1):24.

27. Parsons M, Bailitz J, Chung AS, et al. Evidence-based interventions that promote resident wellness from the council of emergency residency directors. West J Emerg Med 2020;21(2):412–22.

28. Bar-Sela G, Lulav-Grinwald D, Mitnik I. Balint group" meetings for oncology residents as a tool to improve therapeutic communication skills and reduce burnout level. J Cancer Education 2012;27(4):786–9.

29. Karan SB, Berger JS, Wajda M. Confessions of physicians: what systemic reporting does not uncover. J Grad Med Educ 2015;7(4):528–30.

30. Martinelli SM, Chen F, Hobbs G, et al. The use of simulation to improve family understanding and support of anesthesia providers. Cureus 2018;10(3):e2262.
31. Busireddy KR, Miller JA, Ellison K, et al. Efficacy of Interventions to reduce resident physician burnout: a systematic review. J Grad Med Educ 2017;9(3):294–301.
32. Lefebvre DC. Perspective: Resident physician wellness: a new hope. Acad Med 2012;87(5):598–602.
33. Fassiotto M, Simard C, Sandborg C, et al. An integrated career coaching and time-banking system promoting flexibility, wellness, and success: a pilot program at stanford university school of medicine. Acad Med 2018;93(6):881–7.
34. Berg DD, Divakaran S, Stern RM, et al. Fostering meaning in residency to curb the epidemic of resident burnout: recommendations from four chief medical residents. Acad Med 2019;94(11):1675–8.
35. Wang LJ, Tanious A, Go C, et al. Gender-based discrimination is prevalent in the integrated vascular trainee experience and serves as a predictor of burnout. J Vasc Surg 2020;71(1):220–7.
36. Wolpaw JT. It is time to prioritize education and well-being over workforce needs in residency training. Acad Med 2019;94(11):1640–2.
37. Mendelsohn D, Despot I, Gooderham PA, et al. Impact of work hours and sleep on well-being and burnout for physicians-in-training: the resident activity tracker evaluation study. Med Educ 2019;53(3):306–15.
38. Raj KS. Well-being in residency: a systematic review. J Grad Med Educ 2016; 8(5):674–84.
39. Bolster L, Rourke L. The effect of restricting residents' duty hours on patient safety, resident well-being, and resident education: an updated systematic review. J Grad Med Educ 2015;7(3):349–63.
40. Dyrbye L, Shanafelt T. A narrative review on burnout experienced by medical students and residents. Med Educ 2016;50(1):132–49.
41. Howard FM, Gao CA, Sankey C. Implementation of an automated scheduling tool improves schedule quality and resident satisfaction. PLoS One 2020;15(8):e0236952.
42. Levin H, Lim R, Lynch T, et al. Improving resident well-being during shiftwork: are casino shifts the answer? Pediatr Emerg Care 2019;35(12):852–5.
43. Kimo Takayesu J, Ramoska EA, Clark TR, et al. Factors associated with burnout during emergency medicine residency. Acad Emerg Med 2014;21(9):1031–5.
44. Hashimoto DA, Von Hofe JB, McDougall MA. The trainee perspective: what can residency programs do to promote learner well-being? Acad Med 2017;92(1):12.
45. American Board of Anesthesiology. Revised absence from training policy effective July 1, 2019. Available at: https://theaba.org/pdfs/Absence_Training_Policy.pdf. [Accessed 29 September 2021]. Accessed.
46. Stack SW, Jagsi R, Biermann JS, et al. Maternity leave in residency: a multicenter study of determinants and wellness outcomes. Acad Med 2019;94(11):1738–45.
47. Meeks LM, Ramsey J, Lyons M, et al. Wellness and work: mixed messages in residency training. J Gen Intern Med 2019;34(7):1352–5.
48. Salles A, Cohen GL, Mueller CM. The relationship between grit and resident well-being. Am J Surg 2014;207(2):251–4.
49. Mullins CH, Gleason F, Wood T, et al. Do internal or external characteristics more reliably predict burnout in resident physicians: a multi-institutional study. J Surg Educ 2020;77(6):e86–93.
50. Aggarwal R, Deutsch JK, Medina J, et al. Resident wellness: an intervention to decrease burnout and increase resiliency and happiness. MedEdPORTAL 2017;13: 10651.

51. Samuel SE, Lawrence JS, Schwartz HJ, et al. Investigating stress levels of residents: a pilot study. Med Teach 1991;13(1):89–92.

52. Lases SS, Lombarts MJ, Slootweg IA, et al. Evaluating mind fitness training and its potential effects on surgical residents' well-being: a mixed methods pilot study. World J Surg 2016;40(1):29–37.

53. Winkel AF, Tristan SB, Dow M, et al. A national curriculum to address professional fulfillment and burnout in OB-GYN residents. J Grad Med Educ 2020;12(4):461–8.

54. Chung A, Mott S, Rebillot K, et al. Wellness interventions in emergency medicine residency programs: review of the literature since 2017. West J Emerg Med 2020; 22(1):7–14.

55. Ripp JA, Fallar R, Korenstein D. A randomized controlled trial to decrease job burnout in first-year internal medicine residents using a facilitated discussion group intervention. J Grad Med Educ 2016;8(2):256–9.

56. Verweij H, van Ravesteijn H, van Hooff MLM, et al. Mindfulness-based stress reduction for residents: a randomized controlled trial. J Gen Intern Med 2018;33(4):429–36.

57. Goldberg MB, Mazzei M, Maher Z, et al. Optimizing performance through stress training - An educational strategy for surgical residents. Am J Surg 2018;216(3):618–23.

58. Stepczynski J, Holt SR, Ellman MS, et al. Factors affecting resident satisfaction in continuity clinic-a systematic review. J Gen Intern Med 2018;33(8):1386–93.

59. Barnes EL, Ketwaroo GA, Shields HM. Scope of burnout among young gastroenterologists and practical solutions from gastroenterology and other disciplines. Dig Dis Sci 2019;64(2):302–6.

60. Zhou AY, Panagioti M, Esmail A, et al. Factors associated with burnout and stress in trainee physicians: a systematic review and meta-analysis. JAMA Netw Open 2020;3(8):e2013761.

61. Dyrbye LN, Leep Hunderfund AN, Winters RC, et al. The relationship between burnout and help-seeking behaviors, concerns, and attitudes of residents. Acad Med 2021;96(5):701–8.

62. 4 well-being initiatives to tackle pandemic's heightened stress. 2021 The American Medical Association. Available at: https://www.ama-assn.org/practice-management/physician-health/4-well-being-initiatives-tackle-pandemic-s-heightened-stress. Accessed September 29, 2021.

63. Harris E. The retirement savings coach you already know. 2020 The New York Times. Available at: https://www.nytimes.com/2020/07/25/business/retirement-savings-mentor.html. Accessed September 26, 2021.

64. Kemper KJ, Wilson PM, Schwartz A, et al. Burnout in pediatric residents: comparing brief screening questions to the maslach burnout inventory. Acad Pediatr 2019;19(3):251–5.

65. Hattori K, Asamoto M, Otsuji M, et al. Quantitative evaluation of stress in Japanese anesthesiology residents based on heart rate variability and psychological testing. J Clin Monit Comput 2020;34(2):371–7.

66. Eisenach JH, Sprung J, Clark MM, et al. The psychological and physiological effects of acute occupational stress in new anesthesiology residents: a pilot trial. Anesthesiology 2014;121(4):878–93.

67. Martinelli SM, Isaak RS, Chidgey BA, et al. Family comes first: a pilot study of the incorporation of social support into resident well-being. J Educ Perioper Med 2020;22(4):E652.

68. American Board of Anesthesiology. 2019 revised absence from training policy effective. Available at: http://www.theaba.org/ABOUT/Policies-BOI. Accessed August 5, 2021.

Investigating Wellness and Burnout Initiatives for Anesthesiology Resident Physicians

Time for Evidence-Based Investigation and Implementation

Kelsey M. Repine, MD[a,*], Oliver Bawmann, MD[b],
Madelyn Mendlen, BS[c], Steven R. Lowenstein, MD, MPH[d]

KEYWORDS

• Burnout • Well-being • Medical training • Gratitude • Residency

KEY POINTS

- Burnout affects residents and practicing physicians across most specialties, and it is especially widespread in emergency medicine, critical care, and anesthesiology.
- Physicians and residents who have burnout are more likely to be involved in medical errors and suffer lapses in professionalism, which may undermine the medical teamwork dynamic and patient safety.
- Although data from qualitative studies and randomized trials are limited, the available evidence suggests that interventions to reduce burnout and promote resident wellness are most successful when they are led or co-led by residents, and when they have buy-in from both administration and resident leaders.
- Individuals who journal about gratitude report higher positive states of alertness, enthusiasm, determination, attentiveness, and energy compared with individuals who focus on hassles or a downward social comparison.

[a] Anesthesiology Department, University of Colorado School of Medicine, 12401 East 17th Avenue, 7th Floor, Aurora, CO 80045 USA; [b] Internal Medicine-Pediatrics Department, University of Colorado School of Medicine, 12631 East 17th Avenue, 8601, Aurora, CO 80045; [c] University of Colorado School of Medicine, 13001 E 17th Place, Aurora, CO 80045; [d] University of Colorado School of Medicine, 13001 East 17th Place, Campus Box C-290, Aurora, CO 80045, USA
* Corresponding author. Anesthesiology Department, University of Colorado School of Medicine, 12401 East 17th Avenue, 7th Floor, Aurora, CO 80045 USA.
E-mail address: Kelsey.repine@cuanschutz.edu

Anesthesiology Clin 40 (2022) 275–285
https://doi.org/10.1016/j.anclin.2022.01.004
1932-2275/22/© 2022 Elsevier Inc. All rights reserved.
anesthesiology.theclinics.com

INTRODUCTION
Defining and Evaluating Physician Burnout

The foundation of the physician-patient relationship depends, in part, on societal expectations of the ideal physician's characteristics–energetic, enthusiastic, accomplished, and engaged, to name a few.[1] When physician burnout is present, these ideal characteristics may fade and subsequently undermine the physician-patient relationship.[1] Burnout is defined by a triad of high emotional exhaustion (for example, work-related fatigue), low personal accomplishment (feelings of frustration with work-related achievements), and high depersonalization (often a defense mechanism to separate oneself from work).[1–4] This combination is the basis of the Maslach Burnout Inventory scale, which is the gold standard in measuring physician burnout.[1,3–5]

Burnout is the result of chronic interpersonal and environmental stressors that lead to impaired professional development, indifference, and even carelessness.[1–3] Burnout is not a human weakness; rather, it is a prevalent consequence of the increasingly stressful practice of medicine. The World Health Organization has added burnout to the *International Classification of Diagnosis, Eleventh Revision* as an occupational phenomenon.[4,6] Practicing physicians have higher rates of burnout (37.9%) compared with the US general working population (27.8%).[7] The topic of burnout is also documented in the medical literature; many articles describe burnout and pose the question of how to address it. Nonetheless, understanding burnout in medicine, and especially in anesthesiology, requires further investigation.

The prevalence and consequences of burnout in anesthesiology

Information regarding the prevalence and cause of burnout in anesthesiology is limited.[7] A 2017 systematic review focusing on burnout in anesthesiology found only 15 research-based "PICO" (Problem, Intervention, Comparison, Outcome) articles.[2] Nevertheless, the messages were clear: The highest prevalence of burnout in physicians exists among critical care and emergency medicine physicians (55%), closely followed by anesthesiologists (50%).[2,8] This systematic review found that increased work hours and time-intensive and difficult call schedules are associated with increased resident burnout.[2] Systems that modified these 2 factors reported improved resident wellness and decreased burnout; importantly, 49% of residents reported improved patient safety.[2] Other studies report that burnout is increased among younger physicians, female physicians, physicians with children, and physicians who practice in academic centers.[4]

A 2019 repeated cross-sectional survey study published in *Anesthesiology* found that 51% (2531 of 4966) of anesthesiology residents and first-year graduates had a high degree of burnout, 32% (1575 of 4941) were in distress, and 12% (565 of 4840) screened positive for depression.[7] However, burnout is not isolated to the resident anesthesiologist population. Two studies published in *Anesthesiology* and the *Journal of Clinical Anesthesiology* in 2011 investigated burnout among anesthesiology department chairs and program directors and found that moderate burnout was present in approximately 70% of respondents, and high burnout was reported by 20% to 28% of respondents.[4]

The consequences of physician burnout are severe. Physicians who report high levels of burnout make more medication errors than physicians who report lower burnout.[1] Higher levels of burnout are also associated with decreased physician professionalism, as well as an increased risk of developing clinical depression, suicidal ideation, and substance use disorders, as described in later discussion.[1,2]

Burnout and clinical depression are not the same, but they are linked. They coexist, often in the same individuals. Burnout is a pressing concern, as physicians have a higher suicide rate than the general public[1]; in fact, 300 to 400 physicians commit suicide annually.[4] Pointedly and tragically, this means that approximately 1 physician commits suicide each day. The 2 leading causes of death among resident physicians are neoplastic disease and suicide.[4] Although resident physicians are at increased risk of suicide and suicidal ideation, the suicide rate among physicians is highest in late middle age.[1] A 2004 meta-analysis found that male physicians are 1.41 times more likely to commit suicide than age- and gender-matched individuals in the general population. Female physicians are 2.27 more likely to commit suicide compared with the general population.[1,9] Suicide is the result of a combination of biologic, behavioral, and environmental factors.[1] Suicide can be the devastating outcome when burnout is superimposed on these other factors, such as mental illnesses, like depression or bipolar disorder.[1] When characterizing burnout, wellness, and physician suicide, it is critical to remember that the cause of burnout is specifically linked to the workplace, whereas depression does not necessarily have a workplace connection.[2,5,7]

As noted above, although burnout and depression often coexist, they are not the same. Depression is a clinically diagnosed mental illness characterized by changes in mood, anhedonia, weight changes, sleep disturbances, fatigue, feelings of guilt, hopelessness, and helplessness, concentration difficulties, and loss of energy.[1] Depression requires professional evaluation, and treatment often involves medication and therapy. Depression is distinct from burnout, which is situational and career-specific and must be addressed from both an individual perspective and, perhaps more importantly, an organizational level. When addressing well-being, it is vital to distinguish between burnout and depression.

Anesthesiologist well-being and COVID-19
The optimal methods for addressing burnout and promoting well-being are unknown; however, these concepts are gaining traction nationally in anesthesiology, as evidenced by an increasing number of well-being talks and presentations at annual society conferences. For example, 27 presentations on anesthesiologist well-being and burnout were highlighted at the 2016 American Society of Anesthesiology (ASA) meeting, and more than 18 were presented at the 2021 ASA meeting.[1] Indeed, well-being has become even more pertinent and urgent amid the COVID-19 pandemic, which has placed unprecedented stress on anesthesiologists, trainees, nurses, advanced practice providers, and other health care team members and systems.[5,10] A systematic review published in 2019 in the *Archives of Academic Emergency Medicine* found 12 studies focused on the epidemiology and prevention of burnout among health care workers in relationship to COVID-19, but found that low-quality evidence and early-stage research did not provide sound recommendations, and argued for larger, interventional studies to investigate solutions for COVID-19 burnout.[5] In addition, because of the uncertainty regarding the length of the current pandemic, the effects of COVID-19 on burnout on health care workers are speculated to be lasting.[10]

Physician well-being: a medical emergency
Physician well-being is a multidimensional entity that encompasses physicians as individuals and the clinical environments in which physicians work.[1] Individual interventions, such as mindfulness and resilience training, are insufficient if environmental and system-related stressors in the workplace go unaddressed, and if physicians are unable to find meaning in their work. In addition, implementing a "one-size-fits-all" solution is unlikely to be sufficient.[1] There is a need to identify effective systems-level interventions and provide practicing physicians and trainees with necessary support

and accessible resources. We must address environmental and work-related stressors, even as we promote physician self-care.[1] In this way, we can best preserve and build on the espoused characteristics of our profession: skilled, compassionate, energetic, enthusiastic, accomplished, engaged, and responsive, that are at the heart of the physician-patient relationship. Said differently, a comprehensive strategy, with buy-in by hospital and training program leaders, is needed to best care for the caregiver.

Wellness Is not Simply the Lack of Burnout

"Many who have addressed physician wellness imply, by default, that it is a lack of burnout, but this is as inadequate as defining health as a lack of disease."[3]

The concept of wellness is difficult to define, particularly when applied through the lens of medical training. One article from the *Journal of Graduate Medical Education* by Eckleberry-Hunt and colleagues,[3] published in 2009, defined wellness as "...a dynamic and ongoing process involving self-awareness and healthy choices resulting in a successful, balanced lifestyle." This definition incorporates essential components of wellness: protecting the balance between physical, emotional, intellectual, and social aspects of one's life; accomplishment; acceptance; time outside of work; confidence; empowerment; presence; recognition and management of signs of burnout; and physical health.[3] Most importantly, this definition of wellness highlights that wellness is not simply a lack of impairment.[3] Wellness and burnout need to be addressed in a coordinated fashion when conceptualizing how to optimize medical resident training.[3] It is insufficient to simply work toward reducing burnout to promote wellness; we must do both concurrently to achieve lasting improvement in the lives of physicians, including trainees.

Not surprisingly, and similar to physician burnout statistics, resident well-being is consistently lower than general population well-being norms.[11] Improved resident well-being is associated with feelings of control and autonomy, competence (eg, pursuit and achievement of goals, opportunity for learning, increased confidence and mastery), and social relatedness (eg, positive feedback and positive colleague relationships).[11] Adequate sleep and physical activity are also associated with an increase in resident well-being.[11] Promoting well-being of residents is essential, as resident wellness is associated with resident empathy.[11]

The Accreditation Council for Graduate Medical Education (ACGME), in conjunction with the American Board of Anesthesiology (ABA), recently added wellness to the Anesthesiology Milestones Project (effective July 1, 2021).[4] The ACGME and ABA took this important step, citing a "responsibility to maintain [the] personal, emotional, physical, and mental health" of trainees.[4] According to the Milestones Project, "This sub-competency [Professionalism 3: Well-Being] is not intended to evaluate a resident's well-being. Rather, the intent is to ensure that each resident has the fundamental knowledge of factors that affect well-being, the mechanisms by which those factors affect well-being, and available resources and tools to improve well-being."[12]

The inclusion of wellness as a training milestone embodies the ACGME and ABA's commitment to "restoring meaning in medicine" for resident physicians, in addition to the Physician Well-Being Initiative.[13] The initiative centers on providing well-being related sessions at the annual education conference, hosting symposia that unite stakeholders dedicated to improving resident and fellow wellness, and publishing tools and resources for wellness expansion for residents, fellows, and faculty alike.[13] In addition, in 2017, the ACGME revised its Common Program Requirements to emphasize that "psychological, emotional, and physical well-being are critical in the development of competent, caring, and resilient physician."[13]

Key points number 1: Physician burnout

- Burnout affects residents and practicing physicians across most specialties, and it is especially widespread in emergency medicine, critical care, and anesthesiology.
- Burnout is distinct from clinical depression; also, burnout is not an inherent weakness. Rather, burnout is an occupational hazard, the result of multiple stressors in the clinical workplace.
- Physicians and residents who have burnout are more likely to be involved in medical errors and suffer lapses in professionalism, which may undermine the medical teamwork dynamic and patient safety.

A Dearth of Evidence-Based Wellness Initiatives

Published in *Anesthesiology* in 2019, a repeated, nationwide, cross-sectional survey study among anesthesiology residents who were registered with the ABA, including interns and recent graduates, revealed 2 factors that are consistently and statistically correlated with a lower risk of burnout, distress, and depression: (1) the resident physician's perception that their workplace provides sufficient resources to address burnout and depression and the resident's comfort using them (burnout odds ratio = 0.51; distress odds ratio = 0.51; depression odds ratio = 0.52); and (2) the resident physician's perception that they were able to maintain a balance between their work and professional lives (burnout odds ratio = 0.61; distress odds ratio = 0.50; depression odds ratio = 0.58).[7] Importantly, how a residency program advocates, builds, and sustains these 2 qualities in wellness programming is unknown and requires further investigation.

Authors from the Yale University School of Medicine performed a randomized controlled trial within the anesthesiology department of a large teaching hospital of a workplace preventative intervention called *Coping with Work and Family Stress*. The program consisted of sixteen 1.5-hour resident training sessions on how to identify risks for burnout, while simultaneously emphasizing and bolstering protective mechanisms.[8] Specifically, residents learned several key skills, including identification of stressful situations, effective problem-solving, communication skills, and strategies to navigate conflict.[8] The training also included techniques for modifying cognitive processes, stress management, and mitigating avoidance coping.[8] According to the report, anesthesiology residents who participated in this training experienced greater reductions in anxiety compared with those who did not ($P = .02$). In addition, parental role stressors were rated significantly lower ($P = .03$), and residents reported a significant increase in problem-solving coping ($P = .03$) and social support from the workplace ($P = .02$), as well as a nonstatistically significant decrease in alcohol consumption.[8] This randomized trial among anesthesiology residents demonstrated that interventions focused on learning coping strategies can have significantly positive effects on anesthesiology resident well-being during training.[8] However, more research is needed to determine best practices for implementation, evaluation, and sustainability of similar training programs with an eye toward improving the overall well-being of anesthesia residents.

Resident Leaders for Resident Benefit

A traditional top-down approach to resident wellness programming may not be the most efficacious approach. With this in mind, in 2017, the internal medicine residency program at Columbia University piloted a peer-based wellness program known as READ-SG: *Reflect, Empathize, Analyze, and Discuss in Small Groups.*[14] The hypothesis is that a bottom-up approach, led by resident physicians supporting and learning from each other, may foster more wellness and personal growth among residents and, perhaps, prevent burnout and other adverse health and wellness effects of residency training.[14] Other studies show that when driven by resident leaders, implementing well-beingness measures significantly improves resident perceptions in domains, such as perceptions of wellness opportunities ($P<.05$), time for wellness ($P<.05$), satisfaction with work-life balance ($P<.05$), and quality of life ($P<.05$).[15] Perhaps most importantly, these measures show persistent improvement at 6 and 15 months postintervention.[15]

Supporting resident-led well-being programs may be beneficial because resident physicians may have different perspectives regarding pertinent well-being issues during residency compared with program leadership. For example, in 2015, the Council on Resident Education in Obstetrics and Gynecology/Association of Professors in Gynecology Wellness Task force distributed a survey to all obstetrics-gynecology residents and program directors and found that 89.4% of obstetrics-gynecology residents identified either themselves or another colleague as struggling with wellness; at the same time, 33% of surveyed obstetrics-gynecology program directors reported "no known issues" regarding resident wellness within their program.[16] Still, 99% of program directors stated that wellness was a priority in their program.[16] Another US national survey in 2017 demonstrated that academic anesthesiology chairs show a strong interest in burnout counseling; among 75 anesthesiology department chairs, nearly 75% had referred at least 1 member of their department to wellness resources within the past 5 years.[4] These surveys reflect the importance of seeking a variety of perspectives and approaches to advance well-being initiatives, with the caveat that support from faculty and department leaders is essential to meeting the goal of integrating well-being into the culture of residency education.[3]

Despite the focus on interventions led by faculty and resident wellness champions, a recent meta-analysis published in *JAMA Internal Medicine* in 2017 demonstrated that organization-directed interventions (for example, reducing or rescheduling workload requirements and addressing other environmental stresses) are associated with higher treatment effects among physicians when compared with physician-directed interventions (eg, mindfulness-based stress reduction, training focused on building self-confidence, or communication workshops).[2,17] Nonetheless, physician- and trainee-directed interventions still produce significant benefits in reducing burnout.[2] Thus, there is a need for both resident-led, faculty-led, program leadership-led and organization-led commitments to improving wellness among resident and faculty physicians. Although resident-led programming may be the galvanizing force that encourages peer buy-in, organizational and systemic changes are crucial to decrease adverse mental health effects and improve wellness outcomes.

Because of the multifaceted programming required to implement wellness initiatives for residents, using technology may be a promising medium for effecting positive change.

The Role of Technology in Resident Well-Being

Published in the *Journal of Graduate Medical Education* in 2013, a survey of 450 residents in primary care specialties (internal medicine, family medicine, and pediatrics), surgery, and other hospital-based specialties (defined as surgery, other hospital-based specialties, and fellowship training) identified the following barriers to resident participation in wellness programs: time to participate in the program (67%); uncertainty about helpfulness (27%); stigma about participating in a wellness program (27%); concern about being viewed as a "less competent" or "problematic" resident

(27%); and concern about confidentiality (21%).[18] A majority (87%) of resident physicians reported that if a wellness initiative is available, they are "very likely" or "somewhat likely" to use it.[18] The study also found gender, ethnic, and racial differences in accessing wellness programs: male residents and residents who identify as an ethnic or racial minority were less likely to seek counseling, whereas female residents were more concerned about taking time to access services as well as the stigma associated with accessing wellness programs and resources.[18] The aforementioned barriers, stigmas, time pressures, lack of trust, and lack of accessibility, are compounded by the perpetual stressors of microaggressions and stereotyping that underrepresented minority individuals in medicine often face. To effectively implement wellness programming, leadership must acknowledge and address these disproportionate burdens.

Implementing a well-being program via an app on a personal device has the potential to mitigate some of these barriers to trainee participation. Resources can be accessed confidentially at any time, in any location, by the resident physician. This strategy could ease the barriers of accessibility and confidentiality that may prevent resident participation. In 1 study published in *Clinical Psychology Review* in 2009, Internet-based interventions (IBI) for depression and anxiety for the general population generated effect sizes that are comparable to clinician-administered interventions.[19] This study found that individuals who used IBI for mental health services also experienced a decrease in barriers similar to those described above, including stigma, confidentiality, cost, and geographic and time-based barriers.[19]

Key points number 2: Well-being programming data for resident physicians

- *Although data from qualitative studies and randomized trials are limited, the available evidence suggests that interventions to reduce burnout and promote resident wellness are most successful when they are led or co-led by residents, and when they have buy-in from both administration and resident leaders.*
- *Common barriers to accessing and using wellness programming include time, stigma, cost, accessibility, and privacy.*
- *Organization-directed interventions (eg, addressing workload requirements and other environmental stresses) are associated with higher treatment efficacy, when compared with physician-targeted interventions (eg, mindfulness-based stress reduction, training focused on building self-confidence, and communication education).*

The Gratitude Journal App: Using Technology to Promote Resident Wellness

At the University of Colorado School of Medicine, we are developing a novel smartphone app centered on cultivating point-of-care gratitude practice and community building. The app will allow residents to log moments of joy and appreciation throughout each day, and to share their gratitude with members of the health care team and the broader community. The app is easily accessible and applicable to all anesthesiology resident physicians, for example, the night-shift resident physician on a break at 2 AM, the early morning parent tending to their children before going to the operating room at 5 AM, the weekend traveler on a flight out of town, and the day-shift resident on a lunch break.

This concept was introduced with hard-copy gratitude journals presented to incoming medical students at the University of Colorado School of Medicine White Coat Ceremony, beginning in 2019. The students were encouraged to write down 3 things for which they are grateful every day. The formatting of the journal allowed students to see gratitude entries from 1 to 3 years prior on that same day, providing a unique and meaningful opportunity for reflection. In addition, the Gratitude Journals feature quotations from faculty members, researchers, and medical school deans regarding the importance of gratitude in medical training and in the profession of medicine. Anecdotally, multiple students have reflected on the utility and power they find in their daily gratitude practice as they progress through their medical training and clinical rotations.

Why gratitude?

In 2013, psychologists Robert Emmons and Robin Stern[20] from the University of California-Davis published "Gratitude as a Psychotherapeutic Intervention," stating that "…gratitude has one of the strongest links to mental health and satisfaction with life of any personality trait–more so than even optimism, hope, or compassion." Perhaps most pertinent to physicians, Emmons and Stern[20] reported that those who practice gratitude are more effective in coping with stress and demonstrate increased resilience in the face of trauma-induced stress.

They conducted 2 studies where individuals were randomized to using (1) a weekly gratitude journal, or (2) a weekly journal chronicling hassles or travails. Emmons and Stern[20] found that "…persons who are randomly assigned to keep gratitude journals on a weekly basis exercise more regularly, report fewer physical symptoms, feel better about their lives as a whole, and are more optimistic about the upcoming week, compared to those who record hassles or neutral life events." In addition, according to Emmons and Stern,[20] "[a] daily gratitude journal-keeping exercise with young adults resulted in higher reported levels of the positive states of alertness, enthusiasm, determination, attentiveness, and energy compared with a focus on hassles or a downward social comparison." Emmons and Stern also observed that individuals who practice gratitude were more empathetic, forgiving, helpful, and supportive, all essential attributes of a compassionate physician.[21] Interestingly, in another article, Emmons and colleagues[20,21] indicated that individuals who practice gratitude are also more likely to be perceived differently by surrounding peers. They stated: "[n]otably, the family, friends, partners, and others who surround them consistently report that people who practice gratitude seem measurably happier and are more pleasant to be around. Grateful people are rated by others as more helpful, outgoing, optimistic, and trustworthy."[20,21]

Gratitude app development specifics

The new smartphone gratitude app is designed to be user-friendly, community-oriented, and centered on regular gratitude practices. Users can personalize settings and reminders, such as when to log their daily gratitude. Users can flip through their virtual journal to reflect on prior entries. Although users can add as many or as few entries of gratitude as they like, the directive suggests 3 entries per day, aligned with the prior hard copy journals' structure. The app allows users to share gratitude with others in their community (for example, a peer, teacher, consultant, learner, or fellow health care team member). Each user also has a virtual collection of gratitude messages from others that they can save for future reflection. Long-term development goals for the app include department-specific "bulletin boards," where a clinician can share gratitude with all colleagues, and also share photographs to make the entry more visually dynamic and enjoyable.

Although the app is currently in the development phase, an essential next step will be to conduct rigorous studies of the impact of the app on resident wellness. Eventually, randomized, controlled, multi-institutional trials will be needed among various resident cohorts and specialties, along with studies of its efficacy for medical students, trainees, faculty, advanced practice providers, nursing team members, and others.

Dismantling barriers to wellness programming through an app

The gratitude app seeks to address the implementation barriers described above. It is resident- and student-led with support of faculty; it provides "point-of-care" accessibility; it encourages and provides a ready platform for reflection; and it ensures privacy and confidentiality unless users opt to share their gratitude with others. Moreover, as stated earlier, burnout is not unique to physicians; therefore, the app provides a platform that enables clinicians to communicate their gratitude to others: a surgeon expressing gratitude to a scrub technician for being completely present during a long surgery; an anesthesiologist expressing gratitude to a nurse who helped resuscitate a patient; or a junior resident expressing gratitude to a senior resident for assisting and teaching in a difficult clinical situation. These may represent opportunities to strengthen community among all health care workers and generally reduce burnout in the health care setting.

Key points: Gratitude in resident physician training

- *Individuals who journal about gratitude report higher positive states of alertness, enthusiasm, determination, attentiveness, and energy compared with individuals who focus on hassles or a downward social comparison.*
- *Individuals who practice gratitude are rated by their peers as measurably happier, more pleasant to be around, and more helpful, outgoing, optimistic, and trustworthy.*

SUMMARY

During the COVID-19 pandemic, it became even more clear that students and physicians at all levels of training are in need of resources to prevent and address burnout. Even if the current COVID-19 pandemic ends, this need will not disappear. Indeed, effective resident physician wellness programs are urgently needed across all medical specialties. Implementation of wellness programming is limited by the lack of randomized controlled trials that better define the impacts of different interventions among resident physicians. The challenges of implementing interventions are compounded by specific barriers, such as funding, institutional and resident buy-in, time pressures, stigmatization, and resident access. Technology is an underused resource in the development of wellness initiatives. Consequently, this deficit provides a unique opportunity to promote wellness and study various initiatives across training programs. Gratitude practice may be an ideal launching point to promote physician well-being, reduce burnout, and provide opportunities for program evaluation.

As a current anesthesiology resident, an internal medicine-pediatrics resident, a third-year medical student, and a senior faculty physician, we feel gratitude ourselves that we are part of this profession. In this article, we sought to describe the challenges at hand regarding burnout and resident physician wellness for the benefit of our peers, the physicians who will follow us, our patients, and ourselves. Even, or especially, during an unprecedented pandemic, this is an opportune time to describe, implement, and formally evaluate wellness programming for resident physicians. While learning the intricacies of a medical subspecialty, it is imperative that physicians learn self-care. This task should not rest solely on the individual physician. It is the duty of the larger medical community to decrease environmental stressors and promote self-care and positive reflection in an effort to mitigate physician burnout.

DISCLOSURES

None.

REFERENCES

1. Kuhn CM, Flanagan EM. Self-care as a professional imperative: physician burnout, depression, and suicide. Can J Anaesth 2017;64(2):158–68.
2. Sanfilippo F, Noto A, Foresta G, et al. Incidence and factors associated with burnout in anesthesiology: a systematic review. Biomed Res Int 2017;2017: 8648925. https://doi.org/10.1155/2017/8648925.
3. Eckleberry-Hunt J, Van Dyke A, Lick D, et al. Changing the conversation from burnout to wellness: physician well-being in residency training programs. J Grad Med Educ 2009;1(2):225–30.
4. Romito BT, Okoro EN, Ringqvist JRB, et al. Burnout and wellness: the anesthesiologist's perspective. Am J Lifestyle Med 2021;15(2):118–25.
5. Sharifi M, Asadi-Pooya AA, Mousavi-Roknabadi RS. Burnout among healthcare providers of COVID-19; a systematic review of epidemiology and recommendations. Arch Acad Emerg Med 2021;9(1):e7.
6. Burn-out an "occupational phenomenon": International Classification of Diseases. Available at: https://www.who.int/news/item/28-05-2019-burn-out-an-occupational-phenomenon-international-classification-of-diseases. Accessed August 22, 2021.
7. Huaping Sun PD. Repeated cross-sectional surveys of burnout, distress, and depression among anesthesiology residents and first-year graduates. In: David O, Warner MD, Alex Macario MD MBA, et al, editors. Anesthesiology. 2019. p. 668–77.
8. Saadat H, Snow DL, Ottenheimer S, et al. Wellness program for anesthesiology residents: a randomized, controlled trial. Acta Anaesthesiol Scand 2012;56(9): 1130–8.
9. Schernhammer ES, Colditz GA. Suicide rates among physicians: a quantitative and gender assessment (meta-analysis). Am J Psychiatry 2004;161(12): 2295–302.
10. Amanullah S, Ramesh Shankar R. The impact of COVID-19 on physician burnout globally: a review. Healthcare (Basel) 2020;8(4).
11. Raj KS. Well-being in residency: a systematic review. J Grad Med Educ 2016; 8(5):674–84.
12. Education. Anesthesiology milestones. Accreditation Council for Graduate Medical Education (ACGME). Implementation Date: July 1, 2021; Second Revision: November 2020, First Revision: December 2013.
13. Improving physician well-being: restoring meaning in medicine. Chicago (Illinois): Accreditation Council for Graduate Medical Education. Available at: https://www.acgme.org/what-we-do/initiatives/physician-well-being/.
14. Abrams MP. Improving resident well-being and burnout: the role of peer support. J Grad Med Educ 2017;9(2):264.
15. Denise I Garcia AP, Jose G, Donna M, et al. Resident-driven wellness initiatives improve resident wellness and perception of work environment. J Surg Res 2021;258:8–16.
16. Winkel AF. Whose problem is it? The priority of physician wellness in residency training. In: Anh T Nguyen HKM, Valantsevich D, Woodland Mark B, editors. Journal of surgery education. 2017.
17. Panagioti M, Panagopoulou E, Bower P, et al. Controlled interventions to reduce burnout in physicians a systematic review and meta-analysis. JAMA Intern Med 2017;177(2):195–205.

18. Ey S, Moffit M, Kinzie JM, et al. "If you build it, they will come": attitudes of medical residents and fellows about seeking services in a resident wellness program. J Grad Med Educ 2013;5(3):486–92.
19. Amstadter AB, Broman-Fulks J, Zinzow H, et al. Internet-based interventions for traumatic stress-related mental health problems: a review and suggestion for future research. Clin Psychol Rev 2009;29(5):410–20.
20. Emmons RA, Stern R. Gratitude as a psychotherapeutic intervention. J Clin Psychol 2013;69(8):846–55.
21. Mccullough ME, Emmons RA, Tsang JA. The grateful disposition: a conceptual and empirical topography. J Pers Soc Psychol 2002;82(1):112–27.

Antiracism in Health Professions Education Through the Lens of the Health Humanities

Kamna S. Balhara, MD, MA[a],*, Michael R. Ehmann, MD, MPH, MS[a],
Nathan Irvin, MD, MSHPR[b]

KEYWORDS

- Antiracism • Health humanities • Narrative medicine • Health equity
- Graduate medical education

KEY POINTS

- Racism is a public health crisis and poses a critical threat to patients, health professions trainees, and the health professions workforce.
- The health humanities—a transdisciplinary field that incorporates arts, humanities, and social sciences to further health equity and social justice—represents an ideal pedagogical scaffold for antiracist education in the health professions.
- Arts and humanities-based pedagogies such as narrative medicine or Visual Thinking Strategies are especially effective in encouraging self-reflection, critique, and collaboration, which are necessary in antiracist education. Works of art or literature can serve as "third things," which engender psychologically supportive spaces for learning.
- Educators seeking to apply the health humanities toward antiracism in health professions education should consider (1) identifying partners and stakeholders in all aspects of health and health care, (2) focusing on faculty development, (3) setting expectations and making discomfort productive, and (4) adapting such approaches to the specific contexts of their individual teaching and learning environments.

[a] Emergency Medicine Residency Program, Johns Hopkins University School of Medicine, Johns Hopkins Department of Emergency Medicine, 1830 E Monument Street, Suite 6-100, Baltimore, MD 21287, USA; [b] Johns Hopkins University School of Medicine, Johns Hopkins Department of Emergency Medicine, 1830 E Monument Street, Suite 6-100, Baltimore, MD 21287, USA
* Corresponding author.
E-mail address: kbalhar1@jhmi.edu
Twitter: @KamnaBalharaMD (K.S.B.); @MichaelEhmannMD (M.R.E.); @swervinnirvin (N.I.)

Anesthesiology Clin 40 (2022) 287–299
https://doi.org/10.1016/j.anclin.2021.12.002   **anesthesiology.theclinics.com**
1932-2275/22/© 2022 Elsevier Inc. All rights reserved.

INTRODUCTION AND BACKGROUND
Racism: a Public Health Crisis

In 2021, the Centers for Disease Control and Prevention declared racism a serious threat to public health.[1] Racism has long been ingrained in the structures of health and the practice of health care, and this recognition, although belated, underscores the urgent need to address racism in medicine. The racist history of American health care is evident in the indelible examples of inequity that litter its past, including the practice of experimentation and exploitation without consent, disparate access to care, and segregation in hospital wards.[1–4] Racism remains a threat to patients by contributing to rampant disparities in morbidity and mortality, including poor maternal outcomes among Black women, differential care and outcomes in stroke and cardiovascular disease for people of color, and disparities in coronavirus disease 2019 (COVID-19) outcomes.[1] Furthermore, racism also represents a threat to the diversity and inclusivity of the health care workforce. Racist policies such as the early exclusion of Black students from medical schools and of Black physicians from national physician organizations, coupled with the closure of historically Black medical schools as a result of the Flexner report, have contributed to a persistent underrepresentation of Black and indigenous people of color matriculants in medical schools.[4,5] These disparities endure beyond medical school training; racial minorities graduating from US medical schools are less likely to initially secure residency positions compared with their White counterparts even after controlling for differences in test scores, and consequently remain underrepresented in the physician workforce.[4,6] Medical trainees continue to face race-based discrimination and harassment, which threatens their confidence, performance, well-being, and willingness to remain in medicine and academics.[7–10] Finally, the lack of widespread acceptance of race as a social, as opposed to biological, construct continues to hinder medical research and propagate racist myths that can compromise patient care.[11,12] Racism, in all its forms, whether institutionalized, personal, or internalized, must be addressed to mitigate the threats its continued existence poses to patients and health professionals.[1,13] In this context, health professions educators must recognize the common refrain initially expressed by American political activist and scholar, Angela Davis: "In a racist society, it is not enough to be non-racist; we must be anti-racist."

What Does It Mean to be Antiracist in Health Professions Education?

The author and activist Bell Hooks describes how any practical model for social change around racism should include "an understanding of ways to transform consciousness that are linked to efforts to transform structures."[14] Ibram X. Kendi similarly notes that combating racism demands a "reorientation of our consciousness."[15] Focusing on this transformation of individual consciousness, antiracist educational approaches "explain and counteract the persistence and impact of racism using praxis as its focus to promote social justice."[16] Antiracist education includes critical reflection about, and subsequent action on, the impacts of power relations intrinsically tied to race, which represent crucial steps toward the structural change necessary to combat racism in health care. Learners and educators in the health professions have issued urgent calls for antiracism not only to be thoughtfully integrated into health professions education but also to be reimagined as a core competency for any physician-in-training.[17–20] However, antiracist education in the health professions remains remarkably limited, with little scholarly attention paid to teaching the effects of structural racism and studying individual and collective actions to combat it. Moreover, a consensus on effective approaches to achieving these goals is notably lacking.[10,21,22]

Antiracist pedagogy goes beyond the classroom and the clinic, encompassing the incorporation of relevant content in curricula, as well as a reexamination of "*how* one teaches," paired with "an organizing effort for institutional and social change."[17] Antiracist curricular approaches are multifaceted in temporality; they ask educators and learners alike to interrogate the past, reflect on the present, and prepare for the future. Finally, antiracist approaches demand transformation at the individual level, necessitating a critical consciousness of one's own biases and privileges. Traditional approaches in health professions education may be insufficient to meet these needs. Consequently, to successfully integrate antiracism into the fabric of education, it is necessary to explore other disciplines and pedagogies that encourage praxis and partnership beyond hospital walls; incorporate historical, social, and political forces that shape power structures; and create avenues for critical self-reflection.

The health humanities represent an ideal scaffold upon which to build antiracist pedagogy in medical education. The health humanities are a transdisciplinary field that blend the arts and humanities with a commitment to social justice, and look beyond illness to the broader continuum of health and the social, historical, and political forces that impact it.[23,24] While providing means for individual introspection and critique, the health humanities also generate inclusive dialogue and action on crucial issues in health by centering voices that are often minoritized or unheard in traditional medical discourse, such as those of patients and nonphysician health care staff.

The Health Humanities: a Scaffold for Antiracism in Health Professions Education

Broadly, the arts and humanities have been recognized as integral components of medical education by both the Association of American Medical Colleges and the National Academy of Sciences, Engineering, and Medicine.[25,26] Evidence to date has demonstrated the potential impacts of the health humanities on health professions learners across multiple domains including[1] skills-based outcomes (eg, observation and interpretation),[2] relational outcomes (eg, empathy, communication, and tolerance of ambiguity), and[3] transformational outcomes (eg, professional identity formation and resilience).[26–29] Specifically, sociocultural critique, attention to inequitable systems, and subsequent advocacy to address inequality have been posited as among the core functions of the arts and humanities in medical education.[28,30]

Thus, pedagogies within the arts and humanities lend themselves well to antiracist instruction. Narrative medicine, for instance, adopts a biopsychosocial approach to encourage engagement with diverse voices, exploration of personal narratives, and strengthening of collaborative relationships.[31] Another commonly applied approach, Visual Thinking Strategies, uses art to level traditional learning hierarchies to encourage learners to value multiple perspectives and enhance critical thinking, collaboration, intellectual curiosity, and openness to the unfamiliar.[32]

Furthermore, arts- and humanities-based approaches influence skills, competencies, and attributes that are theoretically of value to both educators and learners seeking to meaningfully integrate antiracism in health professions education; these can be considered in the context of the "see, name, understand, and act" framework to antiracism in medical education described by Solomon and colleagues (**Fig. 1**).[20]

Antiracism requires that we first "see," by having a heightened awareness of explicit and subtle manifestations of racism in the world around us, and being cognizant of our blind spots, privilege, and bias. Arts- and humanities-based approaches have been demonstrated to not only enhance observation skills and confer visual literacy among health professions learners, but also represent a means to illustrate racism in structural contexts and to illuminate personal biases via critical consciousness and reflection.[33–38]

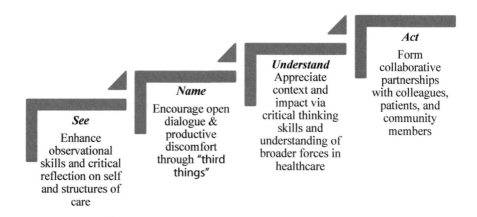

Fig. 1. Examples of health humanities-based skills and tools for each step of the "see, name, understand, act" antiracism in medical education framework.[20]

Once "seen," the ramifications of personal biases and imbalanced structures of power must subsequently be "named" and discussed. This process creates discomfort, vulnerability, and exposure, which can be especially challenging within the hierarchical structures associated with medical training. To help overcome the barriers that this hierarchical structure creates, art has been used successfully both within and outside of medicine as a "third thing." A "third thing" is a work of art or some other object or image that serves as a reflective trigger or conversational mediator that generates a safe space for sharing perspectives.[39,40] Gaufberg and colleagues describe how "third things" can render discomfort palatable or productive:

> Direct confrontation with deep truths can be painful, frightening, even blinding, and third things can open an avenue for 'indirection.' A participant moves from an exploration of the 'third thing' to his or her own story or 'truth.' If one's revelations begin to become too personal or painful, he or she can return to an exploration of the 'thing.' Thus, third things modulate the tension between depth of revelation and emotional safety.

The use of "third things" in medical education allows exploration of assumptions and clarification of values among a group working together. As most arts- and humanities-based approaches to stimulating discussion do not rely upon a differential in "expertise" or "knowledge" of art between teacher and learner, the "third thing" serves to flatten traditional hierarchies and contribute to the development of a shared language among participants.[40] The use of such tools to encourage this exchange of perspectives among learners, a core function of the arts and humanities in health professions education, is especially vital, as such exchanges enhance empathy and develop tolerance of ambiguity. Indeed, art-based educational interventions have been shown to positively impact measures of empathy among health care trainees and faculty and neurobiological research confirms how viewing and discussing art may be linked with empathic responses or embodied cognition.[41–43] In addition, because works of art or literature often lack definitive interpretations, learners are asked to sit with uncertainty. Implementation of arts- and humanities-based curricula among medical students and interprofessional health students has been shown to lead to greater comfort with uncertainty or ambiguity, a vital skill for health care professionals in training.[34,41] Such attributes, supported through the use of structured humanities-based approaches, like the use of a "third thing," may represent important stepping stones for health care learners to identify a safe space to embrace the discomfort and vulnerability that arises from "naming" the racist structures in which they exist.

Once "seen" and "named," it is imperative to subsequently "understand" the causes and effects of racism, by creatively and critically untangling the complex roots and consequences of individual and structural racism. Thinking about art, or esthetic thought, encompasses both critical and creative thinking, with subsequent impacts on observing, speculating, and reasoning based on evidence that is transferable to other settings, including medicine.[44] The ability to think "out of the box" may be key to challenging norms and existing structures. Humanities-based approaches grounded in social, political, community, and historical context may be key to the process of understanding and dismantling what has been seen and named.

Finally, antiracist pedagogies compel us to "act." The humanities encourage collaborative partnerships not only among health professionals at various levels of training from different specialties or disciplines but also with patients, activists, communities, and scholars in fields beyond medicine.[37,38,45,46] These coalitions and partnerships can act collectively to interrupt and rebuild racist structures, systems, and norms. Arts- and humanities-based approaches, specifically health humanities-based approaches, may help nurture individual and institutional relationships that may be key to sustained and effective structural change. The centering of marginalized voices inherent to the health humanities also comprises a key component of antiracist praxis.[47]

DISCUSSION
The Health Humanities at Hopkins Emergency Medicine Initiative

Given the relative paucity of sustained and longitudinal curricula focusing on social justice, and the promising potential of the health humanities as a pedagogical framework for such efforts, we created the Health Humanities at Hopkins Emergency Medicine (H3EM) initiative in 2018. H3EM represents a multidisciplinary initiative that encourages education, scholarship, and innovation in the health humanities and social medicine and aims to provide practitioners of emergency medicine (EM) with the tools to (1) understand and address the human experiences of health and illness and (2) serve the surrounding communities by improving the delivery of patient-centered care built upon cultural humility.

In alignment with the core principles of the health humanities, H3EM was built in partnership with multiple stakeholders in health care, including nurses, faculty, attending physicians, resident physicians, administrative staff, interprofessional EM team members, patients, and caregivers. Efforts to advance social justice demand not only an interdisciplinary team but also a multifaceted approach. H3EM therefore comprises a health humanities-based longitudinal curriculum to help trainees and faculty alike "see," "name," and "understand" the roots and consequences of racism and social injustice paired with initiatives that encourage cross-disciplinary collaborations and antiracist action, including speaker series featuring artists and activists, and seed grants and awards for trainees' innovations within this field.

H3EM Health Humanities-Based Antiracist Curriculum

H3EM's annual longitudinal curriculum is incorporated into weekly EM didactics, which are attended by residents (who are protected from clinical responsibilities during this time), faculty, staff, physician assistant trainees, and medical students.

Additional sessions occur asynchronously outside of scheduled weekly didactics, for a total of 8 to 12 sessions each academic year. In previous iterations of our curriculum, we focused on issues around bias, resilience, and the social determinants of health.[45,46] In 2020, given the significant import of, and lack of formal curricula on, antiracism in health professions education, we sought to create a health humanities curriculum specifically focused on antiracism, with the goal of initiating crucial conversations within our residency and department. The curriculum was grounded in the dual pillars of antiracist education: encouraging thought and supporting action at individual and institutional levels. We adopted an intentional approach that encouraged trainees and faculty to understand their own social positions, while focusing on cognitive aspects of racism to identify and address individual blind spots. The curriculum was designed to be flexible and provide a psychologically supportive space for discussions in response to current events, while creating opportunities for exploring historical contributors to racism at the institutional or systemic level. We also sought to create a collaborative community between educators and learners and to provide avenues for applications of theory into praxis by including patients and health care team members in conversations on how to move forward. This dual structure—thinking and acting at individual and system levels—was replicated within the structure of each individual session. Our curriculum comprised 8 sessions, which wove the arts and humanities with an understanding of historical context and critical reconsideration of current practices. During each session, principles of narrative medicine and visual thinking strategies were used to generate individual reflection and collaborative conversation on thematically relevant visual art, literature, poetry, nonfiction, and podcasts; this was paired with opportunities for exploring and deconstructing past or current racist structures or practices by understanding key historical events, discussing evidence-based practices in antiracism, and engaging in discussion with patients, health care team members, artists, and activists.

The overall objectives of the curricula were 4-fold: (1) to engage in reflection on the ways in which racism affects our patients, our colleagues and ourselves; (2) to critique the systems and institutions in which we work, live, and interact to build a heightened awareness of structural racism and its underpinnings; (3) to encourage action toward interrupting and dismantling racist ideas, systems, and practices; and (4) to develop skills to support others when they have been harmed by racist acts.

The curriculum highlighted important topics in antiracist praxis.[17,47,48]

Recognizing that past is prologue, one session focused on the historical documentation of racism in medical care and research to understand its current-day repercussions, whereas another explored the painful past of xenophobia in pandemics to help contextualize ongoing anti-Asian rhetoric amid the COVID-19 pandemic. We also sought to generate critical reflection, and subsequent action, on microaggressions toward clinicians and patients. For instance, in a session focused on microaggressions in the workplace, we introduced learners to the different types of microaggressions experienced by health care team members and engaged in a discussion of the ways in which they or their colleagues are affected by them. We paired this discussion with a reading and discussion of Dr. Damon Tweedy's[49] experiences as detailed in his novel, *Black Man in a White Coat,* followed by techniques for combating or responding to such instances. In another session, we used audio podcasts and essays to demonstrate the harms that can occur when patients are victims of epistemic or emotional microaggressions. Other sessions used works of art, poetry, and fiction to discuss topics such as structural racism or stigmatizing language in medical communication. In many instances, the incorporation of these "third things" or reflective triggers was instrumental in creating safe spaces for engaging in these powerful yet uncomfortable conversations. Descriptions of some of the sessions comprising the H3EM curriculum are provided in **Table 1**.

In addition to the synchronous sessions, we supplemented our curriculum with an asynchronous speaker series featuring individuals working at the nexus of the arts and antiracism. Our initial speaker was LaToya Ruby Frazier, a renowned photographer and visual artist known for using her platform to bring attention to, and advocate for, communities that have been ravaged by poverty, racism, and environmental exploitation. In her session, she shared evocative photographs chronicling injustice, racism, and disinvestment in Braddock, Pennsylvania, and Flint, Michigan, combined with a powerful narrative of her own experiences of racism as a caregiver navigating the hospital setting. We also hosted Kondwani Fidel, a poet and spoken word artist

Table 1
Descriptive examples of sessions included in Health Humanities at Hopkins Emergency Medicine antiracism curriculum in emergency medicine

Session Title	Session Objectives	Works of Art or Literature Used in Session
Social Justice and Racism	• Develop common vocabulary around race and antiracism • Confront historical and present complicity of medicine in racism • Recognize productive value of discomfort	• Robert Colescott's painting, "Emergency Room" • Ross Gay's poem, "A Small Needful Fact"
Words Hurt: "Micro"aggressions • Macroimpact	• Understand and recognize different types of microaggressions • Explore stories of harm experienced by clinicians due to microaggressions • Gain comfort with frameworks for responding to microaggressions and being an upstander instead of a bystander	• Excerpt from Dr. Damon Tweedy's book, *Black Man in a White Coat*
Microaggressions: The Harm We Inflict on Patients	• Explore specific categories of microaggressions faced by patients • Discuss how to recognize and avoid epistemic, emotional, and self-identity microaggressions[53]	• Podcast/story of Alan Pean • Joe Fassler's essay, "How Doctors Take Women's Pain Less Seriously"
Past is Present: The Germs of Racism in Pandemics	• Explore parallels of xenophobia and racism in past pandemics with current events • Recognize how medicine has been co-opted, or been complicit, in furthering racist agendas • Understand xenophobia's impacts on patients, public health measures, and clinicians	• Images from Angel Island immigration center • Physicians' nonfiction narratives from popular media

who took participants on a journey, both historical and anecdotal, of how racist policies created and sustained inequity in Baltimore. Both sessions highlighted the importance of confronting racism on systemic and personal levels.

Important Impacts of the H3EM Curriculum

The H3EM initiative has been impactful for our department and residency. Formal feedback from resident learners on H3EM curricular programming has highlighted how this humanities-based approach has been transformational to departmental culture; they specifically highlight its impact on encouraging perspective sharing; improving communication with patients, colleagues, and other nonphysician colleagues; and raising awareness of, and creating commitment to, interrupting bias and systematic racism.[46] Learners believe that the initiative is critical to well-being and resilience and has given them an opportunity to start engaging with or reengaging with the arts and humanities more regularly. Learners also spoke on the impact of intentionally protected time and space to process and reflect on some of the powerful events, circumstances, and challenges experienced as physicians, allowing them to uphold their own humanity as well as that of their colleagues and patients.[50]

The antiracist curriculum has created opportunities for learners and faculty alike to unburden themselves and share experiences of racism that they have encountered. A session focusing on a discussion of Robert Colescott's painting "Emergency Room" spurred residents to request that we create an anonymous online forum in which clinicians could share their own experiences with discrimination.[50] These accounts of racism were then actively integrated into subsequent sessions for discussion on how to address these issues in a transparent fashion. Creating a safe forum for residents to share their own experiences within the workplace sparked an awareness of, and empathy for, the lived realities of colleagues and created sources of support for those who previously had thought they had to shoulder these burdens alone.

Since the inception of the H3EM curriculum, residents have committed themselves to reflecting and processing their own experiences and sharing these experiences in essays, poetry, or other artistic media, some of which has been disseminated to the nearly 500-person department at large and published in the peer-reviewed literature.[51] The beneficiaries of the H3EM curriculum are not limited to physicians alone; organized sessions have often been joined by other members of the health care team, including nurses and those working in community outreach who have conveyed safety in sharing their experiences and perspectives.

Given that a core tenet of antiracism is action, our curriculum actively encourages residents to become advocates and catalysts for change. To help support their work, we developed an innovation grant to fund projects targeted toward interrupting the social forces that hinder patients and community members from reaching their full potential. Our current grantee is exploring the downstream effects of structural racism; this project involved collaboration with a reentry program to understand the health needs and gaps for individuals exiting the carceral system in hopes of developing solutions to overcoming these gaps.

Teaching this curriculum and exploring these important antiracist concepts has also been profoundly affecting for us as educators. It has challenged us to look beyond simply creating an antiracism-focused curriculum and to consider how our broader residency curriculum, itself, can be antiracist. Our health humanities-based antiracism curriculum has generated sufficient momentum to encourage educational leaders in our department to review the curriculum to identify areas in which refinement and further integration of antiracist praxes can occur. To date, specific measures taken by this taskforce include ensuring that presentations on clinical content do not conflate race, ethnicity, and genetic origins when discussing disease; systematically incorporating discussions around health disparities into all core content; ensuring appropriate representation in clinical vignettes; and ensuring that invited guest speakers reflect our department's values of highlighting diverse people and perspectives.

Tips for Implementation and Lessons Learned

We believe that similar humanities-based antiracist curricula can be implemented in any health professions educational setting. Faculty interested in developing a curriculum like H3EM should start by identifying stakeholders and experts at their local level. This group may include those within the institution, including faculty in other departments or disciplines, as well as other health professional staff such as nurses or pharmacists, and patient or family councils or advisory groups. Trainees should be recruited as design partners to enhance engagement and responsiveness to learner needs. Partners should also be sought outside of the health professions, especially if faculty need additional support or expertise with humanities frameworks. Potential collaborators include humanities scholars (eg, historians and anthropologists), museum-based educators, community organizers, artists, or activists. These partners should be engaged in all aspects of curriculum design and implementation.

Antiracist transformation requires buy-in at all levels within a department, including among the faculty leading the department and training the residents, and requires reflection into *how* we teach. Given the role faculty play not only in education but also in establishing and perpetuating the culture and norms in the health care and educational environments that may propagate racism and inequity, it is critical that they receive instruction on antiracism and are afforded safe spaces to assess their own socialization and worldviews.[17,48] Although this process may potentially be uncomfortable, faculty cannot ask residents to critically reflect on these issues if they themselves are unwilling to do so.

As the content and format of humanities-based antiracist educational sessions may be unfamiliar and potentially uncomfortable for many learners, all sessions should be prefaced with a declaration of ground rules or community practices to set expectations. In doing so, faculty should consider their goals and objectives. Specific statements to consider may include reminding participants that each session represents a space where diverse perspectives are encouraged, although no one is obligated to participate, in recognition that the content may spark strong emotions or discomfort. However, it is also important to highlight that discomfort may be expected and can be productive because it represents a core aspect of learning and transformation. Participants should also be reminded that there is no prerequisite expertise or knowledge of the arts and humanities required for successful participation, and that in discussing open-ended works of art or literature, there is no "right" or "wrong" interpretation.

When planning and implementing antiracist curricula via a health humanities approach, it is crucial for educators to meet learners where they are. Faculty and trainees alike may have variable needs or expectations and may be in different "zones" in the process of becoming antiracist.[52] Such "zones" include the "fear zone," characterized by avoidance or denial; the "learning zone," where increased discomfort is tolerated and accompanied by openness to vulnerability, self-critique, and diverse perspectives; and the "growth zone," wherein one starts to assume responsibility and engage in advocacy and education. Learners' readiness and receptiveness may vary, and those leading the curriculum may need to adapt to their specific learners and learning environment. Studies of antiracism curricula among medical students have shown that students of color and White students have differing needs or experiences when participating in such curricula. Students of color at one institution, for instance, expressed a constant awareness of racism that impacted medical training; they highlight the importance of having time to not only talk about content and skills relevant to antiracism but also to debrief and address the emotional burden of discussing racism.[10] As such, Ona and colleagues[10] suggest that when designing and implementing such curricula, educators should respect polyvocality and the existence of multiple struggles. Debriefs and check-ins with learners should be conducted, and appropriate resources or outlets for debriefing or counseling should be made available to all participants. Educators must make it a priority to ensure that the content of sessions minimizes risks of retraumatization, or vicarious or secondary traumatization, of faculty and participants alike.

Last, it is important to remember that racism has shaped many of our systems and institutions for generations; it will take widespread, dedicated, and persistent effort to dismantle racism and its vestiges. There is no panacea and no individual training or one-time initiative will suffice to overcome the threat that racism continues to pose to public health in the twenty-first century. Being an antiracist is, therefore, not defined by a single action, but instead represents an iterative, sustained, and multifaceted effort. Most importantly, words without action are of limited utility; it is important to pair these discussions with actions that address the issues and concerns that are unveiled through conversation.[17,48]

SUMMARY

Racism represents a critical threat to patients, learners, and clinicians alike; this multi-dimensional problem demands a multidimensional solution. In addition to sustained institutional and systemic change, expanding our arsenal of educational techniques to include the health humanities represents an important step toward an antiracist future in medicine. In centering all voices in medicine and adopting a transdisciplinary approach, the health humanities may help equip those engaged in health care with the tools to understand, critique, and transform our health systems into equitable, antiracist, and healing-centered structures of care for all.

CLINICS CARE POINTS

- Racism is a critical threat to patients, health professions learners and trainees, and the health professions workforce.

- Antiracism involves identifying, critiquing, and transforming elements of individual consciousness along with systems and structures, yet antiracism remains lacking in health professions education.

- The health humanities, a transdisciplinary field that incorporates arts, humanities, and social sciences toward a mission of social justice, represents an ideal pedagogical scaffold for antiracist education in the health professions.

- Educators seeking to apply the health humanities toward antiracism in health professions education should consider (1) identifying partners and stakeholders in all aspects of health and health care, (2) focusing on faculty development, (3) setting expectations and making discomfort productive, and (4) adapting such approaches to their individual teaching and learning environments.

- Incorporate multiple voices and stakeholders to understand the polyvocality of individuals' experiences with racism and its intersections with other "-isms."

- Dismantling racism requires iterative and deliberate efforts to understand how racism manifests and to combine this understanding with plans of action to facilitate meaningful forward progress.

DISCLOSURE

The authors have nothing to disclose.

REFERENCES

1. Racism and health. Centers for Disease Control and Prevention. 2021. Available at: https://www.cdc.gov/%20healthequity/racism-disparities/index.html. Accessed September 1, 2021.
2. White RM. Unraveling the Tuskegee study of untreated syphilis. Arch Intern Med 2000;160(5). https://doi.org/10.1001/archinte.160.5.585.
3. Wailoo K. Historical aspects of race and medicine. JAMA 2018;320(15):1529.
4. The Sullivan Commission on Diversity in the Healthcare Workforce. Missing Persons: Minorities in the Health Professions. Available at: https://campaignforaction.org/wp-content/uploads/2016/04/SullivanReport-Diversity-in-Healthcare-Workforce1.pdf. Accessed Sept 1 2020.
5. Lett LA, Murdock HM, Orji WU, et al. Trends in racial/ethnic representation among US medical students. JAMA Netw Open 2019;2(9). https://doi.org/10.1001/jamanetworkopen.2019.10490.
6. Sondheimer HM, Xierali IM, Young GH, et al. Placement of us medical school graduates into graduate medical EDUCATION, 2005 through 2015. JAMA 2015;314(22):2409.
7. Osseo-Asare A, Balasuriya L, Huot SJ, et al. Minority resident physicians' views on the role of race/ethnicity in their training experiences in the workplace. JAMA Netw Open 2018;1(5). https://doi.org/10.1001/jamanetworkopen.2018.2723.
8. Strayhorn TL. Exploring the role of race in black males' sense of belonging in medical school: A qualitative pilot study. Med Sci Educator 2020;30(4):1383–7.
9. Dyrbye LN, Satele D, West CP. Association of characteristics of the learning environment and us medical STUDENT Burnout, empathy, and career regret. JAMA Netw Open 2021;4(8). https://doi.org/10.1001/jamanetworkopen.2021.19110.
10. Ona FF, Amutah-Onukagha NN, Asemamaw R, et al. Struggles and tensions in antiracism education in medical school: Lessons learned. Acad Med 2020; 95(12S). https://doi.org/10.1097/acm.0000000000003696.
11. Witzig R. The medicalization of race: Scientific legitimization of a flawed social construct. Ann Intern Med 1996;125(8):675.
12. Ioannidis JP, Powe NR, Yancy C. Recalibrating the use of race in medical research. JAMA 2021;325(7):623.
13. Jones CP. Levels of racism: A theoretic framework and a gardener's tale. Am J Public Health 2000;90:1212–5.
14. hooks b. Killing rage: ending racism. New York: Henry Holt and Company; 2006.
15. Kendi IX. How to Be an antiracist. London: Vintage; 2021.
16. Blakeney AM. Antiracist pedagogy: Definition, theory, and professional development. J Curriculum Pedagogy 2005;2(1):119–32.
17. Kishimoto K. Anti-racist pedagogy: From faculty's self-reflection to organizing within and beyond the classroom. Race Ethn Educ 2016;21(4):540–54.
18. Sharda S, Dhara A, Alam F. Not neutral: Reimagining antiracism as a professional competence. Can Med Assoc J 2021;193(3). https://doi.org/10.1503/cmaj.201684.
19. Ahmad NJ, Shi M. The need for anti-racism training in medical school curricula. Acad Med 2017;92(8):1073.

20. Solomon SR, Atalay AJ, Osman NY. Diversity is not enough. Acad Med 2021. https://doi.org/10.1097/acm.0000000000004251.
21. Paul DW, Knight KR, Campbell A, et al. Beyond a moment — reckoning with our history and embracing antiracism in medicine. N Engl J Med 2020;383(15): 1404–6.
22. Neff J, Holmes SM, Knight KR, et al. Structural competency: Curriculum for medical students, residents, And INTERPROFESSIONAL teams on the structural factors that Produce health disparities. MedEdPORTAL 2020;16(1). https://doi.org/10.15766/mep_2374-8265.10888.
23. Crawford P, Brown B, Baker C, et al. In: Health humanities. London: Palgrave-Macmillan; 2015.
24. Klugman CM, Lamb EG, editors. Research methods in health humanities. Oxford: Oxford University Press; 2019.
25. National Academies of Sciences, Engineering, and Medicine. The Integration of the Humanities and Arts with Sciences, Engineering, and Medicine in Higher Education: Branches from the Same Tree. Washington, DC: The National Academies press; 2018.
26. Howley L, Gaufberg E, King B. The fundamental role of the arts and humanities in medical education. Washington, DC: AAMC; 2020.
27. Mangione S, Chakraborti C, Staltari G, et al. Medical students' exposure to the humanities correlates with positive personal qualities and reduced burnout: A multi- institutional U.S. survey. J Gen Intern Med 2018;33(5):628–34.
28. Dennhardt S, Apramian T, Lingard L, et al. Rethinking research in the medical humanities: a scoping review and narrative synthesis of quantitative outcome studies. Med Educ 2016;50(3):285–99.
29. Ousager J, Johannessen H. Humanities in undergraduate medical education: a literature review. Acad Med 2010;85(6):988–98.
30. Moniz T, Golafshani M, Gaspar CM, et al. The prism model: Advancing a theory of practice for arts and humanities in medical education. Perspect Med Educ 2021; 10(4):207–14.
31. Charon R. Narrative medicine: honoring the stories of illness. New York: Oxford University Press; 2008.
32. Research and theory. Visual Thinking Strategies. Available at: https://vtshome.org/research/. Accessed July 1, 2020.
33. Naghshineh S, Hafler JP, Miller AR, et al. Formal art observation training improves medical students' visual diagnostic skills. J Gen Intern Med 2008;23(7):991–7.
34. Klugman CM, Peel J, Beckmann-Mendez D. Art rounds: Teaching interprofessional students visual thinking strategies at one school. Acad Med 2011; 86(10):1266–71.
35. Gurwin J, Revere KE, Niepold S, et al. A randomized controlled study of art observation training to improve medical student ophthalmology skills. Ophthalmology 2018;125(1):8–14.
36. Griffith DM, Semlow AR. Art, anti-racism and health equity: "don't ask me why, ask me how. Ethn Dis 2020;30(3):373–80.
37. Zeidan A, Tiballi A, Woodward M, et al. Targeting implicit bias in medicine: Lessons from art and archaeology. West J Emerg Med 2019;21(1):1–3.
38. Marr B, Baruch J. The weight of Pain: What does a 10 on the pain scale MEAN? An innovative use of art in medical education to Enhance pain Management (fr482a). J Pain Symptom Manage 2016;51(2):381–2.
39. Gaufberg E, Batalden M. The third thing in medical education. Clin Teach 2007; 4(2):78–81.

40. Gaufberg E, Olmsted MW, Bell SK. Third things as inspiration and artifact: A multistakeholder qualitative approach to understand patient and family emotions after harmful events. J Med Humanit 2019;40(4):489–504.
41. Bentwich ME, Gilbey P. More than visual literacy: Art and the enhancement of tolerance for ambiguity and empathy. BMC Med Educ 2017;17(1).
42. Potash JS, Chen JY, Lam CLK, et al. Art-making in a family medicine clerkship: How does it affect medical student empathy? BMC Med Educ 2014;14(1). https://doi.org/10.1186/s12909-014-0247-4.
43. Kesner L, Horáček J. Empathy-related responses to depicted people in art works. Front Psychol 2017;8. https://doi.org/10.3389/fpsyg.2017.00228.
44. Housen AC. Aesthetic thought, critical thinking and transfer. Arts Learn Res J 2001-2002;18(1):121.
45. Balhara K, Irvin N. A community mural tour: Facilitating experiential learning about social determinants of health. West J Emerg Med 2021;22(1). https://doi.org/10.5811/westjem.2020.9.48738.
46. Balhara K, Irvin N, Regan L. Teaching outside the box: A Health Humanities-based curriculum to teach social determinants of health. West J Emerg Med 2020;21(4.1):559.
47. Ford CL, Airhihenbuwa CO. The public health critical race methodology: Praxis for antiracism research. Soc Sci Med 2010;71:1390e1398.
48. Wear D, Zarconi J, Aultman JM, et al. Remembering Freddie Gray: Medical education for social justice. Acad Med 2017;92:312–7.
49. Tweedy D. Black man in a white Coat: a Doctor's reflections on race and medicine. New York: Picador; 2016.
50. Balhara KS, Irvin N. "The guts to really look at It"—Medicine and race in Robert Colescott's emergency room. JAMA 2020. https://doi.org/10.1001/jama.2020.20888.
51. Morse K, Balhara K, Irvin N. I am... Acad Emerg Med 2021. https://doi.org/10.1111/acem.14212.
52. Becoming Anti-Racist. A Surgeon's Journey Through Research &; Design. Available at: https://www.surgeryredesign.com/. Accessed January 5, 2021.
53. Freeman L, Stewart H. Microaggressions in clinical medicine. Kennedy Inst Ethics J 2018;28(4):411–49.

It Takes a Village
A Narrative Review of Anesthesiology Mentorship

Albert H. Tsai, MD[a],*, Natalie J. Bodmer, MD[a], Kush Gupta, BS[b],
Thomas J. Caruso, MD, MEd[a]

KEYWORDS

- Mentoring • Anesthesia • Medical student • Resident • Fellow • Faculty

KEY POINTS

- Mentorships are crucial to the career success and well-being of an anesthesiologist.
- Mentoring needs differ based on the stage of training and career.
- Mentorships should be structured and evidence-based, but tailored to the specific needs of its subjects.

FOREWORD

I first met Dr. Robert Gaiser in 2009 as a bright-eyed first-year medical student at an anesthesiology career interest talk and asked to shadow him because of the promise of a job whereby "you can wear pajamas to work every day" seemed too good to be true. A career in medicine had been a lifelong dream for as long as I could remember, but I had not given serious thought to a specific career path, and naively believed that simply graduating from medical school would lead to a fulfilling professional life, irrespective of specialty choice. I vividly remember donning scrubs for the first time as Dr. Gaiser showed me how to tie my surgical mask, with the same fondness that a child might recall his father teaching him to tie his shoelaces. The first stop of our tour of the operating rooms was a patient on cardiopulmonary bypass. "Look! This patient has no pulse, but he is still alive, isn't that cool?" Dr. Gaiser remarked as I peeked through the operating room window and seriously pondered my career choice for the first time. "This might be too intense for me, but it is very cool," I replied, staring in awe of the team and machines working in unison. Later that day, Dr. Gaiser bought me coffee at the cafeteria and thanked me for showing interest in anesthesiology. "What advice

[a] Department of Anesthesiology, Perioperative and Pain Medicine, Stanford University School of Medicine, 300 Pasteur Drive, Room H3580, MC 5640, Stanford, CA 94305, USA; [b] Class of 2022, Stanford University School of Medicine, 300 Pasteur Drive, Room H3580, MC 5640, Stanford, CA 94305, USA
* Corresponding author.
E-mail address: ahtsai@stanford.edu

Anesthesiology Clin 40 (2022) 301–313
https://doi.org/10.1016/j.anclin.2022.01.005

can you give me?" I asked. "My only advice at this point is to enjoy medical school. I will help you through the application process if you're still interested next year. If you ever want to hang out again, let me know," he replied with a grin.

Twelve years later, I cannot help but feel overwhelmed with gratitude for mentors like Dr Gaiser who guided me on the path toward my dream job: a cardiac anesthesiologist at a renowned academic medical center. As I progressed through the unique challenges of medical school, residency, fellowship, and now navigating an academic career as an early career faculty member, I have had the incredible privilege of establishing lasting relationships with my mentors that have provided invaluable support, coaching, and advocacy. Dr Gaiser not only introduced me to the specialty that I have come to love but has also been an integral presence in both my professional and personal lives. Another mentor, Dr Max Kelz, instilled the joys of scientific inquiry during our shared time working on a Foundation for Anesthesia Education and Research (FAER) medical student internship; he has similarly become a close friend and confidante. Additionally, Drs Jonathan Gavrin, Daryl Oakes, Ethan Jackson, and Tom Caruso have shaped me into a clinician, educator, and trainee advocate far more talented and passionate than I could have achieved otherwise. I am indebted to them all and inspired to pay it forward. How might I best draw on my mentorship experiences and strive to provide similar opportunities for others? In this piece—a mentorship roadmap of sorts—we will review current literature, paradigms, and practices in medical student, resident, fellow, and early career faculty mentorship models in anesthesiology. We will highlight the unique characteristics, needs, and challenges at each stage of career development and propose evidence-based frameworks for implementing successful mentoring programs in anesthesiology.

In gratitude, Albert Tsai, M.D.

BACKGROUND
A historical perspective

Medical training is historically built on an apprenticeship model, relying on experiential learning by pairing a trainee with an experienced clinician, particularly in the surgical and procedural subspecialties.[1] Bolstered by William Steward Halsted, M.D. of Johns Hopkins University who introduced the German model of graded responsibility in 1889, the hierarchical nature of medicine still exists today[2]. The success of this training structure relies on effective mentorships throughout all levels of medical education, from medical students to faculty. Despite the integral role of mentorship in medical training, the expectations and responsibilities of the mentor–mentee relationship remain vague.[3,4]

Defining mentorship

Although various definitions for mentors exist, we define a mentor as a supporting person who provides 2 broad categories of service to another individual: career enhancement and psychosocial support.[5,6] Career enhancement prepares the mentee for advancement and relies on the sponsorship and protection of the mentee, provision of exposure, provision of challenging assignments, and transmission of professional ethics. Psychosocial support enhances the mentee's sense of competence, identity, and work-role effectiveness. It includes role modeling, providing a sense of acceptance and confirmation, offering counseling, and friendship (**Table 1**).[5] Because the specific career enhancement and psychosocial needs vary depending on the mentee and their stage of training and career (**Table 2**), this definition provides the flexibility and personalization of each mentor–mentee relationship within a structured framework.

Table 1
Domains of effective mentorship

Career Enhancement	Psychosocial Support
Sponsorship	Role Modeling
Protection	Sense of Acceptance and Confirmation
Provision of Exposure and Visibility	Counseling
Provision of Challenging Assignments	Friendship
Transmission of Ethics	

Essential Functions of Mentors to Mentees.
Adapted from Johnson WB. The Intentional Mentor: Strategies and Guidelines for the Practice of Mentoring. Prof Psychol Res Pract. 2002;33(1):88 to –96.

CURRENT PRACTICES AND COMMENTARY
Medical student mentorship

Medical school requires students to navigate an incredibly complex learning environment. Medical students are tasked with acquiring a vast foundation of knowledge, while also attuning to the art of patient care and determining their career trajectory.[7] This period is demanding and stress-inducing, and has contributed to the increasing incidence of medical student burnout in recent years.[8] The combined pressures of academic performance and self-discovery in medical school highlight the role of mentorship for psychosocial growth and career development. A successful medical school mentorship model may improve academic performance and productivity, reduce burnout, and provide a sense of competence and career identity.[9–12]

The importance of near-peer mentoring

The cultivation of near-peer relationships—residents or senior medical students who are at similar stages of training to the medical student mentee—has been proposed as an effective mentorship model due to its ability to offer social congruence.[13–15] In near-peer relationships, residents and senior medical students provide emotional support, coping strategies, and counsel to their mentees based on their ability to relate to their shared experiences.[16] These student-guided programs may decrease anxiety, stress, and burnout,[13–15] as well as offer equivalent or even superior teaching experiences compared with that of senior faculty instructors.[17] This may be due to the near-peer mentor's greater scheduling accessibility and ability to meet the needs of medical students, in the form of more frequent, organic, one-on-one interactions as opposed to sporadic, formal meetings with assigned mentors.[17]

Limited exposure to anesthesiology

Anesthesiologists have long recognized the inconsistent exposure of medical students to learning opportunities in anesthesiology throughout medical school. Fewer than 22% of American medical schools have mandatory anesthesiology clerkships, and nearly 10% of senior medical students report no learning resources for anesthesiology.[18,19] As a result of the paucity of formal anesthesiology exposure, medical student impressions may be inordinately influenced by fleeting impressions, stereotypes in popular culture, and incomplete information from physicians in other specialties.[20,21] Perhaps not surprisingly, medical students desire greater formal interaction with anesthesiologists and exposure to the discipline.[20,21]

Table 2 Variable Mentorship needs			
	Medical Student	**Resident/Fellow**	**Faculty**
Clinical Skills & Knowledge	Physiology Basic Procedures (ie, IVs) Examination Preparation	Anesthesiology Knowledge Examination Preparation Procedural Competency	Consolidation of Clinical Skills Supervision of Trainees
Psychosocial Needs	Self-Discovery	Avoidance of Isolation Sense of Confidence	Sense of Purpose Establishing Reputation
Career Advancement Needs	Exposure to Anesthesia	Specialty Selection Postresidency Career Path	Networking Academic Productivity

Examples of how skills/knowledge, psychosocial, and career needs evolve through medical training.

Increasing exposure to anesthesiology through near-peer mentoring

While incorporating anesthesiology as a core clinical rotation in the medical student curriculum may be an effective strategy toward greater exposure and increased interest in the field, doing so requires substantive administrative and at times, political, efforts. Alternatively, the near-peer mentoring model can be implemented to increase our specialty exposure at the medical school level. At Stanford University School of Medicine, residents across departments are actively involved in mentoring medical and high school students. In addition to participating in the medical school's anesthesiology interest group, anesthesia residents volunteer with Project Lead the Way and the California Society of Anesthesiologists and travel to local high schools to discuss careers in anesthesiology. Residents also participate in international outreach through a robust global health program. The Anesthesia Diversity Council, comprised of Stanford residents and faculty, recruits underrepresented minority medical students from around the country to participate in our clerkship experience through the Stanford Clinical Opportunity for Residency Exposure (SCORE) program, which provides further opportunity for near-peer mentoring partnerships. When initiated early in medical student learning, these structured programs facilitate relationship building and networking in anesthesiology, particularly if a medical school lacks a formal anesthesia clerkship.

ANESTHESIOLOGY TRAINEE MENTORSHIP

While the near-peer mentorship model is well-suited toward undergraduate and medical students, anesthesiology residency represents a distinct set of needs that benefit from complementary mentorship models. Residents must acquire new clinical and technical skill sets, work rigorous schedules, and care for critically ill patients.

Resident/fellow mentoring needs in anesthesiology

The structure of anesthesiology training can be uniquely isolating. Anesthesiology residents mostly work in operating rooms, independently of their peers; conversely, most specialties are scaffolded with teams of interns, residents, and fellows, all learning from one another. This lack of peer feedback may lead residents to question their progress and lead to decreased self-confidence. Faculty mentors are critical to ensure that residents are provided with sufficient feedback and adequate psychosocial, academic, and career support.[22–24] Trainees from programs with formal mentorship programs report higher overall satisfaction with their training experience and feel better prepared for their future careers.[25,26] Residents who decide to work in academic medicine are more likely to have had a mentor, which is correlated with more peer-reviewed publications and obtaining grants.[27]

Anesthesiology trainees also experience high-stress situations at work, including intraoperative deaths, hemodynamic instability, and difficult airways. 51% of anesthesiology residents report burnout, 32% report feeling distressed, and 12% report depression during their training.[28] Furthermore, anesthesiologists have a 2-fold increased risk of substance abuse-related mortality and suicide compared with other specialties.[29] This reinforces the need for mentors who can foster an open and trusting environment, in which mentees feel safe asking for help. The mentor's role includes supporting mentees through the social-emotional aspects of training that transcend discussions of career and research. The mentor should remain cognizant of their own limitations and know when to connect the trainee with the appropriate resources if they recognize signs of burnout and depression beyond their scope of professional expertise.

Establishing mentorship

As adult learners, residents should reflect on past experiences and examine their goals when choosing a mentor.[30] Mentoring is more likely to be successful when the mentee chooses a mentor, rather than being assigned to one.[31] However, the residency program is responsible for actively initiating mentor relationships by connecting faculty and trainees with common interests.[32] Anesthesiology training in the United States is relatively short. With fellowship applications due before the end of CA-2 year, identifying a mentor is time-sensitive. However, efforts to quickly establish mentorship should be weighed against the time required for residents to identify the optimal mentor to foster their specific growth and development.[33]

The ideal mentor

There are common qualities among effective mentors. Generally, the ideal mentor fosters a resident's professional growth and mitigates feelings of isolation.[34] Residents may prefer mentors who are nonjudgmental, calm, and approachable.[35–38] A successful mentor should be skilled at providing constructive feedback, offer professional networking opportunities, and have the mentee's best interests at heart.[30,39] While residents may prefer a mentor of similar gender and ethnicity, doing so is not always feasible. It is beneficial to engage in a mentor relationship that is open to topics of gender and ethnic differences in an understanding and nonjudgmental manner.[40] It should be emphasized that while no faculty will possess every desired quality, there are certain individuals who lack the core requisites of effective mentorship and thus are ill-suited to serve in the role. Those individuals should not be pressured to mentor trainees.

The ideal mentee

The mentee must also accept active responsibilities, such as a willingness to be communicative and open about their goals, challenges, and mentorship expectations. Additionally, as with the mentor, the mentee should strive to be open-minded and recognize their own unconscious biases to cultivate a trusting relationship. This is especially true in relationships that do not share common genders or ethnicities.

Ultimately, the mentor–mentee relationship is a bidirectional, symbiotic relationship and for it to be successful, both parties must be open and actively engaged.

The academic village

Given the multifaceted demands of anesthesiology residency, the multiple opportunities for initiating mentorship, and the extensive qualities required of successful mentors, residents often identify more than one mentor by the conclusion of their training. For example, female and underrepresented minority residents may seek out multiple mentors, usually one in the subspecialty they are pursuing and another with a shared background.[41–44] The concept of an "academic village" describes the importance of mentoring networks toward the development of a trainee into an academic faculty member.[32] For example, a mentee may look to one mentor for academic support, another for clinical teaching, and another for psychosocial support. Together, these relationships harmonize to produce a safe, confidential space for the trainee to openly ask questions, seek advice, and receive feedback.[45–48]

Changing dynamics and limitations

The timbre of any mentoring relationship is constantly evolving. Initial mentorship topics may center on clinical strategies to succeed as a trainee, whereas later focus may be devoted toward career planning. The relationship should adapt to the challenges the resident faces throughout their training experience. Although some mentorships thrive beyond the intended timeframe, providing natural opportunities for the relationship to end may minimize the risk of unnecessary or fractured mentor relationships that linger beyond their utility. Although successful mentorships may lead to lifelong friendships, it is not a requirement. Many impactful mentorships are career-oriented, and those who prefer the compartmentalization of the personal and professional often gravitate toward such arrangements.

Mentoring relationships should be able to come to a natural close without coercion or fear of retribution due to the power dynamics that invariably exist between faculty and trainee. Defined reassessments of formal mentor relationships provide low-risk opportunities for the mentee and mentor to terminate. The option to extend the current relationship should also exist if both parties are amenable. This opt-in structure relinquishes pressure to continue an ineffective mentorship without fear of retaliation.

EARLY CAREER FACULTY MENTORSHIP

The misconception that faculty can only serve as mentors, not mentees themselves, is as common as it is insidious. Early career attendings must consolidate their teaching skills, establish favorable reputations within their practice, and surmount a host of other challenges. Their need for mentorship is abundant.

Early career mentoring in academic anesthesiology

Early career faculty mentorship results in increased professional satisfaction, improved confidence, enhanced academic productivity, expedited promotional advancement, and greater retention[49–53]. Although the definition of scholarly activity for anesthesiologists has expanded to curriculum development, quality improvement, health care access, global health, and informatics, many institutions continue to emphasize "traditional" metrics of academic productivity such as basic research grants and scientific publications[54]. This discrepancy contributes to the ongoing need for early career development mentorship.[30] Successful faculty mentors should tailor their approaches to the career goals of the mentee that account for specific promotion criteria of each institution to ensure that nonclinical efforts are optimally contributing to career advancement.

Aligning goals, but paving different paths

The mentorship dynamic at the faculty level is intrinsically different from that of medical school and residency, and may present unique challenges as both mentor and mentee are fully trained attending physicians. The near-peer model of mentorship that is ideal at the medical school level may not be as applicable at this career stage as many near-peer faculty share similar professional development challenges. However, successful mid-career and senior faculty have the experience to adequately support and advocate for early career faculty. Unlike faculty-to-resident mentorship, faculty-to-faculty mentorship has a distinct set of aspirations. The mentor and mentee should align career objectives and devise a plan in which both parties can achieve their respective goals while supporting each other along similar yet distinct paths. This form of parallel mentoring allows for guidance and advocacy while avoiding cloning, or leading the mentee to become a miniature version of the mentor, which deprives the early career faculty of establishing their own identity and may strain the relationship. Successful mentorship at the faculty level is characterized by a sense of reciprocity, mutual respect, clear expectations, and shared values.[39] Effective mentors to early career faculty will guide, rather than lead their mentee toward their desired career goals and provide the support necessary to achieve them.

DISCUSSION
Strategies for success

Though well-intentioned, most mentoring initiatives are poised to fail from random and forced assignments of mentor–mentee pairings, leading to a lack of relationship foundation and trust.[5] Consequently, the implementation of a successful mentoring program must be thoughtfully executed within an organized framework. We have characterized this framework by proposing a 5-step mentorship plan, which is highlighted by the identification of program rationale, provision of mentee education, design of tailored programs, development of mentor profiles, and the fostering of mentor relationships[10].

Identification of program rationale

The first step to the implementation of a successful mentoring program is to identify effective, volunteer mentors through didactics and interactive sessions on the benefits and requirements of successful mentorships. By highlighting the core characteristics of ideal mentors, faculty candidates can assess their own desire and suitability to serve as mentors. This self-selecting approach ensures mentors are motivated and may avoid forced or ineffective mentorships.

Provision of mentee education

Mentee indifference is often cited by mentors as a reason for losing interest in the relationship[55]. It is crucial to educate mentees on their active role in cultivating successful mentorships. Mentees should be proactive and engaged, follow-up on assigned tasks, solicit feedback, and prepare for conversations with mentors. Goals, values, and action items must be built into the dialogue to achieve both the mentee and mentor's career trajectories.

TOM CARUSO, MD, MED

Residency:
☐ Anesthesiology: Massachusetts General Hospital 2009–2012

Fellowship:
☐ Pediatric anesthesiology: LPCH Stanford 2012–2013

Board certifications:
☐ Anesthesiology 2012
☐ Pediatric Anesthesiology 2013

Years on Staff at LPCH: 8 y

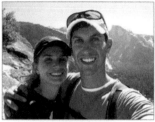
Tom with his wife, Erika

Pediatric anesthesia interests: Developing safe transitions of care between the OR and PACU/ICUs. Using IT and analytics to ensure appropriate pre operative antibiotic administration. Virtual Reality for preoperative anxiety.

Other work related interests: Quality improvement issues including decreasing our local SSI and CLABSI rates. Graduate medical education – presently work with GME to implement mentor programs throughout residency programs here at Stanford. Mobile app development for GME and SOM.

What I enjoy doing outside of work: Grilling, cycling, happy hour.

Words other people use to describe me: Enthusiastic, persistent, energetic.

Fig. 1. Sample mentor profile for assisting mentees with mentor selection.

Development of mentor profiles

Because the identification of a faculty mentor is best conducted early in the course of a relatively short anesthesiology residency, development of mentor profiles can serve as a useful source for mentor identification and selection (**Fig. 1**). This resource allows the trainee to evaluate the potential fit of mentorship and is another way to optimize pairings.

Fostering mentor relationships

Given the rigors of residency and fellowship training, time commitment has been identified at our institution as one of the largest barriers to successful mentorships. Programs should provide integrated time to foster mentorship relationships. We

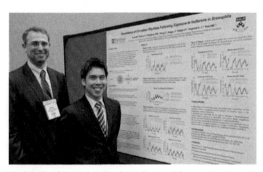

Fig. 2. Albert Tsai, MD (author) as a medical student with mentor Max Kelz, MD, PhD at ASA 2011 in Chicago.

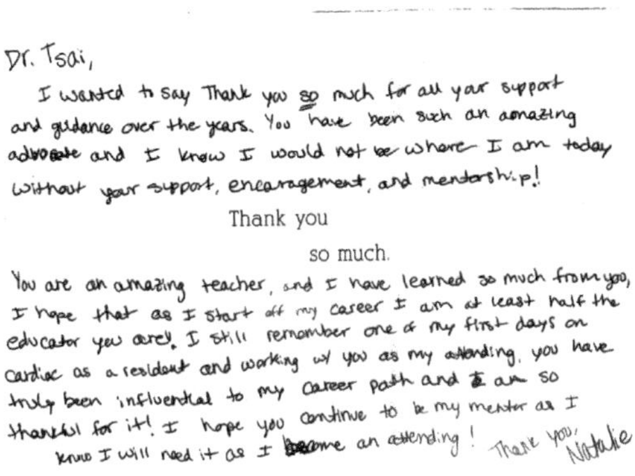

Dr. Tsai,

I wanted to say Thank you so much for all your support and guidance over the years. You have been such an amazing advocate and I know I would not be where I am today without your support, encouragement, and mentorship!

Thank you

so much.

You are an amazing teacher, and I have learned so much from you. I hope that as I start off my career I am at least half the educator you are. I still remember one of my first days on cardiac as a resident and working w/ you as my attending, you have truly been influential to my career path and I am so thankful for it! I hope you continue to be my mentor as I know I will need it as I become an attending! Thank you, Natalie

Fig. 3. Letter from a mentee.

recommend meetings at least every 4 months, which may be creatively facilitated by using protected lecture time, hosting structured mentoring social events in lieu of Grand Rounds, and pairing the mentor and mentee to work together in the operating room whenever feasible.

SUMMARY

In a recent opinion piece, "Mentoring Matters," Max Kelz, MD, PhD, describes how adopting a new mentee is much like raising a child: the commitment can last for decades, and he shares in his mentees' struggles and accomplishments (**Fig. 2**).[56] As a new father of two daughters, I have been blessed with a newfound appreciation for this sentiment in a way that I likely took for granted when I first met the instrumental figures that would constitute my academic (and personal) village. Much like parenting and the practice of anesthesiology, there is no singular way to mentor. Genuine compassion must lie at the core of these relationships; with proper guidance and cultivation, mentors can profoundly shape careers and lives.

I recently found an envelope addressed to me on the anesthesia machine of the operating room in which I was working (**Fig. 3**). It was from a trainee who I have known for the past 5 years and someone whose compassion, resilience, and work ethic have always been a source of my own inspiration. We were never formally assigned as a mentor and mentee, but had organically developed an enduring mentorship bond encompassing all of the characteristics of a successful mentoring relationship. After reading the heartfelt note, I could not help but feel that of all the accolades I have been encouraged to pursue throughout my career in medicine, this informal, often overlooked aspect of my job would lead to my most cherished accomplishment to date. Later that day, I bought her coffee at the cafeteria and thanked her for the wonderful letter. With 3 short months between her and graduation, she asked, "What advice can you give me?" "My only advice at this point is to enjoy the remainder of fellowship. If you ever need help, just know that you are surrounded by a wonderful village," I replied with a grin.

CLINICS CARE POINTS

- Mentors provide career enhancement and psychosocial support through various essential functions, including sponsorship and protection, provision of exposure and challenging

assignments, transmission of professional ethics, role modeling, offering acceptance, confirmation, counseling, and friendship.
- Effective mentoring leads to greater career satisfaction, personal fulfillment, academic productivity, and promotional advancement.
- Mentorship needs vary between individuals and evolve through the various stages of medical training. Successful mentors are effective in using different mentoring strategies to ensure continued support of the mentee regardless of changing goals and challenges.
- Common mentoring pitfalls include random or forced pairings, mentor and/or mentee apathy or distrust, and cloning of the mentee.

DISCLOSURE

The authors have nothing to disclose.

REFERENCES

1. Bishop WJ. The early history of Surgery. New York: Barnes & Noble, Inc; 1960.
2. Sadideen H, Kneebone R. Practical skills teaching in contemporary surgical education: how can educational theory be applied to promote effective learning? Am J Surg 2012;204(3):396–401.
3. Merriam S. Mentors and proteges: A critical review of the literature. Adult Education Q 1983;33:161–73.
4. Bogat GA, Redner RL. How mentoring affects the professional development of women. Prof Psychol Res Pr 1985;16:851–9.
5. Johnson WB. The intentional mentor: strategies and guidelines for the practice of mentoring. Prof Psychol Res Pract 2002;33(1):88–96.
6. Arthur MB. Review of Mentoring at Work: Developmental Relationships in Organizational Life. Admin Sci Quart 1985;30(3):454–6.
7. Cruess RL, Cruess SR, Boudreau J, Donald MD, et al. MHPE; Steinert, Yvonne PhD Reframing Medical Education to Support Professional Identity Formation. Acad Med 2014;89(11):1446–51. https://doi.org/10.1097/ACM.0000000000000427.
8. Ishak W, Nikravesh R, Lederer S, et al. Burnout in medical students: a systematic review. Clin Teach 2013;10(4):242–5.
9. Frei E, Stamm M, Buddeberg-Fischer B. Mentoring programs for medical students–a review of the PubMed literature 2000-2008. BMC Med Educ 2010;10:32.
10. Caruso TJ, Steinberg DH, Piro N, et al. A Strategic Approach to Implementation of Medical Mentorship Programs. J Grad Med Educ 2016;8:68–73.
11. Hirsch AE, Agarwal A, Rand AE, et al. Medical Student Mentorship in Radiation Oncology at a Single Academic Institution: A 10-Year Analysis. Pract Radiat Oncol 2015;5:e163–8.
12. Fares J, Al Tabosh H, Saadeddin Z, et al. Stress, Burnout and Coping Strategies in Preclinical Medical Students. N Am J Med Sci 2016;8(2):75–81.
13. Chang E, Eddins-Folensbee F, Coverdale J. Survey of the Prevalence of Burnout, Stress, Depression, and the Use of Supports by Medical Students at One School. Acad Psychiatry 2012;36:177–82.
14. Ragins B, Kram E. The handbook of mentoring at work: theory, research and practice. California: Sage Publications Inc.; 2007.

15. Akinla O, Hagan P, Atiomo W. A systematic review of the literature describing the outcomes of near-peer mentoring programs for first year medical students. BMC Med Educ 2018;18:98. https://doi.org/10.1186/s12909-018-1195-1.
16. Benè KL, Bergus G. When Learners Become Teachers: A Review of Peer Teaching in Medical Student Education. Fam Med 2014;46(10):783–7.
17. Barker JC, Rendon J, Janis JE. Medical Student Mentorship in Plastic Surgery: The Mentee's Perspective. Plast Reconstr Surg 2016;137(6):1934–42.
18. Percentage of medical schools with separate required clerkships by discipline: anesthesiology. Association of American Medical Colleges. Available at: www.aamc.org/data-reports/curriculum-reports/interactive-data/clerkship-requirements-discipline. Accessed September 21, 2021.
19. Henschke SJ, Robertson EM, Murtha L, et al. Survey of medical students' knowledge and perceptions of anesthesiology at one Canadian university: pre-clerkship and during clinical clerkship, a cohort study. Can J Anesth/j Can Anesth 2018;65:325–6.
20. Naik VN. Pre-clerkship teaching: Are we missing an opportunity? Can J Anesth/j Can Anesth 2017;64:6–9.
21. Ly EI, Catalani BS, Boggs SD, et al. The Anesthesiology Clerkship: A Requisite Experience in Medical Education. Ochsner J 2020;20(3):250–4. https://doi.org/10.31486/toj.20.0094.
22. Genuardi FJ, Zenni EA. Adolescent medicine faculty development needs. J Adolesc Health 2001;29:46–9. Stubbe DE. Preparation for practice: child and adolescent psychiatry graduates' assessment of training experiences. J Am Acad Child Adolesc Psychiatry. 2002;41:131-139.
23. Coleman VH, Power ML, Williams S, et al. Racial and gender differences in obstetrics and gynecology residents' perceptions of mentoring. J Contin Educ Health Prof 2005;25:268–77.
24. Leppert PC, Artal R. A survey of past obstetrics and gynecology research fellows. J Soc Gynecol Investig 2002;9:372–8.
25. Sciscione AC, Colmorgen GH, D'Alton ME. Factors affecting fellowship satisfaction, thesis completion, and career direction among maternal-fetal medicine fellows. Obstet Gynecol 1998;91:1023–6.
26. Ramanan RA, Taylor WC, Davis RB, et al. Mentoring matters. Mentoring and career preparation in internal medicine residency training. J Gen Intern Med 2006;21:340–5.
27. Berk RA, Berg J, Mortimer R, et al. Measuring the effectiveness of faculty mentoring relationships. Acad Med 2005;80:66–71.
28. Sun H, Warner DO, Macario A, et al. Repeated Cross-sectional Surveys of Burnout, Distress, and Depression among Anesthesiology Residents and First-year Graduates. Anesthesiology 2019;131(3):668–77.
29. Rodrigues JVDS, Pereira JEG, Passarelli LA, et al. Risk of mortality and suicide associated with substance use disorder among healthcare professionals: A systematic review and meta-analysis of observational studies. Eur J Anaesthesiol 2021;38(7):715–34.
30. Straus SE, Chatur F, Taylor M. Issues in the mentor-mentee relationship in academic medicine: qualitative study. Acad Med 2009;84:135–9.
31. Yehia BR, Cronholm PF, Wilson N, et al. Mentorship and pursuit of academic medicine careers: a mixed methods study of residents from diverse backgrounds. BMC Med Educ 2014;14:26.
32. Neelankavil J, Goeddel LA, Dwarakanath S, et al. Mentoring Fellows in Adult Cardiothoracic Anesthesiology for Academic Practice in the Contemporary Era-

Perspectives From Mentors Around the United States. J Cardiothorac Vasc Anesth 2020;34(2):521–9.

33. Jackson VA, Palepu A, Szalacha L, et al. Having the right chemistry": a qualitative study of mentoring in academic medicine. Acad Med 2003;78:328–34.

34. Sinai J, Tiberius RG, de Groot J, et al. Developing a training program to improve supervisor–resident relationships, step 1: Defining the types of issues. Teach Learn Med 2001;13:80–5.

35. Kotta Prasanti Alekhya, Jamie Sin Ying Ho. Residents' Perspectives on the Mentor-Mentee Relationship. JACC: Case Rep 2021;3(Issue 9):1244–6.

36. Busari JO, Weggelaar NM, Knottnerus AC, et al. How medical residents perceive the quality of supervision provided by attending doctors in the clinical setting. Med Educ 2005;39:696–703.

37. Kenton K. How to teach and evaluate learners in the operating room. Obstet Gynecol Clin North Am 2006;33:325–32.

38. Levy BD, Katz JT, Wolf MA, et al. An initiative in mentoring to promote residents' and faculty members' careers. Acad Med 2004;79:845–50.

39. Straus SE, Johnson MO, Marquez C, et al. Characteristics of Successful and Failed Mentoring relationships: a qualitative study across two academic health centers. Acad Med 2013;88:82–9.

40. Koopman RJ, Thiedke CC. Views of family medicine department Chairs about mentoring junior faculty. Med Teach 2005;27:734–7.

41. Amonoo HL, Barreto EA, Stern TA, et al. Residents' Experiences with Mentorship in Academic Medicine. Acad Psychiatry 2019;43(1):71–5.

42. Pfund C, House SC, Asquith P, et al. Training mentors of clinical and translational research scholars: a randomized controlled trial. Acad Med 2014;89(5):774–82.

43. Brown JB, Thorpe C, Paquette-Warren J, et al. The mentoring needs of trainees in family practice. Educ Prim Care 2012;23(3):196–203.

44. McNamara MC, McNeil MA, Chang J. A pilot study exploring gender differences in residents' strategies for establishing mentoring relationships. Med Educ Online 2008;13:7.

45. Hekelman FP, Blase JR. Excellence in clinical teaching: The core of the mission. Acad Med 1996;71:738–42.

46. Kram KE. Mentoring at work. Glenview, ill: Scott. Foresman and Company; 1985.

47. Markakis KM, Beckman HB, Suchman AL, et al. The path to professionalism: Cultivating humanistic values and attitudes in residency training. Acad Med 2000;75:141–50.

48. Hauck F, Zyzanski S, Alemagno S, et al. Patient perceptions of humanism in physicians: Effects on positive health behaviors. Fam Med 1990;2:447–52.

49. Sambunjak D, Straus SE, Marusić A. Mentoring in academic medicine: a systematic review. JAMA 2006; 296:1103–1115

50. Efstathiou JA, Drumm MR, Paly JP, et al. Long-term impact of a faculty mentoring program in academic medicine. PLoS ONE 2018;13(11):e0207634.

51. Holliday EB, Jagsi R, Thomas CR, et al. Standing on the shoulders of giants: results from the radiation oncology academic development and mentorship assessment project (ROADMAP). Int J Radiat Oncol Biol Phys 2014;88:18–24.

52. Levy AS, Pyke-Grimm KA, Lee DA, et al. Mentoring in pediatric oncology:a report from the children's oncology group young investigator committee. J Pediatr Hematol Oncol 2013;35:456–61.

53. Morrison LJ, Lorens E, Bandiera G, et al. Impact of a formal mentoring program on academic promotion of department of medicine faculty: a comparative study. Med Teach 2014;36:608–14.

54. Hindman BJ, Dexter F, Todd M. Research, Education, and Nonclinical Service Productivity of New Junior Anesthesia Faculty During a 2-year Faculty Development Program. Anesth Analg 2013;117-1:194–204.
55. Zerzan JT, Hess R, Schur E, et al. Making the most of mentors: a guide for mentees. Acad Med 2009;84(1):140 144.
56. Max B. Kelz; Mentoring Matters. ASA Monitor 2021;85:44.

Early-Career Physician Burnout

Leelach Rothschild, MD[a], Ciera Ward, MD[b],*

KEYWORDS

- Early career • Burnout • Physician satisfaction • Depersonalization • Career stages
- Compassion • Gender differences

KEY POINTS

- Burnout syndrome, which is more prevalent among physicians than the general population, is characterized by emotional exhaustion, depersonalization, and low sense of personal accomplishment.
- Early-career anesthesiologists are faced with significant work, family, personal, and career demands, which may lead to increasing work-life challenges and conflicts.
- Burnout rate among early-career anesthesiologists has not yet been studied and could help target programming and education during residency training.

INTRODUCTION

Burnout, first described in pediatric mental health workers who experienced emotional depletion and disengagement, continues to plague physicians across medical specialties, and the field of anesthesiology is no exception.[1] A recent study by Afonso and colleagues demonstrated that workplace factors, specifically the lack of feeling supported, led to high risk for both burnout and burnout syndrome.[2] Burnout is a state of work exhaustion characterized by the following 3 components: (1) A continual breakdown of one's emotional framework resulting in emotional exhaustion, (2) Cynicism concerning the loss of idealistic expectations and values of one's profession (depersonalization), and (3) Doubt related to one's ability to capably perform well within the role (personal accomplishment).

The prevalence of burnout among physicians ranges widely from 28% to 75% globally, but few studies have looked at the origins of burnout for anesthesiologists and at the prevalence of burnout among different career stages of anesthesiologists.[3] Considerable focus has been placed on retaining physicians and minimizing burnout in more seasoned anesthesiologists. The authors review the literature to better understand drivers of burnout for early-career physicians, and specifically for

[a] University of Illinois Hospital and Health Sciences System, 1740 West Taylor Street, Suite 3200, Chicago, IL 60612, USA; [b] Christus Mother Frances Hospital, Attn: Dr Ciera Ward w/ Anesthesia, 800 East Dawson Street, Tyler, TX 75701, USA
* Corresponding author.
E-mail address: cierakaylynn@gmail.com

Anesthesiology Clin 40 (2022) 315–323
https://doi.org/10.1016/j.anclin.2021.12.003
1932-2275/22/© 2022 Elsevier Inc. All rights reserved.

anesthesiology.theclinics.com

anesthesiologists. They attempt to uncover and elucidate contributors to early-career burnout and explore possibilities for mitigating burnout so that it has a less significant impact on our physicians.

Early-career anesthesiologists are faced with a plethora of challenges as they transition from a very regimented schedule with little autonomy in residency training to a private practice or academic setting. Early-career anesthesiologists must integrate into a new system whereby they may not initially have a strong presence. Recent graduates must also quickly learn to navigate new and complicated organizational networks within their hospitals and institutions. These professional challenges often overlap with intersecting personal and financial stressors as graduates start families, manage housing relocation pressures, and take on medical student financial debt burden. It is common for this transition to not be supported with any vacation time even if relocating to a new state is required; as such, recent graduates often do not have the necessary support in place to help them acclimate before starting into their new jobs.

DEFINING THE EARLY-CAREER PHYSICIAN AND ANESTHESIOLOGIST

"Early career" has been used to describe a variety of stages of medical practice. Some investigators have defined early career as medical student trainees through the early postgraduate resident training years.[4] In this article, the authors align with Dyrbye and colleagues,[5] who define early career as the first 10 years of practice after completing residency. Early-career anesthesiologists face distinct challenges as they transition from supervised residency training into a workforce of significant autonomy in either academic medicine or private practice.

RESIDENTS AND BURNOUT: THE SEEDS ARE PLANTED

Dyrbye and colleagues[6] suggest that burnout appears to peak during medical training, where overall burnout, depersonalization, and fatigue are most prevalent and occur with an increased incidence relative to the similarly aged US population.[6] Despite current work hour restrictions for medical students and trainees, fatigue is still a commonly cited factor contributing to burnout.[6] However, Dyrbye and colleagues[6] found that overall burnout, high levels of depersonalization, and high fatigue were most prevalent during training and improved for the early-career physician; interestingly, emotional exhaustion peaked during training and was least prevalent in the early-career stage. Despite higher quality-of-life indicators in the early-career group of physicians, at least 51% were burned out, and 40% reported having at least 1 symptom of fatigue, with a higher prevalence of high emotional exhaustion, high depersonalization, and burnout as compared with their US population control sample.[6] Initial attempts are underway to better understand burnout factors in residents and to mitigate their impact to prevent further progression into the early physician career years.

The high rate of burnout in resident trainees has also gained significant attention and concern because of the link to patient safety.[7] Residency training is a "time of temporary imbalance," where residents are required to adapt and cope with extreme disruptions to work-life balance.[8] The well-being of anesthesiology residents is critical, as it supports quality patient-centered care in the perioperative space. Anesthesiology residency, however, is fraught with unique workplace stressors. Residents are required to adapt to operating room dynamics and acute patient care scenarios that arise. Stressful clinical emergencies may undermine resident confidence, which may be further compounded by isolation and other negative factors specific to anesthesiology.

Anesthesiology residents, like all trainees, experience disrupted sleep schedules, which alter normal restorative sleep cycles and greatly impact well-being. In addition, anesthesiology residents are part of a teams-based approach to patient care in the operating room and must learn to adapt to this multifaceted model. Residents must also continuously adapt to constantly changing anesthesiology faculty preferences, equipment modifications, and new rotation and clinical site schedules and demands. Cumulatively, this challenging work milieu limits a trainee's capacity to address stressors at home or those pertaining to self-care.

Anesthesiology residents are typically in their mid to late twenties and early thirties, often balancing the demands of fulfilling their training requirements while tending to expanding families and obligations at home. These 2 pressures are contextualized within a specialty that does not necessarily lend itself to the camaraderie and benefits of a close-knit workplace community to bolster one's sense of belonging and support. Anesthesiology residents, by nature, work independently in the operating room for long hours with minimal interaction from fellow anesthesia residents and colleagues. In other specialties, residents may round together in the morning and have opportunities to share meals over grand rounds and department conferences. Conversely, anesthesiology residents experience relatively more isolation because of limited opportunities to mingle and interact with peers, leading to feeling less supported in their respective residency experiences.

COMPASSION AND BURNOUT: CAN WE INTERCEPT EARLY?

When physicians overidentify with the suffering of their patients, they may begin to feel overwhelmed and, paradoxically, exhibit callousness toward others. Such behaviors define depersonalization, which is one of the 3 hallmark signs of burnout, and a primary contributor to physician distress. Empathic distress occurs when providers have a self-oriented response to others' suffering, which causes detachment from a situation to protect oneself from negative feelings. There is a very strong and direct correlation between empathic distress and burnout. Medical schools and graduate medical education programs have not yet focused attention on teaching physicians how to care for their patients and simultaneously tend to their own complex emotional experiences and pain that may ensue from witnessing pain and suffering in others. Research with trauma therapists demonstrates that well-developed empathy and compassion help both clinicians and patients and provide protection against burnout.[9] Excessive sharing of others' negative emotions, especially when vicariously experiencing their pain, may lead to aversive feelings and maladaptive behaviors and cause a decreased desire to help others, ultimately resulting in empathic distress.[10]

Compassion is defined as a feeling of concern for others' suffering and a desire to alleviate that suffering.[11] Compassion training is a resource to decrease empathic distress, improve well-being, and mitigate burnout.[11] One study demonstrated that medical students who chose "patient-remote" specialties, such as radiology, had lower empathy scores, which could be considered a surrogate marker for empathic distress and burnout.[12] Anesthesiology is similarly not heavily patient-facing and can be considered "patient-remote." As new graduates leave anesthesiology training with a potentially limited capacity to digest and process emotional pain related to patient care, they would likely benefit from compassion training. Additional challenges that may incur empathic distress and burnout for early-career anesthesiologists include the hidden curriculum of medical school and residency. Billings and colleagues[13] found that exposure to unprofessional conduct and cynicism during internal medicine residency training was associated with higher burnout and cynicism scores.

As early-career physicians leave a training culture that breeds cynicism, they are prone to a loss of empathy and decreased humanism.[14] A humanism curriculum pilot study for internal medicine residents and obstetrics and gynecology residents found that participants had decreased burnout rates and improved compassion scores.[15] Compassion training is now offered at multiple academic and medical centers across the country as an antidote to burnout and to improve resiliency and increase well-being. Incorporating compassion training into resident anesthesiology curricula may improve early-career anesthesiologists' ability to manage emotional stressors and mitigate cynicism and early-career burnout.

MENTAL HEALTH AND BURNOUT IN EARLY-CAREER ANESTHESIOLOGISTS

Early-career physician well-being is closely correlated to the state of residents' mental health during their training. Over 4 years of training, anesthesiology residents must gain proficiency in both technical and cognitive skills, while learning to have presence and become a leader in the perioperative space. The potential for psychological and emotional challenges are ubiquitous during residency and naturally persist as residents transition to an independent practitioner. This occupational stress may lead to adverse mental health challenges.[16] A cross-sectional survey by Sun and colleagues[17] among anesthesiology residents and first-year graduates found that after 1 year of residency, approximately half of anesthesiologists reported burnout, half reported distress, and one in 8 positively screened for depression. Depression is a known risk factor for suicide, particularly when coupled with poor sleep quality, limited psychosocial supports, and anxiety. Sun and colleagues provided evidence of high depression in an anesthesiology cohort and described that the rate of suicidal ideation is similar to adults with major depressive disorder in the lay community.[18]

THE TRANSITION FROM RESIDENCY: NEW CHALLENGES

Recent anesthesia graduates must learn to work within completely new health systems to supervise teams of clinicians, manage divisions and departments, and interact with administration and leadership circles.[19] In addition to these vital tasks, postgraduates must continue preparation for the American Board of Anesthesiologists written and applied board examinations. Apart from board preparation, anesthesiology residency training does not provide a specific curriculum to address the critical issues that impact the growing and flourishing needs and opportunities within a resident's first years out of training.

Organizational psychology may be an instrumental resource for early-career physicians, as they begin to function more autonomously as leaders within a department or health system, develop their clinical styles, and nurture their work-life integration.[19] Anesthesiology residency programs may benefit from providing training in various aspects of organizational psychology to nurture the development of strong leaders. Cordova and colleagues[19] state that organizational psychology's "emphasis on principles of motivation, team development, communication, alignment of organizational and professional values, and diversity, equity, and inclusion supports this function."

Previous studies have demonstrated an inverse relationship between burnout and physician age; indeed, younger members of the clinical anesthesia workforce experience burnout at a higher rate.[3] Although anesthesiology residents develop resilience and learn to manage stress during their training, some may rely more heavily on survival mode tactics. They idealize a future career of autonomy and less stress, where their efforts are ultimately rewarded. However, as anesthesiology residents transition into attendings, they move from one set of challenges to another. As a new physician in practice, whether in academics or private practice, recent graduates need to adapt to a new environment, learn the business aspects of medicine, and establish themselves within a new workplace. These realities may not align with expectations of a recent graduate and may incur additional stress.

PHYSICIAN STRESSORS IN THE EARLY-CAREER YEARS

Evidence from a 2017 study supports an increased rate of burnout in new graduates who completed their training in the preceding 11 months, increasing from 28% to 75%.[4] Early-career physicians have many work-related demands. Here, the authors review the Job Demands Resources Model (JD-R) as described by Hariharan and Griffin[20] to provide a conceptual framework for early-career burnout. The JD-R model breaks down work stressors and personal qualities into work-related demands and resources (eg, individual coping mechanisms), respectively. The JD-R model has been used to describe burnout in early-career physicians to better understand the unique stressors of this subgroup.[20] Within this model, the potential for positive outcomes for both work-related and individual-related demands relies solely on the ability to best use available coping resources. Hariharan and Griffin[20] differentiate work-related from person demands, which the authors apply to the field of anesthesiology.

Work-Related Demands

It is well known that a strong association exists between increased patient load, time constraints, long work hours through on call or overtime, and symptoms of burnout. Many, if not all, of these demands are experienced within the first few years following residency training. The medical culture can foster a competitive and hierarchical nature, which dissuades expressions of vulnerability.[20] Newly independent physicians may combat imposter syndrome with the increase in responsibility and liability found in their new role as an autonomous practitioner. This may lead to a sense of needing to prove oneself to new colleagues and subsequently suppress disclosing concerns or fears. Additional stressors, such as bad outcomes, an absence of camaraderie among new colleagues, or insufficient support from administration, may cumulatively contribute to early burnout.

Personal Demands

As humans caring for other humans, physicians may minimize the impact that non-work-related demands can have on work-related activities, job satisfaction, and clinical outcomes. Notably, major life events, both positive and negative (eg, serious illness, birth of a child, death of a loved one), can lead to burnout and are repeatedly reported in the literature.[20] Other stressors specifically encountered by early-career physicians include but are not limited to concern for the future, generalized stress, and work-related stress. Hariharan and Griffin[20] stated one of the strongest predictors of burnout in early-career physicians is mental health disorders, such as posttraumatic stress disorder, which is commonly found in conjunction with burnout. Higher rates of burnout are also associated with imposter syndrome, self-reported anxiety, and perfectionism. An individual's response to negative events may further contribute to the likelihood of burnout, with women showing greater rates of self-blame compared with their male colleagues.

WORK-RELATED ENVIRONMENTS: PRIVATE PRACTICE VERSUS ACADEMIC PRACTICE IN EARLY-CAREER ANESTHESIOLOGISTS

There is a lack of evidence in the literature to suggest a significant difference between types of anesthesia practice that may impact rates of burnout for early-career physicians. Academic anesthesiologists have specific challenges, and it has been suggested that there may be inattention to the humanistic values of faculty that may contribute to low retention.[21] Academic programs may benefit from programming and support to help guide early-career anesthesiologists to engage in personal reflection to focus on their strengths, passions, and values in an effort to direct their careers toward meaningful work. Based on work by Lieff,[21] this approach is also applicable to career planning and development of academic anesthesiologists and may help with retention of anesthesiology faculty.

Private practice varies in management complexities within individual practice groups as well as by region. Partnership tracks have the added burden of learning how to join and eventually manage a business in addition to all other forms of expected knowledge to newly graduated anesthesiologists. Many private practice anesthesiology groups must travel to multiple facilities within a certain region, which disrupts one's daily routine through the dissimilarities between different locations. Private practice groups can reduce these burdens with shared workloads, mentorship, and schedule flexibility.

GENDER DISPARITIES AND PARENTAL STATUS AMONG EARLY-CAREER PHYSICIANS

As a larger percentage of women enter medicine and become part of the workforce, it is critical to understand the drivers of gender gaps for this new generation of women physicians. Frank and colleagues[22] followed a cohort of physicians who completed training to better understand how the role of family may contribute to female workforce attrition and, in this case, possible burnout in a physician's early career. Women physicians were more likely to hold part-time positions as compared with their male counterparts, and these differences were more pronounced in women with children. Frank and colleagues[22] found that there was a 9.6% gender gap in full employment within the first year of training, growing to 38.7% by 6 years after completion of training. This gender-gap disparity likely contributes to inequities in compensation and promotion as well as leadership roles. Dyrbye and colleagues[6] demonstrated that an early-career male physician was associated with lower odds of experiencing fatigue. In addition, Sun and colleagues[17] found that being a woman was associated with a higher risk of distress among anesthesiology residents and first-year graduates. Starmer and colleagues[23] also found that female gender, although not associated with higher rates of burnout, was associated with lower likelihood of career satisfaction and work-life balance.[23] Gender inequity should receive widespread acknowledgment in both academia and private practice. It is imperative that women anesthesiologists experience similar retention and advancement as men counterparts. Policies, such as paid parental leave, scheduling flexibility, and lactation support, to name a few, should reflect a supportive culture that values both women and men anesthesiologists equally.

EARLY BURNOUT IN NONANESTHESIOLOGISTS: ARE THERE SIMILARITIES OR COROLLARIES?

Many specialties have studied early-career burnout rates and professional engagement in the literature; the authors review several articles that focused on surgical fields, oncology, emergency medicine, and primary care fields to better understand the determinants of early-career physician burnout that may apply to anesthesiology. Anesthesia training programs are similar to other specialty programs in that they focus on clinical competencies and skills development and do not tend to other aspects of career development, such as business and administrative aspects of medical practice management. Firdouse and colleagues[24] investigated the challenges facing recent Canadian surgical graduates, specifically assessing their competency in managing their own practice.[24] They found that 68% of surgical graduates were not comfortable with the business aspects of a practice, specifically, coding and billing for services. Interestingly, 98% of this cohort also perceived that they did not receive any formal training to prevent burnout.[24]

Zhang and colleagues[25] studied early- and mid-career breast surgeons and found that breast surgeons who had been in practice for 5 to 9 years had significantly higher rates of burnout that were attributed to a variety of practice and personal factors. Conversely, earlier literature work found that midcareer, defined as physicians in practice from 11 to 20 years, had the highest rate of burnout, which was not aligned with the trends in breast surgeons.[5] In pediatrics, multivariable modeling showed that excellent or very good health of the physician, peer support, and patient care resources were associated with lower prevalence of burnout and a higher likelihood of career and life satisfaction.[23]

Hall and colleagues[26] surveyed emergency department physicians and found that they had a "ten-year survival rate" of 84.9%, akin to an attrition rate of 15.1% after 10 years. Emergency medicine physicians may turn to early retirement because of their increased workload intensity, lack of emergency room safety, and age.[27] Early retirement can usually be attributed to a mismatch of work-related stress and a high-pressure working environment that lead to burnout. The similarities between anesthesiology and emergency medicine owing to the chaotic nature and high acuity and intensity of clinical cases should prompt anesthesiologists to study similar trends within our field.

MITIGATING EARLY-CAREER BURNOUT AND NEXT STEPS

The best strategy to address early-career burnout in anesthesiologists is prevention, namely, in promoting personal and professional engagement through the utilization and maximization of organizational support and resources. Many organizational resources exist to help the early-career physician. The American Society of Anesthesiologists (ASA) Well-Being Resources Web site (https://www.asahq.org/advocating-for-you/well-being) launched in 2020 and offers a variety of multitiered resources delineated for the individual, organization, society, and culture, COVID-19 pandemic related, and others. In addition, the Accreditation Council for Graduate Medical Education (ACGME) has prioritized the well-being of trainees through milestones and program requirements. The recently launched ACGME AWARE project (https://dl.acgme.org/pages/well-being) includes a suite of on-demand resources designed to promote well-being among trainees, including digital workshops, podcasts, and a downloadable app for easy access to these tools.

Furthermore, an anesthesiologist's personal and professional support networks are crucial for ensuring success and minimizing unhealthy stressors. Mentorship, connection, and community with peers and colleagues who can relate to similar stressors may decrease the odds of burnout. Assessing and ensuring appropriate work-life integration and balance allows individuals to derive meaning from their professional life, which promotes engagement both within and outside of the workplace. Fostering holistic health inclusive of physical, mental, emotional, spiritual, financial, and so forth is essential.

MOVING FORWARD AND LOOKING AHEAD

Although the authors continue to track metrics and gather data in an effort to better understand the vast importance of this topic, there is still much left to be discovered.

For this reason, many organizations, including the ASA, have made significant strides in addressing issues related to burnout in anesthesiology, particularly amid the current pandemic. In 2021, the ASA conducted a national burnout survey among anesthesiology trainees. The results are pending but will undoubtedly provide valuable information regarding the specific stressors and coping mechanisms currently experienced by our early-career physicians and generate new ideas to promote a healthier and happier future for our specialty.

CLINICS CARE POINTS

- Early career anesthesiologists are faced with a plethora of challenges as they transition from residency training where they had a very regimented schedule with little autonomy and move into private or academic practice.

- Burnout often develops during medical training, but studies show that implementing humanism curricula into residency training resulted in decreased burnout rates and improved compassion scores.

- There is a great need for further research in early-career burnout as few studies have looked at the origins and prevalence of burnout among different career stages of anesthesiologists.

- Many organizational resources are available to anesthesiologists in every stage of their career including, but not limited to, the Accreditation Council for Graduate Medical Education (ACGME) (https://dl.acgme.org/pages/well-being) and the American Society of Anesthesiologists (ASA) (https://www.asahq.org/advocating-for-you/well-being).

DISCLOSURE

C. Ward does not have any commercial or financial conflicts to disclose. L. Rothschild does not have any commercial or financial conflicts to disclose.

REFERENCES

1. Freudenberger HJ. The staff burn-out syndrome in alternative institutions. Psychotherapy: Theor Res Pract 1975;12(1):73–82.
2. Afonso AM, Cadwell JB, Staffa SJ, et al. Burnout rate and risk factors among anesthesiologists in the United States. Anesthesiology 2021;134(5):683–96.
3. Shanafelt TD, Boone S, Tan L, et al. Burnout and satisfaction with work-life balance among US physicians relative to the general US population. Arch Intern Med 2012;172(18):1377–85.
4. Monrouxe LV, Bullock A, Tseng HM, et al. Association of professional identity, gender, team understanding, anxiety and workplace learning alignment with burnout in junior doctors: a longitudinal cohort study. BMJ Open 2017;7(12): e017942.
5. Dyrbye LN, Varkey P, Boone SL, et al. Physician satisfaction and burnout at different career stages. Mayo Clin Proc 2013;88(12):1358–67.
6. Dyrbye LN, West CP, Satele D, et al. Burnout among U.S. medical students, residents, and early-career physicians relative to the general U.S. population. Acad Med 2014;89(3):443–51.
7. West CP, Tan AD, Habermann TM, et al. Association of resident fatigue and distress with perceived medical errors. JAMA 2009;302(12):1294–300.
8. Ratanawongsa N, Wright SM, Carrese JA. Well-being in residency: a time for temporary imbalance? Med Educ 2007;41(3):273–80.

9. Kearney MK, Weininger RB, Vachon ML, et al. Self-care of physicians caring for patients at the end of life: "being connected... a key to my survival. JAMA 2009; 301(11):1155–64. E1151.

10. Klimecki OM, Leiberg S, Ricard M, et al. Differential pattern of functional brain plasticity after compassion and empathy training. Soc Cogn Affect Neurosci 2014;9(6):873–9.

11. Singer T, Klimecki OM. Empathy and compassion. Curr Biol 2014;24(18):R875–8.

12. Neumann M, Edelhauser F, Tauschel D, et al. Empathy decline and its reasons: a systematic review of studies with medical students and residents. Acad Med 2011;86(8):996–1009.

13. Billings ME, Lazarus ME, Wenrich M, et al. The effect of the hidden curriculum on resident burnout and cynicism. J Grad Med Educ 2011;3(4):503–10.

14. Dyrbye LN, Thomas MR, Shanafelt TD. Medical student distress: causes, consequences, and proposed solutions. Mayo Clin Proc 2005;80(12):1613–22.

15. Dotters-Katz SK, Chuang A, Weil A, et al. Developing a pilot curriculum to foster humanism among graduate medical trainees. J Educ Health Promot 2018;7:2.

16. Eisenach JH, Sprung J, Clark MM, et al. The psychological and physiological effects of acute occupational stress in new anesthesiology residents: a pilot trial. Anesthesiology 2014;121(4):878–93.

17. Sun H, Warner DO, Macario A, et al. Repeated cross-sectional surveys of burnout, distress, and depression among anesthesiology residents and first-year graduates. Anesthesiology 2019;131(3):668–77.

18. Cho Y, Jeon Y, Jang SI, et al. Family members of cancer patients in Korea are at an increased risk of medically diagnosed depression. J Prev Med Public Health 2018;51(2):100–8.

19. Cordova MJ, Gimmler CE, Osterberg LG. Foster well-being throughout the career trajectory: a developmental model of physician resilience training. Mayo Clin Proc 2020;95(12):2719–33.

20. Hariharan TS, Griffin B. A review of the factors related to burnout at the early-career stage of medicine. Med Teach 2019;41(12):1380–91.

21. Lieff SJ. Perspective: the missing link in academic career planning and development: pursuit of meaningful and aligned work. Acad Med 2009;84(10):1383–8.

22. Frank E, Zhao Z, Sen S, et al. Gender disparities in work and parental status among early-career physicians. JAMA Netw Open 2019;2(8):e198340.

23. Starmer AJ, Frintner MP, Freed GL. Work-life balance, burnout, and satisfaction of early-career pediatricians. Pediatrics 2016;137(4).

24. Firdouse M, Chrystoja C, de Montbrun S, et al. Transition to independent surgical practice and burnout among early-career general surgeons. Surg Innov 2021. 15533506211039682.

25. Zhang JQ, Dong J, Pardo J, et al. Burnout and professional fulfillment in early and early-mid-career breast surgeons. Ann Surg Oncol 2021;28:6051–7.

26. Hall KN, Wakeman MA, Levy RC, et al. Factors associated with career longevity in residency-trained emergency physicians. Ann Emerg Med 1992;21(3):291–7.

27. Shin J, Kim YJ, Kim JK, et al. Probability of early retirement among emergency physicians. J Prev Med Public Health 2018;51(3):154–62.

Anesthesiology Residency and Relationship Health

A Psychological Approach

Jo M. Vogeli, PhD[a],*, Daniel Abraham, MD[b]

KEYWORDS

- Relationships • Residency training • Biopsychosocial model • Optimism bias
- Cognitive dissonance • Social comparison theory • Self-efficacy

KEY POINTS

- Anesthesia residency can take a significant toll on personal and professional relationships.
- There is an escalating focus on anesthesia training programs attempting to address burnout and well-being.
- Burgeoning research is demonstrating the benefit of fostering personal and professional relationships in avoiding burnout.
- This article takes a theory-based approach using total well-being and psychological concepts to gain an understanding of the influence of anesthesia residency on relationships.

INTRODUCTION

Humans have an intrinsic need for connection and belongingness on a physical and emotional level.[1] We are a social species and as such engaging with others promotes well-being and is protective against physiologic and psychological stressors. Social connectedness and personal relationships are key elements of the 3 domains of the biopsychosocial model of health. The biopsychosocial model was developed by psychiatrist George Engel, MD in 1977 in response to perceived shortcomings in the traditional biomedical model that only considers physical or physiologic factors of illness. The biopsychosocial clinical approach attends to biological factors in addition to psychological (eg, thoughts, emotions, behaviors) and social (eg, economic, environmental, and cultural) dimensions and the interconnectedness among the 3 domains to promote health.[2,3]

[a] Department of Anesthesiology Wellbeing Program, University of Colorado School of Medicine, Anschutz Medical Campus, 12631 East 17th Avenue, Mailstop 8202, Suite L15-2007, Aurora, CO 80045, USA; [b] Department of Anesthesiology and Critical Care, Perelman School of Medicine at the University of Pennsylvania, 3400 Spruce Street, 6 Dulles Building, Philadelphia, PA 19104, USA
* Corresponding author.
E-mail address: Jo.Vogeli@cuanschutz.edu

Anesthesiology Clin 40 (2022) 325–336
https://doi.org/10.1016/j.anclin.2022.01.006
1932-2275/22/Published by Elsevier Inc.

Building relationships and connecting to others, whether it be friendships, familial, or romantic partners, are key components of a healthy life. Individuals in committed relationships produce less cortisol when faced with psychological stressors.[4] In addition to benefiting from a physiologic stress buffer, we mirror the health behaviors of those around us. When we surround ourselves with healthy lifestyles, we too are more likely to eat healthy diets, engage in physical exercise, and are less likely to smoke.[5] Conversely, an imbalance in any component of our biopsychosocial makeup can result in lower levels of functioning in all areas. Ample research demonstrates that a strong social support system is known to improve both physical and mental health.[6–8] However, when the human requirement for connection, social companionship, and understanding are unavailable, a sense of thwarted belongingness arises. Thwarted belongingness has deleterious effects on mental health, and of primary concern, thwarted belongingness is one of the primary factors involved in suicidal ideation and behaviors.[9] Anesthesia training can be a stressful and profoundly lonely experience. The physical boundaries of an anesthesiologist's working environment—the sterile drape separating the singular anesthesiologist from the surgical team—coupled with long, unpredictable hours often spent alone can render significant mental and emotional strain. Further, it is not uncommon for the clinician to veer toward isolation after an unexpected or adverse perioperative event out of fear of professional litigation or critique from peers and colleagues.[10] This level of isolation is problematic, as satisfying the need for belongingness requires (1) frequent, positive interactions with the same individuals and (2) engaging in these interactions within a framework of long-term, stable care and concern.[1] Considering the timing of residency within the spectrum of adulthood and its potential to disrupt personal relationships, there is added concern for anesthesiology residents' immediate and long-term well-being. The benefits of relationships for health and well-being during residency are clear; conversely, a lack of support either at work or at home is linked to poor physical and emotional health.[11] As such, anesthesiology residents are uniquely positioned to significantly benefit from intact personal relationships and a sense of belonging, yet this basic human need can often be ignored or superseded by the demands and rigors of anesthesia training.

Personal relationships and a sense of belonging are essential elements of a meaningful life. A sense of purpose acts as a protective factor against stress and burnout on the job and promotes positive health as we age. The impact of this protective factor is even greater when strong relationships are developed early in adulthood.[12]

In recent years, much research has been done related to resident well-being and burnout during residency.[13–16] Although we have gained a better understanding of efficacious interventions, institutional changes, and resident education programming, the research seeking to understand the implications of residency on personal relationships is lacking. Preliminary research suggests that fostering professional and social relationships can reduce loneliness and levels of burnout both at work and at home.[17] Given that the mental health, physical wellness, and work performance of a physician are deeply entwined in the quality of interpersonal relationships, we closely examine the stressors of anesthesia residency and its potential harm to relationships through a biopsychosocial lens. Personal anecdotes are used, with permission from the individual, to illustrate 4 key cognitive processes: optimism bias, cognitive dissonance, social comparison, and self-efficacy. The authors would like to thank those who provided their personal experiences with relationships during their anesthesiology residency. All individuals asked for anonymity, and the authors respected that request.

OPTIMISM BIAS

I matched. It was a great day and a great year that followed. My [partner] and I were thrilled for our new adventure. We planned where we would go for date nights and get-aways on my days off. When moving day came, we packed up the car with all our be-longings and our dog. We took photos of our drive along the way for memories. I was two months into residency when I realized this was not the adventure we anticipated.

Humans are subject to many biases, and one of the more prominent biases relates to optimism. The optimism bias is holding a steadfast and often unrealistic belief that future events will be positive and stressors related to the future event will be less impactful than they are.[18] Research shows that the likelihood of an outcome has no effect, and when faced with equal probability of either a negative or positive outcome, individuals will almost always report that the positive outcome is more likely to occur.[19,20] This optimistic fallacy in thinking has evolutionary roots.[20] Optimism promotes motivation and prompts us to set goals and take preemptive steps to ensure a positive outcome.[21,22] This works well when the goal is likely to have a positive outcome or evidence shows that an experience is likely to be positive. However, when less favorable information is provided about a desired outcome, focalism, or the cognitive process of attending to positive information and viewing negative information as less salient, is often used.[23]

The loss of family and friends, our support—we missed it more than we anticipated. This was especially true for my [partner] who was home all day with the baby. It was so much more difficult than either of us expected.

Overall, the optimism bias sets us up for better outcomes. When we maintain a positive outlook, we have a greater sense of control. However, optimism bias can have adverse effects. When compared with counseling education for doctoral candidates and their spouses, physician residents and their spouses scored higher on shared marriage values but scored lower on realistic beliefs.[24] During residency, expectations about time, energy, and professional identity can be quickly defeated, and a lack of preparation along with unrealistic perceptions of manageable stress thresholds can cause discord in personal relationships.[25]

If I could have done one thing differently, I would have created a better support system around my [partner]. I would have invested in pre-emptive marriage counseling. Childcare is also a huge issue. It's so expensive and unreliable. I wish I had been more aware of all of this.

Having a more realistic understanding of the burdens of residency is important; encouraging residents and their partners to be aware of optimism bias may be helpful. Awareness that focalism shifts attention toward positive information and discounts less favorable information can create better communication patterns both before and during residency. An understanding of optimism bias can guide anesthesiology residency programs toward developing pragmatic initiatives geared toward preparing residents and their partners on what to expect before the start of CA1 year.

What can be done? Training programs can develop an anticipatory guidance program that taps into each biopsychosocial domain. Guidance could include information on where to live, childcare resources, how to eat healthy on a limited budget, and options for exercise/recreational activities in the area. Including "hindsight guidance" from current and recently graduated residents may provide further insight. Current and past residents can share their thoughts and experiences to help better prepare residents and partners. Pairing up residents with a current resident before they arrive can serve as a peer support system available throughout residency. Including options to pair up partners/spouses of current residents with incoming partners/spouses would provide an additional social support network. These are all options that would better prepare residents and their partners/spouses with realistic expectations and offer support to manage potential struggles throughout residency.

COGNITIVE DISSONANCE

Residency is challenging, with long hours and emotionally exhausting experiences. I had always leaned on my friendships to serve as a reservoir of happiness; our shared experiences would buoy me in times of stress. But I was finding that the seemingly endless time commitment of residency was changing me. I have always believed that my emotional responses kept me in tune with my own experiences and the world around me. But I suddenly worried I was losing that side of myself. Years of putting my career ahead of most things, including my friendships, caused me to turn to pragmatism and isolation in an effort to shield myself from disappointment and sadness.

Cognitive dissonance is a psychological process whereby an individual experiences distress due to incongruence between personal values and a competing external force.[26] Loss of autonomy, a divide in home life situation, exhaustion, and negative social comparison are driving forces for depression, anxiety, and burnout.[17] These factors are also known to create dissonance in one's identity.[27] Often, this cognitive dissonance can infiltrate and cause discontent in personal relationships. Interestingly, the stronger the personal relationship, the greater the dissonance. Individuals are more likely to feel safe expressing negative moods around those they trust the most despite the potential consequences this may have on a relationship.[28] Professional identity formation and the demands of residency training are pivotal factors that affect personal relationships. In previous research, residents reported that this transition in identity led them to believe they needed to place greater emphasis on professional expectations and subsequently deprioritize personal relationships.[29] Such shifts in relationship prioritization can create resentment for both the resident and those closest to them, leading residents to experience an internal struggle due to the misalignment of actions and personal values. This incongruence in work and home elicits higher levels of anxiety and burnout, and in turn, cognitive dissonance. For the individual to protect themselves from experiencing any negative emotion, shifting the blame to an intimate partner can be common, and residents can inadvertently damage their relationship due to cognitive dissonance.

Our relationship struggled. My [partner] told me I was one person at work and another at home. This perception that I was two different people (i.e., at work versus at home) was key. By the time I graduated, we were in a better place, but it did take time to understand how I had changed.

When residents prioritize their professional identity over personal relationships, this can create a phenomenon known as surface acting, which is closely related to cognitive dissonance.[30] Surface acting is amplifying the professional way one presents themselves on the job despite the individual's true emotional experience. An individual believes they cannot express thoughts and emotions or behave in a manner aligned with their true selves at work, and this misalignment creates a disingenuous experience for the individual. Surface acting leads to negative emotions and anxiety, and this high arousal state leads to a narrow mindset, undue critical thinking, avoidance, and has been identified as a predictor of marital discord.[30] Surface acting is not exclusive to individuals in medical residency; however, it may be more prevalent in this demographic. An essential component of surface acting is the suppression of emotion and belief that the expression of emotions is unprofessional and undesirable during residency is a common perception.[31] As such, residents may use surface acting as a form of self-regulation.

My [partner] is not in medicine and neither of us came from families in medicine so we didn't know what to expect during residency. I always felt guilty for how long I worked. When we had a child, my guilt increased.

A significant other's occupation can affect relationship dissonance during residency.

Relationship satisfaction during residency tends to be higher when both partners are physicians

or physician trainees. Variances in professional roles (eg, physician vs nonphysician) are associated with lower levels of marital satisfaction. Women resident physicians who are also mothers report lower levels of marital satisfaction regardless of their partner's role; this discontent is higher when the male partner is a nonphysician.[32–35] To manage the dissonance between personal and professional relationships, a resident may distance themselves from their closest relationships. When surveyed, residents shared that they prioritized relationships with those in medicine to help navigate opposing emotions they experienced in relationships with those outside of medicine.[29] The effort to resolve conflicting emotions may have immediate benefits but ultimately decreases an overall sense of social support, leaving the resident more prone to depression, anxiety, and other health-related problems.

The negative effects of cognitive dissonance and surface acting are bidirectional, causing counterintuitive behaviors at home and a reduction in work performance. Residency workload, scheduled hours, and educational demands may feel heightened, sleep becomes deprived, and mood spillover at home can occur. Negative mood spillover is known to result in withdrawal, avoidance, and antagonistic interactions with intimate partners characterized by greater expressions of criticism and disapproval, thereby threatening the supportive relationship.[36] Strife at home creates further emotional and physical exhaustion, leading to diminished physical and cognitive resources available at work. Dissonance also causes an emotional disturbance that can result in anxiety at work, known as professional dissonance.[37,38] Because of a heightened state of exhaustion and anxiety, a resident may conserve resources by reducing their work efforts to avoid a negative perception by peers, attendings, and leadership. This cycle can seem neverending for a resident, and a common thought for individuals caught in this cycle is to either end the marriage or leave their training position.[30,36] In other words, this discordance in thoughts, actions, and values can disrupt the very relationships that ideally fortify resident well-being and contribute to an optimal training experience.

What can be done? The best approach to mitigating cognitive dissonance is to focus on the values driving the dissonance. Values are guides we ascribe to accomplish goals; identifying how a value relates to long- and short-term goals is an important first step. There are a variety of empirically supported, value-directed writing exercises and activities that can help improve professional identity and resolve conflict between emotions and behaviors. Using the services of psychologists or wellness or well-being coaches within the department or the institution's well-being programs to implement these values-based training approaches would be most beneficial.

SOCIAL COMPARISON THEORY

It was mid-CA2 year when I realized I made a mistake. I should have gone into computer programming. My friends were all at home, in homes they owned, and making plans to go to the lake for the weekend. There was also the group trip to Europe that I had to say "no" to. I wanted their success and all I felt I had was my failure. I wanted out of medicine forever. Now my friends say they want my life, though I could not imagine that being the case during CA2 year.

Before residency, medical students typically experience success at the same level or often greater than peers. The ultimate goal as a medical student is successfully matching for residency. However, once an individual begins residency, a shift in identity can take place. [29,38] Anesthesiology residency is filled with evaluative methods, including social comparison. The social comparison theory was developed by psychologist Leon Festinger in 1954 and proposed that an individual is unable to accurately appraise one's own abilities and opinions without relying on a relational comparison to others.[39] The social comparison theory has since expanded beyond emphasis on abilities and opinions to include emotions, levels of satisfaction, and overall well-being. Self-evaluation, self-improvement, and self-enhancement are identified as the 3 drivers for social comparisons and deriving one's aspiration.[40] Individuals are in a constant state of self-evaluation, with approximately 10% of all thoughts involving some element of comparison (eg, intelligence, success, possessions, looks). These comparisons are used to determine information about oneself and establish self-worth and esteem.[41]

Residency was emotionally complicated as I was older than some of my attendings and at the same life stage as many junior faculty but with different expectations and financial situations.

There was a lot of delayed gratification, as we would always say that "once we are attendings, we can do x, y, z …."

Social comparison can be beneficial for motivation and positive change when individuals compare themselves with others to promote personal development and create a more positive self-image. However, the "who" you are comparing with is important for a positive outcome, and the definition of a peer is important in this regard. Social comparison is likely beneficial to most before anesthesiology residency. Finding similarities in general life directions, abilities, and financial standing among same-age peers is an easy task. However, when residency starts, other nonphysician, same-age peers may be graduating with advanced degrees, and likely buying a house, engaging in activities of choice on weekends, and going on vacations without extensive scheduling restrictions. In general, these same-age peers are experiencing an increase in independence, whereas residents are seeing more restrictions in their levels of autonomy. It is important to understand that social comparison is only appropriate and beneficial when comparing oneself with others currently in similar or attainable situations.[39] The residency training period creates a temporary imbalance in life situations between individuals that were once at an equal stage in life trajectory, and residents may have difficulty pivoting comparison away from those individuals.

The direction of comparison is an important component of the social comparison theory. We engage in either upward comparison (ie, someone whose life situation is perceived to be preferable) or downward comparison (ie, someone whose life situation is perceived to be less desirable). Upward social comparison is more common, as a goal of comparison is to elicit motivation.[39] Although upward comparison can be a strong driver for motivation, vast differences in abilities can reverse this effect. When upward comparison occurs with an unequal baseline, an individual is at risk of excluding those they are inappropriately comparing themselves with from their social network or they may seek to isolate themselves due to the defeating nature of the comparison.[42] This retreat from social support often leads to feelings of inferiority, negative emotions such as depression and anxiety, and regret for life choices despite the likelihood of a promising outcome.[43]

Regardless of obvious inequities in lifestyle, residents are prone to engage in upward social comparison with peers of the same age, increasing the risk for relationship problems, diminished social support, and doubting one's abilities and willingness to continue in the training program. This variance in biopsychosocial functioning can skew perceptions of future success due to a lack of motivation and belief in one's ability to overcome the hardships of residency training. *What can be done?* Because social comparison during anesthesiology residency often revolves around financial factors, independence, and life choices, incorporating programming related to these topics would be beneficial. Some residency programs offer presentations about career and financial trajectories for graduating senior residents. Inviting seasoned career anesthesiologists to discuss their experiences along with salary expectations and general differences between academic versus private practice would be beneficial. In addition, discussions about loan repayment options, insurance options (eg, health, life, disability), as well as other financial investment advice may also be helpful. These salient topics may yield a wealth of practical advice for residents as well as give them hope for their own future career and financial success. Having early and midcareer anesthesiologists present each year starting CA1 year could be more beneficial. In day-to-day interactions, residents can see that no one attending is destitute, but it can be difficult for the resident to see this for themselves because the negative social comparison to same-age peers skews realistic perception. Hearing multiple real-life anecdotes on a regular basis is the best way to assuage this misperception and reinforces the transience of residency. Residents can then begin to compare themselves on a more realistic level.

SELF-EFFICACY

In all my years of training, I never felt less competent as I did during my CA2 year. I was exhausted and felt like I lost the support of all my friends and family. Then I was involved in a medication error. Even though everyone tried to assure me they could have easily made the same mistake in the same situation, I had a difficult time accepting this. I didn't just question why I went into medicine, I questioned whether I had what it took to be an anesthesiologist.

In 1977, psychologist Albert Bandura coined the phrase self-efficacy, a well-researched concept based on insight and perceived control. Self-efficacy involves an individual's perception of their abilities and skills to succeed in a future-oriented situation.[44] Perception is a key component of self-efficacy, and stressful situations can skew an individual's realistic perception of abilities and skills. Self-efficacy is influenced by mastery experiences, past experiences of success, vicarious experiences, making comparisons by observing others' success, social persuasion, receiving feedback from others regarding one's potential, and current emotional states. Higher levels of self-efficacy are related to health and well-being benefits including increased resilience, healthy lifestyle habits, greater educational achievement, and higher levels of satisfaction in relationships.[45]

Vicarious experience occurs when one observes others close to them successfully achieving a goal. This success translates to a thought and perception that the observer may also have the cognitive or physical resources to achieve a similar goal. For example, an individual's siblings and friends graduate from college, thus reinforcing the individual's belief that they could also graduate from college. The more similar a current life situation is, the more likely one interprets the success of others as personal capability, thereby increasing self-efficacy. A decline in self-efficacy may occur for residents involved in intimate partner relationships.[46] One possible explanation for this decline connects vicarious experiences with the social comparison theory. Typical goal achievement for their stage in life (eg, owning a house, travel, financial stability) may currently be unattainable. Vicarious experience for goal achievement feels subpar, and a resident may begin to question their ability to achieve desired goals.

During my first months as an early-career attending, a colleague approached me with concern regarding the amount of call shifts I was volunteering for. I couldn't help myself. I felt like I would never catch up on my medical school debt and couldn't get over the feeling that I had ruined my [partner's] life.

Guilt and shame can affect self-efficacy. Residents may experience heightened levels of self-blame and embarrassment due to seemingly insurmountable student loan debt relative to their training-level income, as it may be inadequate to support household needs. Work schedules and demands can also exacerbate the disparity in the division of household responsibilities, including childcare; this can worsen feelings of guilt and shame, particularly for residents who are parents.[47]

My partner started to resent me, and, in turn, I resented [them] for resenting me.

Self-efficacy is influenced by both encouragement and discouragement pertaining to an individual's performance or ability to perform.[48] Residents may shift their primary source of positive encouragement to the training program, where continually exceeding expectations is rewarded.[49] This shift leaves little room for intrinsic reward and can conflict with home life expectations, causing negative reinforcement and discouragement in personal relationships. Guilt, shame, and an imbalance in household responsibilities can perpetuate negativity and resentment in the relationship. In turn, residents may question their ability to succeed in relationships, at work, or both. This lowered level of self-efficacy can lead to lower levels of perceived control, depression, anxiety, and eventual burnout, and these emotional states can continue to suppress levels of self-efficacy.[36,45] Such disruption in emotional states and relationship health creates significant imbalance in all biopsychosocial domains. *What can be done?* When attendings and leadership humanize themselves, this gives the resident permission to acknowledge their own vulnerability. Good Grief Rounds is an evidence-based program in which storytelling is used to share experiences related to difficult patient cases. Attendings share a difficult case and how they processed the experience. Residents are invited to share their own difficult case experiences in small groups or pairs. Good Grief Rounds participants report an increased sense of community and greater meaning in their work.[50] Another similar example is Confession Sessions, attending-facilitated meetings where the residents anonymously share events, mistakes, or concerns on type-written pieces of paper and discussions ensue related to the statements. Confession Sessions are an opportunity for residents to safely gain feedback on errors and for attendings to demonstrate compassion for errors.[51]

These programs are cost-efficient and easy to implement. Incorporating Good Grief Rounds, Confession Sessions, Peer-to-Peer support, or similar programming brings humanness to medicine, and residents learn to be less critical of themselves. The openness and vulnerability embodied in these programs allows the resident to understand they can experience difficult emotions and continue to be well-qualified professionals. These types of programs also help residents process difficult emotions in a growth manner. Emotion-focused programs promote an increase in self-efficacy and in turn help to protect personal and professional relationships from the negative effects of lower levels of self-efficacy.

SUMMARY

All relationships, whether friendships, familial, or romantic, will be affected in some way during the residency training period. Given the importance of social connectedness and relationships for overall health and well-being, it is insufficient to simply sustain relationships. Anesthesiology residency programs need to invest in well-being initiatives that promote thriving in all aspects of a trainee's life, including relationships; this can be achieved with pragmatic measures before residency begins as well as thoughtful, supportive programming throughout training. Relationships encompass each domain of the biopsychosocial model and provide residents with life-long coping skills and improved well-being. Perhaps most importantly for training programs, strong personal and professional relationships shape a "well resident" who can thrive in their learning environment and more fully contribute to the mission and culture of the department.

By taking an approach to understand psychological processes that affect relationships, work performance, and well-being, a deeper level of understanding occurs beyond that of simply understanding anxiety, depression, and burnout as negative and unwanted mood experiences. Understanding the cognitive and psychological underpinnings is an essential move toward recognizing the all-encompassing biopsychosocial impact of medical residency on personal relationships, particularly the unique aspects of anesthesiology residency. The physiologic impact of stress does not work alone, and thought processes, moods, and social and environmental factors influence each other and can work as a protective factor against deleterious effects of stress. To prevent unfavorable crossover in biopsychosocial factors, program leadership and the residents have an opportunity to mitigate disruption in personal and professional relationships, gain a better sense of control for both expected and unexpected stressors during residency, and create an optimal training experience for all.

CLINICS CARE POINTS

- Personal relationships are an essential element of physical, emotional, and social health.
- Anesthesiology residency poses unique barriers to fostering the health of personal relationships, and this can affect professional relationships and engagement in the optimal training experience.
- Anesthesiology resident training programs would benefit from including preemptive and ongoing strategies that include a focus on relationship health as part of well-being initiatives.
- Understanding the psychological underpinnings of personal experience and relationship health provides a good foundation for well-being program development.
- Gaining an understanding of psychological concepts that influence personal and professional relationship health can aid leadership to feel better prepared to address the issue of potential pitfalls in relationships during anesthesiology residency.

DISCLOSURE

The authors have nothing to disclose.

REFERENCES

1. Baumeister RF, Leary MR. The need to belong: desire for interpersonal attachments as a fundamental human motivation. Psychol Bull 1995;117(3):497–529.
2. Engel GL. The need for a new medical model: a challenge for biomedicine. Science 1977;196(4286):129–36.
3. Borell-Carrió F, Suchman AL, Epstein RM. The biopsychosocial model 25 years later: principles, practice, and scientific inquiry. Ann Fam Med 2004;2(6):576–82.
4. Maestripieri D, Klimczuk ACE, Seneczko M, et al. Relationship status and relationship instability, but not dominance, predict individual differences in baseline cortisol levels. PLoS one 2013;8(12):e84003.

5. Mozaffarian D, Afshin A, Popkin BM, et al. Population approaches to improve diet, physical activity, and smoking habits: a scientific statement from the American Heart Association. Circulation 2012;126(12):1514–63.

6. Myers DG. The funds, friends, and faith of happy people. Am Psychol 2000;55(1): 56–67.

7. Amati V, Meggiolaro S, Rivellini G, et al. Social relations and life satisfaction: the role of friends. Genus 2018;74(1). https://doi.org/10.1186/s41118-018-0032-z.

8. Wang J, Mann F, Lloyd-Evans B, et al. Associations between loneliness and perceived social support and outcomes of mental health problems: A systematic review. BMC Psychiatry 2018;18(1). https://doi.org/10.1186/s12888-018-1736-5.

9. Chu C, Buchman-Schmitt JM, Stanley IH, et al. The interpersonal theory of suicide: a systematic review and meta-analysis of a decade of cross-national research. Psychol Bull 2017;143(12):1313–45.

10. Bachiller PR, Vinson AE. One is the loneliest number: social isolation as an occupational hazard of anesthesiology. ASA Monitor 2019;83(12):12–5.

11. Masi CM, Chen HY, Hawkley LC, et al. A meta-analysis of interventions to reduce loneliness. Personal Social Psychol Rev 2011;15(3):219–66.

12. Hill PL, Turiano NA. Purpose in life as a predictor of mortality across adulthood. Psychol Sci 2014;25(7):1482–6.

13. Raj KS. Well-being in residency: a systematic review. J Grad Med Educ 2016; 8(5):674–84.

14. West CP, Dyrbye LN, Shanafelt TD. Physician burnout: contributors, consequences and solutions. J Intern Med 2018;283(6):516–29.

15. Janosy NR, Beacham A, Vogeli J, et al. Well-being curriculum for anesthesiology residents: development, processes, and preliminary outcomes. Pediatr Anesth 2021;31(1):103–11.

16. Thornton KC, Sinskey JL, Boscardin CK, et al. Design and implementation of an innovative, longitudinal wellness curriculum in an anesthesiology residency program. A&A Pract 2021;15(2):e01387.

17. Rogers E, Polonijo AN, Carpiano RM. Getting by with a little help from friends and colleagues: Testing how residents' social support networks affect loneliness and burnout. Can Fam Physician 2016;62(11):e677–83.

18. Sharot T. The optimism bias. Curr Biol 2011;21(23). https://doi.org/10.1016/j.cub. 2011.10.030.

19. Lench HC, Smallman R, Darbor KE, et al. Motivated perception of probabilistic information. Cognition 2014;133(2):429–42.

20. Haselton MG, Nettle D. The paranoid optimist: an integrative evolutionary model of cognitive biases. Personal Social Psychol Rev 2006;10(1):47–66.

21. Lench HC, Levine LJ, Dang V, et al. Optimistic expectations have benefits for effort and emotion with little cost. Emotion 2021;21(6):1213–23.

22. Lench HC, Ditto PH. Automatic optimism: biased use of base rate information for positive and negative events. J Exp Social Psychol 2008;44(3):631–9.

23. Kruger J, Burrus J. Egocentrism and focalism in unrealistic optimism (and pessimism). J Exp Social Psychol 2004;40(3):332–40.

24. Powers AS, Myers JE, Tingle LR, et al. Wellness, perceived stress, mattering, and marital satisfaction among medical residents and their spouses: implications for education and counseling. Fam J 2004;12(1):26–36.

25. McNulty JK, Karney BR. Expectancy confirmation in appraisals of marital interactions. Personal Social Psychol Bull 2002;28(6):764–75.

26. Festinger L. Cognitive dissonance. Scientific Am 1962;207(4):93–106.

27. Aronson E. The theory of cognitive dissonance: a current perspective. In: Berkowitz L, editor. Advances in experimental social psychology, vol. 4. New York: Academic Press; 1969. p. 1–34.
28. McNulty JK. Should spouses be demanding less from marriage? A contextual perspective on the implications of interpersonal standards. Personal Social Psychol Bull 2016;42(4):444–57.
29. Law M, Lam M, Wu D, et al. Changes in personal relationships during residency and their effects on resident wellness: A qualitative study. Acad Med 2017;92(11): 1601–6.
30. Krannitz MA, Grandey AA, Liu S, et al. Workplace surface acting and marital partner discontent: Anxiety and exhaustion spillover mechanisms. J Occup Health Psychol 2015;20(3):314–25.
31. Martín-Brufau R, Martin-Gorgojo A, Suso-Ribera C, et al. Emotion regulation strategies, workload conditions, and burnout in healthcare residents. Int J Environ Res Public Health 2020;17(21):1–12.
32. Jovanovic A, Wallace JE. Lean on me: an exploratory study of the spousal support received by physicians. Psychol Health Med 2013;18(5):543–51.
33. Dyrbye LN, Shanafelt TD, Balch CM, et al. Physicians married or partnered to physicians: a comparative study in the American College of Surgeons. J Am Coll Surg 2010;211(5):663–71.
34. Sobecks NW, Justice AC, Landefeld CS, et al. When doctors marry doctors: a survey exploring the professional and family lives of young physicians. Ann Intern Med 1999;130(4 Part 1):312–9.
35. Warde CM, Moonesinghe K, Allen W, et al. Marital and parental satisfaction of married physicians with children. J Gen Intern Med 1999;14(3):157–65.
36. Pluut H, Ilies R, Su R, et al. How social stressors at work influence marital behaviors at home: an interpersonal model of work–family spillover. J Occup Health Psychol 2021. https://doi.org/10.1037/ocp0000298.
37. Agarwal SD, Pabo E, Rozenblum R, et al. Professional dissonance and burnout in primary care: a qualitative study. JAMA Intern Med 2020;180(3):395–401.
38. Chang LY, Eliasz KL, Cacciatore DT, et al. The transition from medical student to resident: A qualitative study of new residents' perspectives. Acad Med 2020; 95(9):1421–7.
39. Festinger L. A theory of social comparison processes. Hum Relations 1954;7(2): 117–40.
40. Gibbons F, Buunk B. Individual differences in social comparison: Development of a scale of social comparison orientation. J Pers Soc Psychol 1999;76(1):129–42.
41. Gerber JP, Wheeler L, Suls J. A social comparison theory meta-analysis 60+ years on. Psychol Bull 2018;144(2):177–97.
42. van de Ven N. Envy and admiration: emotion and motivation following upward social comparison. Cogn Emot 2017;31(1):193–200.
43. Fang J, Huang X, Zhang M, et al. The big-fish-little-pond effect on academic self-concept: a meta-analysis. Front Psychol 2018;9:1569.
44. Bandura A. Self-efficacy: Toward a unifying theory of behavioral change. Psychol Rev 1977;84(2):191–215.
45. Shoji K, Cieslak R, Smoktunowicz E, et al. Associations between job burnout and self-efficacy: a meta-analysis. Anxiety, Stress and Coping 2016;29(4):367–86.
46. Milam LA, Cohen GL, Mueller C, et al. The relationship between self-efficacy and well-being among surgical residents. J Surg Education 2019;76(2):321–8.
47. Walsh A, Gold M, Jensen P, et al. Motherhood during residency training: challenges and strategies. Can Fam Physician 2005;51(7):990–1.

48. Bandura A. Self-efficacy mechanism in human agency. Am Psychol 1982;37(2): 122–47.
49. Sotile WM, Sotile MO. The medical marriage: Sustaining healthy relationships for physicians and their families. Revised edition. Chicago: American Medical Association Press; 2000.
50. Morrison K, Rondinelli N, Jensen W, et al. Palliative care team does good! good grief rounds facilitated across disciplines in an academic hospital improves factors shown to alleviate burnout. J Pain Symptom Manage 2020;59(2):542–3.
51. Karan SB, Berger JS, Wajda M. Confessions of physicians: what systemic reporting does not uncover. J Graduate Med Education 2015;7(4):528–30.

Physician Coaching

Laura K. Berenstain, MD, FASA, ACC[a],*, Scott D. Markowitz, MD[b,c],
Stephanie I. Byerly, MD[d]

KEYWORDS

- Coaching • Leadership • Professional Development • Well-being
- Positive psychology

KEY POINTS

- Coaching differs from mentoring or sponsorship by its emphasis on mindset and future growth and potential, as well as by viewing the individual as a whole person.
- Coaching may be conducted on an individual, group, or team basis.
- Coaching can facilitate the acquisition of important leadership skills including emotional intelligence, adaptability, conflict management, and negotiation that are often not taught in training environments.
- Coaching has been shown to enhance performance, efficacy, and well-being for physicians.
- Coaching skills and techniques can be learned and used as a part of a leadership style.

The more the world around us is in flux the more we as individuals must be certain about what matters in our lives: how we spend our time, who we are connected to, and where we are going. A coach is someone who can evoke passion and purpose in others, within the dissolving and reconstituting environments of our times.
— -Frederic Hudson, 1995

INTRODUCTION

The practice of anesthesiology requires comprehensive medical knowledge, a robust clinical skill set, and the ability to navigate complex social situations on a daily basis. While medical school and residency training serve as preparation for the first two, training in emotional intelligence, conflict management, negotiation skills, and leadership is often deficient or nonexistent. Additionally, professional development is not always adequately emphasized, resulting in a lack of professional fulfillment for many

[a] Cincinnati Children's Hospital Medical Center, Cincinnati, OH, USA; [b] Washington University School of Medicine in St. Louis, St. Louis, MO, USA; [c] Department of Anesthesiology, Washington University School of Medicine, Campus Box 8054, 660t South Euclid Avenue, St. Louis, MO, USA; [d] Department of Anesthesiology and Pain Management, University of Texas Southwestern, 5323 Harry Hines Boulevard, Dallas, TX 75390, USA
* Corresponding author. 7255 Beech Road, Ambler, PA 19002.
E-mail address: lberenstainmd@gmail.com

Anesthesiology Clin 40 (2022) 337–348
https://doi.org/10.1016/j.anclin.2022.01.007
1932-2275/22/© 2022 Elsevier Inc. All rights reserved.
anesthesiology.theclinics.com

physicians along with inequities in promotion and leadership opportunities for women and underrepresented minorities.[1–3] In addition to the challenges inherent in being a physician, life itself presents changes and transitions that necessitate continual self-assessment, renewal, and learning.

Coaching has been successfully used for both personal and leadership development in the business world for several decades, and now a growing body of evidence is demonstrating its applicability in medicine.[4–6] The International Coaching Federation (ICF) defines coaching as "partnering with a client in a thought-provoking and creative process that inspires the client to maximize their personal and professional potential."[7] Modern coaching began with the partnership of Sir John Whitmore and Timothy Gallwey, Harvard educator and the author of *The Inner Game of Tennis*. As a tennis coach, Gallwey recognized the impact of internal dialogue and negative thinking on performance and learning.[8] While earlier coaching theories developed from psychology and adult learning and development theories, positive psychology, mindfulness, and neuroscience are now increasingly important influences.

> When I decided to become certified as a life coach, my goal was to work with women physicians who were experiencing struggles in life with resultant burnout. I was raised by a single mother who had severe mental illness and I experienced many types of abuse and traumatic experiences as a child. As a result, I made the conscious decision as a young adult that my adult life would be very different from my childhood. From an early age I said I was going to be a doctor, believing that somehow, I could create a perfect life. I married another physician, but after the marriage ended in divorce, I found myself a single parent with primary financial responsibility. The combined responsibilities of full-time parenthood and a career as a full-time academic anesthesiologist led, over years, to burnout. At that time burnout was not openly discussed, and I often wondered if I could keep working as an anesthesiologist for several more decades.
>
> An event in my life about 4 years ago forced me to work on the traumas I had suffered as a child and adult. The work proved transformational, helping me understand how these traumas had impacted my decision-making. The desire to help other women physicians who were suffering led me to coaching school. Coaching school helped me realize that despite my personal growth work and progress there was more work to do, and different tools to use. The tools I learned have subsequently transformed every conversation, situation, and relationship in my personal and professional life.

HOW IS COACHING DIFFERENT? (BOX 1)

Coaching is a unique process that has the potential to fill existing deficiencies for anesthesiologists at the intersection of personal and professional well-being and career development. Through a process involving inquiry, increased self-awareness, reflection, and discovery, it can facilitate growth for individuals, groups, and teams. Rather

---

Box 1
Coaching principles

- Coaching is future and goal-oriented
- Coach and client are equal partners
- The coachee is a "whole" person and does not require fixing
- Clients are resourceful and able to create their own solutions
- Agenda and goals for each session are set by the coachee
- Skilled questions allow the client to discard assumptions and limiting beliefs

than dispensing advice, a coach listens intently, explores with the client (or "coachee"), and asks questions meant to spark insight and facilitate growth. Most importantly, coaching allows the coachee to identify and discard limiting beliefs or assumptions that are often holding them back, allowing them to initiate desired changes and shift their mindset. Coaching can be especially powerful for physicians who suffer from impostor syndrome. Coaching often results in a renewed sense of hope, optimism, and empowerment in the coachee, furthering personal and professional development. Interestingly, the act of coaching can also produce similar beneficial outcomes for the coach, demonstrating the effectiveness of compassion and empathy for others as a self-help tool.

Mentorship and sponsorship have been the most used professional development tools for physicians. Although peer mentoring is gaining traction, traditional mentoring relationships typically involve a more experienced practitioner—usually within the same field—offering guidance to a less experienced individual who is seeking advancement or achievement of a specific goal. Advice is dispensed regarding specific topics or needs, with the mentor acting as a content expert or facilitator: the mentor leads, and the mentee "follows." Sponsorship occurs when a more senior or influential individual creates or supports an opportunity for a junior colleague, personally vouching for them and promoting their career. To differentiate sponsorship from professional coaching, a protégé will receive introductions or opportunities at the behest of the sponsor, while a coachee will determine if and how they will seek introductions and identify opportunities beyond the coaching conversation. (**Fig. 1**).

Coaching also differs from therapy or counseling, although they both offer confidential, supportive, and nonjudgmental relationships that ultimately strive to enable clients to improve or enhance their life experiences. Therapy or counseling is often a long-term process in which a client works with a licensed therapist or counselor who aids in resolving personal or psychological challenges, and clients seeking therapy or counseling are more likely to be persistently distressed than those seeking coaching. Coaching and counseling/therapy are very distinct professions, and it is not uncommon for individuals to have both a therapist and a coach. Coaching is more often a time-limited process of 6 months to a year with a professional who is usually not a licensed health care professional. Perhaps the most important distinction is that in coaching the client is assumed to be "whole," and they can identify and create

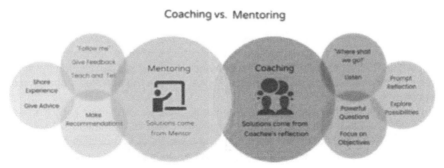

Fig. 1. Distinguishing coaching and mentoring. Mentoring is an established paradigm in medicine. The application of coaching skills, which are distinct from mentoring, can also significantly advance the field of anesthesiology. (*From Schwartz et al, Coaching for the Pediatric Anesthesiologist: Becoming our best selves. Pediatric Anesthesia 2021;31:85*)

their own solutions with the assistance of the coach. Unlike therapy, which explores past experiences, coaching is intrinsically future- and goal-oriented.

While mentorship, sponsorship, training, and coaching are all valuable professional development tools, only coaching views all aspects of the coachee's life and creates space for the exploration of both personal and professional aspirations. Coaching is also a partnership of equals whereby the coachee is regarded as resourceful and able to solve their own problems; they do not need to be "fixed." In many coaching relationships, the coach is not a content expert in the coachee's field. Coaching provides a unique opportunity to focus on the client's strengths, resourcefulness, and the creation of solutions rather than the analysis of problems.

Benefits of coaching

Broadly speaking, coaching can be effective for developing new skills and performance, enhancing personal and professional development, and increasing efficacy with shifts in mindset or worldview. For many physicians, the elements of perfectionism and impostor syndrome become a fixed mindset that leaves them dissatisfied with their trajectory. Others may increase their leadership potential by improving self-awareness, emotional intelligence, and communication skills. Learning to discard limiting beliefs and acquiring new skill sets often leads to an increased sense of hope and empowerment, improving life and career satisfaction, as well as overall well-being. Several studies have shown the benefits of coaching in reducing elements of burnout in physicians and increasing well-being.[5,6]

Responsibilities of the coach and client

During training to become a coach reference is frequently made to "use of self" as an instrument. This phrase means that it is the responsibility of the coach to continue their own self-growth, cultivating self-awareness, empathy, and emotional intelligence to be maximally effective for their clients. The client's responsibility is to be "coachable"; in other words, to seek and be open to change. Coaching may not be a good fit for those who are unwilling to receive feedback or consider change.[9]

Coaching skills–the "coach-approach"

Two crucial elements for success in a coaching relationship are trust and the quality of the coaching. In evaluating the success of coaching relationships, the most important factor has been shown to be the quality of the relationship between coach and coachee.[10] Mutual trust creates psychological safety for the coachee, enabling them to share freely and think aloud during coaching sessions. Adherence to ethical guidelines such as those established by the ICF is essential for the maintenance of this trust.[11] The coaching relationship is further strengthened by the coach's provision of confidentiality, nonjudgment, and acceptance. At times this can include the willingness of the coach to remain in the engagement despite the coachee's challenges or occasional discomfort.

Successful coaches also use evidence-based principles and there is no single universally accepted coaching method; multiple theoretic frameworks have been described. A skillful coach will often combine a variety of approaches best suited to the individual client's needs. However, coaching principles universally include relationship and trust-building, listening, asking powerful questions, challenging assumptions, and being nonjudgmental and nondirective. It is essential that the coach retains the ability to be highly self-aware and respect the values, viewpoints, and perspectives of their clients.

The creation of *a **trusting and confidential relationship between equals*** is a defining characteristic of coaching. Beyond coaching skills and process, the coach is often trained in leadership and communication competencies. Excellent interpersonal and listening skills serve a coach well in fostering a trusting relationship with the coachee. This trust helps the coachee share challenging elements of their life situation or goals which they may not have previously revealed to others. Expressing vulnerability is difficult for many physicians and speaking one's mind can potentially have negative consequences in other venues, hence trust and confidentiality are paramount. As the coachee becomes more open in conversation, the coach can challenge the coachee's limiting beliefs or assumptions, thus creating the opportunity for deeper and more meaningful insights. The presence of a supportive and confidential coaching relationship has been shown to positively affect stress and anxiety for coachees.[12]

One of the key skills in a coach's repertoire is ***active listening***. Coaches learn and practice this skill in formal training. Intent and effective listening enable a coach to detect in tone, cadence, facial expression, and body language the full message conveyed by the coachee. Often a coach will note a change in facial expression or body position that belies the words being spoken. Recognizing a coachee's commitment or discomfort within the conversation, the coach may then ask clarifying questions or challenge assumptions. Effective listening also enables a coach to "read between the lines," often leading to an "Aha!" moment for the coachee. To ensure clarity and facilitate understanding, coaches often paraphrase or summarize what the client has just said. Paraphrasing also allows the client to mirror, or hear themselves, offering validation and the opportunity for reflection. Lastly, the act of intentional and compassionate listening is in itself valuable to the coachee, validating their efforts and acknowledging the challenges that they face.

Coaching skills include ***asking "powerful" or thought-provoking questions.*** These are used to allow the coachee to clarify their thoughts or to challenge assumptions or mindset. They can also help a coachee understand the considerations in their present challenges and select a path toward a future goal. Powerful questions can prompt insights into values and priorities which may have remained hidden behind a complicated series of assumptions. For this reason, coaching questions generally begin with "What" or "How," as opposed to "Why?" In formulating a question, the coach remains nonjudgmental regarding any answer, and to what, if any, insight is needed for the coachee to move forward. An open-ended question can help a coachee discover a previously unforeseen path or conclusion, whereas a leading question could unintentionally influence the coachee, thereby reducing autonomy and the opportunity to create empowerment.

A skilled coach helps increase self-awareness for clients, encouraging goal setting and accountability. Potential becomes unlimited, rather than constrained. Over time, limiting beliefs are examined and left behind. Clients see from a new perspective and become aware of new ways of meeting challenges or overcoming obstacles. This can often take the form of thinking aloud to restructure ideas. The client can determine who they would like to be and how that "way of being" opens possibilities for ongoing learning and forward motion. The end of a coaching session often includes an invitation for the client to summarize what he has learned about himself, along with the next steps for action. **Box 1**

TYPES OF COACHING

Several coaching subcategories exist, all of which share the fundamentals of a coach approach. They differ mainly in the nature of the interpersonal relationship or coaching focus. Although coaching has been used in the past for remediation or to address disruptive or unprofessional behavior, it is now most frequently used to maximize career development and potential. From an organizational perspective, coaching may be provided by either internal coaches, used by the organization, or external coaches serving as consultants. When a coach is used directly by an organization the coaching goals may be performance-oriented or emphasize skill acquisition and often serve the organization as well as the client. The coach is, in effect, working for 2 parties. Many physicians or trainees may choose to use a personal coach outside their institution as well.[13]

Coaching for medical students and residents is being used by some academic departments and medical schools to foster the development of professional identity and specific skillsets.[4] Academic centers using coaching as part of their curriculum or professional development may have either professionally trained coaches and/or department or faculty members who have received specialized training in coaching techniques. For physicians, **peer coaching** generally implies being coached by someone who is also a physician; the coach may have formal training as a professional coach or informal training in coaching techniques. Evidence exists that physicians prefer being coached by physicians, and programs using peer coaching for physicians have been effective at improving physician retention.[14,15]

Individual or one-on-one coaching occurs between a coach and a single coachee. A one-on-one relationship enables the work of coaching to specifically address the unique personal and professional challenges of the coachee, enabling more confidential discussions. Although most coaching has traditionally been conducted in person, virtual sessions or "e-coaching" have been increasingly used due to growing interest in coaching, the global nature of business, and the COVID-19 pandemic. Roughly half of all coaching relationships are now conducted virtually.[16] Coaching sessions may also be conducted by telephone without a visual component, as many experienced coaches believe this facilitates improved listening and detection of voice inflection. In a review of 17 workplace coaching studies, the coaching modality (eg, face-to-face or e-coaching) did not impact the efficacy of coaching.[17]

Team and group coaching serve multiple clients simultaneously. Specific training courses exist for coaches who wish to develop expertise in facilitating team or group coaching. **Team coaching** focuses on creating high-functioning teams or working with existing teams to maximize performance or incorporate change. Goals can include fostering a collective growth mindset, managing team conflict, or decreasing organizational resistance to change. **Group coaching** involves small groups of like-minded individuals with an identified common interest, such as women leaders exploring work–life balance. Group coaching may also provide a more affordable price point for organizations and individuals.

Executive coaching is one of the best-known and longest established branches of coaching. It is defined as "a helping relationship between a client with supervisory authority or responsibility in an organization and a coach, helping the client achieve a mutually defined set of goals with the aim of improving professional performance, well-being, and effectiveness of the organization."[18] Some knowledge of, or experience with, organizational behavior is often useful for executive coaches. Executive coaching clients are often leaders in complex, competitive environments who may lack a touchstone for brainstorming or expanding their perspectives. Executive coaches who are external to the organization offer the benefit of unbiased support to the client as the coach does not have a vested interest in the business or organization. Executive coaches often work with teams as well as individuals. A standard engagement may last 6 months to a year to engender lasting changes in performance and mindset. Examples of common goals in executive coaching relationships include ensuring smooth transitions, managing a new position, navigating complex relationships, and development of "stretch" goals.

Leadership coaching involves managers and team leaders and can be considered a subset of executive coaching. In the corporate environment, leadership coaches are often employees of the organization or business for which they are coaching. Increasingly, business leaders are being encouraged to develop a "coaching approach" as part of their own leadership style to encourage self-confidence and resourcefulness in those who report to them. Leadership development is now recognized as important at all organizational levels. In medicine, leadership coaching can guide preparation for academic promotion, transition to a new role, or leadership within a private practice by developing skill sets including negotiation, conflict management, and emotional intelligence.

My coaching story begins with transitions. I was transitioning from being a junior faculty member to a recruited expert; from being an excellent follower to a novice leader; and from a hospital in one region of the United States to one in a different geographic region. I felt pressure to prove myself worthy of being recruited, but it was not going well. Although I was doing everything I had been taught, I was now receiving messages of nonsuccess. Recognizing my struggles as a hindrance to reaching my potential in the new environment, I engaged a coach and began the hard work of change.

It would be years later before I decided to become a coach myself, in part due to my growing awareness of my colleagues' suffering. With the help of my coach, I found my own path through the feelings of inefficacy and the false security of depersonalization. I wanted to facilitate such change for others. During my training, I learned that what my coach had conducted was not magic, but instead, a combination of science and art.

Life coaches work with clients to attain greater fulfillment in all aspects of their personal and professional lives by enhancing hope, well-being, and resilience. They assist clients in identifying goals, the obstacles preventing them from achieving these goals, and strategies for overcoming these obstacles. Life coaching can take place individually or in group settings, allowing members to energize each other and benefit from collective learning and experiences. Characteristic topics in life coaching include personal insights and self-reflection, identification of negative thought patterns and limiting beliefs, reframing of past experiences with the intent to reshape the present and future, enhancement of well-being and self-esteem, mitigating procrastination, and enhancing motivation. Life coaches can be general coaches that work with clients in every area of their lives, or they may have specific niches such as career management, relationships, diet or fitness, addiction, sports, or financial management. Life coaching can also be used to enhance diversity initiatives, with a focus on awareness and inclusion, generational differences, and cross-cultural styles.

COACHING IN THE WORKPLACE

Medical leadership traditionally has been hierarchal, but leadership styles are gradually shifting to a more distributive approach, with everyone perceived as a potential leader and contributor. The development and use of coaching skills in the workplace can promote this evolution. (**Box 2**). In "A Blueprint for Organizational

> **Box 2**
> **Useful workplace coaching techniques**
>
> *BE CURIOUS and NONJUDGMENTAL*
> - Ask "what" or "how" questions
> - Avoid questions with "yes" or "no" answers
> - Explore potential options
>
> *LISTEN DEEPLY and SUMMARIZE OFTEN*
> - Listen for tone
> - Watch body language
>
> *BE WILLING TO EXPLORE*
> - "What else is possible?"
> - "What if there were no obstacles?"
>
> *THINK POSITIVELY*
> - Assume success
> - The past is less important than the future

Strategies to Promote the Well-being of Health Care Professionals," Shanafelt and colleagues[19] advocate for coaching in the clinical workplace as a fundamental component of leadership development and healthcare worker well-being programming. Learning to ask open-ended questions and practicing active listening as a leader helps people feel valued and contributes to increased employee engagement. The use of coaching techniques and models can be used to strengthen leadership styles and daily workplace interactions, even for those without formal coaching training.

A basic coaching model and useful framework for restructuring conversations and encouraging active listening is the "GROW" model developed by Whitmore.[20]

- **G: Goal. Establish a goal for a particular interaction**. At the outset of the conversation, a typical question might be "What would you like to come away with after this conversation?"
- **R: Reality**. Ask questions to encourage the speaker to focus on specific facts, or the "What" and "How." Questions beginning with "Why" should be avoided due to the tendency to evoke self-justification or defensiveness. Questions might include "What are the key things that we need to know?" or "What really matters here?" Listen carefully for the response and summarize if necessary to ensure understanding.
- **O: Options**. Encourage broad thinking. Questions such as "If there were no obstacles, what would you do?" and "If you had a magic wand, what would you do?" allow the speaker to conceptualize new ideas and potential solutions.
- **W: Will**. "Will" can be used in several ways. "What will you do next?" yields action steps. "On a scale of 1 to 10, how likely is it that you will do this?" helps the speaker define their level of motivation. If action steps are not formed, or the motivation to proceed is low, the process can be repeated.

COACHING AND WELL-BEING

Coaching outcomes can be measured using assessments that focus on workplace performance, well-being, coping, affect, and behavior.[21] Validated instruments include the Satisfaction with Life Scale, Psychological Well-Being, Affect Temperament Scales, and rating of positive and negative affect (PANAS).[22] The Summative

Coaching Evaluation assesses the quality of coaching. Using coaching and follow-up assessment with validated instruments has demonstrated specific improvements in a wide range of industries, including health care.[5,6] In 2009, the Institute of Coaching (IOC) at McLean Hospital, a Harvard Medical School affiliate, was founded to further the scientific underpinnings of coaching by encouraging research and establishment of best practices. The IOC has a Coaching in Health care subgroup and sponsors a yearly Coaching in Health care conference.

Burnout, which is characterized by emotional exhaustion, depersonalization, and reduced perceptions of personal efficacy, is far more common in physicians than the general U.S. population.[23,24] A recent survey of American Society of Anesthesiologists members found 59% at high risk for burnout and 13.8% meeting the criteria for burnout.[25] Several studies investigating coaching interventions for physicians have demonstrated efficacy in mitigating burnout. A randomized coaching intervention for family medicine and pediatric physicians in the Mayo Clinical Health system identified improvements in burnout, emotional exhaustion, quality of life, and resilience compared with physicians who did not receive coaching.[5] McGonagle and colleagues studied 59 early and mid-career primary care physicians, using the Maslach Burnout Inventory and the Workplace PERMA Profiler (positive emotion, engagement, positive relationships, meaning, and achievement) to assess burnout and workplace well-being. Half of the study participants received 6 coaching sessions with a professional coach who had experience with health care professionals. In the conclusion, the coaching cohort reported increased work engagement, psychological capital, and job satisfaction along with decreased burnout. Of note, these results were sustained at the 6-month follow-up. The researchers recommended that health care organizations make coaching available to promote well-being for primary care providers. Some of the coaches who participated in this study anecdotally described the benefits of a similar positive psychology coaching approach with other medical specialties, including anesthesiology. Areas for future study include specific effects of coaching in different medical subspecialties, genders, and career stages.[6]

> My coaching story embodies professional development and well-being. I seemed to "have it all" – a challenging, successful career and 3 beautiful children. Academic promotion was continually delayed though, and when once again I was not put forward for promotion by my department it seemed to confirm my own internal fear that, despite my continually growing CV and achievements, I was never going to be good enough. I increasingly struggled with sadness and burnout, but as the sole support for my family, I could not consider stepping away from my career. After learning about coaching, I decided to try it. Over time, challenged by my coach, I began to identify my strengths and learned to refute my internal critic and limiting beliefs. I decided it was time to redefine my ideas of success and be true to myself. Ultimately that journey led me to become a coach to help and empower others to reach their potential and find their best self.

COACHING, LEADERSHIP, AND EQUITY

In June 2018, the Women's Empowerment and Leadership Initiative (WELI) was founded by the Society for Pediatric Anesthesia with the mission of "empowering highly productive women to achieve promotion, leadership, and equity in pediatric anesthesiology."[26] WELI seeks to promote career development and leadership opportunities for women faculty by offering established leaders in the field the opportunity to learn coaching skills and techniques and then matching them to women faculty seeking promotion and leadership. Although all WELI protégés - are women, the advisors (ie, mentorcoaches) are both men and women. A structured 2-year coaching curriculum has been developed to further support growth in leadership skills and well-being, offering topics such as team management, networking, difficult conversations, and time management at biannual workshops. An early outcome assessment of WELI's efficacy at 2 years found that most members (58%) felt more optimistic about their professional future and 44% thought that WELI contributed positively to their overall quality of life. Notably, surveyed WELI mentor-coaches also emphasized an appreciation for their new skill set, demonstrating a benefit for participants at all career levels.[27,28]

SUMMARY

Anesthesiologists face daily challenges that require emotional intelligence and adaptability. Coaching is commonly used in multiple industries and evidence suggests that coaching can provide benefits in both well-being and professional development for physicians. Coaching differs from training, mentoring, or sponsorship and can add a valuable dimension to professional development and well-being by increasing self-awareness, clarifying personal values, and developing important skill sets for success. Coaching can empower physicians to create a life with goals that are both personally and professionally meaningful and satisfying.

CLINICS CARE POINTS

- *Coaching is a relationship that employs a specific process to facilitate professional and personal development and can be used in one-on-one, group, or team settings.*
- *Coaching can be provided either internally by organizations or externally by consultants or private coaches. External coaches may have very specific niches to help clients.*
- *Anesthesiologists are at high risk for burnout, and coaching interventions have been shown to decrease burnout and positively impact psychological capital.*
- *Anesthesiologists work in intense environments in which emotional intelligence and communication skills are necessary and coaching is an effective method for developing these skillsets.*
- *Even without formal coaching training anesthesiologists can develop coaching skills and use a "-coachapproach" for the benefit of peers and themselves.*

DISCLOSURE

The authors have nothing to disclose.

REFERENCES

1. Bissing MA, Lange EM, Davila WF, et al. Status of women in academic anesthesiology: a 10-year update. Anesth Analg 2019;128:137–43.
2. Richter KP, Clark L, Wick JA, et al. Women physicians and promotion in academic medicine. N Engl J Med 2020;38:2148–57.
3. Toledo P, Duce L, Adams J, et al. Diversity in the american society of anesthesiologists leadership. Anesth Analg 2017;124:1611–6.
4. Cameron D, Dromerick LJ, Ahn J, et al. Executive/life coaching for first year medical students: a prospective study. BMC Med Educ 2019;19:163.

5. Dyrbye LN, Shanafelt TD, Gill PR, et al. Effect of a professional coaching intervention on the well-being and distress of physicians: A pilot randomized clinical trial. JAMA Intern Med 2019;179:1406–14.

6. McGonagle AK, Schwab L, Yahanda N, et al. Coaching for primary care physician well-being: a randomized trial and follow-up analysis. J Occup Health Psychol 2020;25:297–314.

7. International Coaching Federation. Available at: https://coachingfederation.org. Accessed November 30, 2021.

8. Gallwey WT. The inner game of tennis. the classic guide to the mental side of peak performance. New York: Random House; 1974.

9. Diller SJ, Frey D, Jonas E. Coach me if you can! Dark triad clients, their effect on coaches, and how coaches deal with them. Coaching 2021;14:110–26.

10. Graßmann C, Schölmerich F, Schermuly CC. The relationship between working alliance and client outcomes in coaching: a meta-analysis. Hum Relations 2020;73(1):35–58.

11. Goldvarg D, Mathews P, Perel N. Meeting ethical guidelines and professional standards. In: Professional coaching competencies the complete guide. Arroyo Grande: Executive College Press; 2018. p. 5–43.

12. Myers DG. Close relationships and quality of life. In: Kahneman D, Dierner E, Schwartz N, editors. Well-being: the foundations of hedonic psychology. New York: Russell Sage Foundation; 1999. p. 374–91.

13. Parsons AS, Kon RH, Plews-Ogan M, et al. You can have both: coaching to promote clinical competency and professional identity formation. Perspect Med Educ 2021;10:57–63. https://doi.org/10.1007/s40037-020-00612-1.

14. Hu YY, Fix ML, Hevelone ND, et al. Physicians' needs in coping with emotional stressors: the case for peer support. Arch Surg 2012;147:212–7.

15. Maguire M. Peer coaching can relieve physician burnout. Today's Hospitalist; 2020. Available at. https://www.todayshospitalist.com/peer-coaching-relieve-physician-burnout. Accessed September 23, 2021.

16. ICF global coaching survey 2020. Available at. http://coachingfederation.org. Accessed September 26, 2021.

17. Jones RJ, Woods SA, Guillaume YR. The effectiveness of workplace coaching: a meta-analysis of learning and performance outcomes from coaching. J Occup Organiz Psych 2016;89:249–77.

18. Kilburg RR. Toward a conceptual understanding and definition of executive coaching. Consult Psychol J 1996;48:134–44.

19. Shanafelt T, Stolz S, Springer J, et al. A blueprint for organizational strategies to promote the well-being of health care professionals. NEJM Catalyst 2020;1(6). https://doi.org/10.1056/CAT.20.0266.

20. Whitmore J. Coaching for performance. 4th ed. London: Brealey; 2009.

21. Theeboom T, Beersma B, van Vianen AE. Does coaching work? A meta-analysis on the effects of coaching on individual level outcomes in an organizational context. J Posit Psychol 2014;9:1–18.

22. Greif S. Advances in research on coaching outcomes. Int Coach Psychol Rev 2007;2:222–49.

23. Maslach C, Jackson SE. Burnout in organizational settings. J App Soc Psychol Annu 1984;5:133–53.

24. Shanafelt TD, West CP, Sinsky C, et al. Changes in burnout and satisfaction with work-life integration in physicians and the general US working population between 2011 and 2017. Mayo Clin Proc 2019;94:1681–94.

25. Afonso AM, Cadwell JB, Staffa SJ, et al. Burnout rate and risk factors among anesthesiologists in the United States. Anesthesiology 2021;134:683–96.
26. Women's empowerment and leadership initiative. Available at. http://weli. pedsanesthesia.org/.Accessed. Accessed September 23, 2021.
27. Schwartz JM, Wittkugel E, Markowitz SD, et al. Coaching for the pediatric anesthesiologist: becoming our best selves. Pediatr Anesth 2021;31:85–91.
28. Schwartz JM, Markowitz SD, Yanofsky SD, et al. Empowering women as leaders in pediatric anesthesiology: methodology, lessons, and early outcomes of a national initiative. Anesth Analg 2021;133(6):1497–509.

Nutritional Wellness for the Busy Health Care Provider
Small Everyday Wins

Alan Robert Bielsky, MD[a],*, Carolyn Berger Foley, MD[b]

KEYWORDS

• Wellness • Nutrition • Mindfulness • Emotional health

KEY POINTS

- Health care providers are at risk of poor diet and nutrition
- Diet and nutrition are associated with well-being
- Solutions to poor diet and nutrition rely on intentional choices and forethought
- Resources are available to help guide personal choices and institutional efforts to advance nutritional wellness for physicians

INTRODUCTION

The focus of health care provider wellness to date has been heavily biased toward mindfulness, stress reduction techniques, and emotional support. While vital and noble, there is a marked dearth of information and strategies that address the contribution of nutrition to comprehensive wellness. As health care providers, we are, to varying extents, susceptible to similar barriers to adequate nutrition that are found in vulnerable populations such as the elderly, school children, and families suffering from food insecurity. This article aims to describe the relationship between physician nutrition and physician well-being, barriers to nutrition encountered by health care providers, and hopefully benefits physician well-being on an individual and population health basis.

Physicians and Wellness

Working in medicine is a mentally and physically strenuous job, requiring years of training, odd hours, immense stress, and competing demands. As such, it is often

[a] University of Colorado School of Medicine, Children's Hospital Colorado, Anesthesia Box 090, 13123 East 16th Avenue, Aurora, CO 80045, USA; [b] Department of Anesthesiology, University of Colorado School of Medicine, Anesthesia Box 090, Children's Hospital Colorado, Aurora, CO 80045, USA
* Corresponding author.
E-mail address: Alan.bielsky@childrenscolorado.org

Anesthesiology Clin 40 (2022) 349–357
https://doi.org/10.1016/j.anclin.2022.01.008
1932-2275/22/© 2022 Elsevier Inc. All rights reserved.
anesthesiology.theclinics.com

the personal health of physicians is often ignored.[1] In turn, this can lead to decreased performance as well as decreased sustainability and satisfaction with practicing medicine.[2,3]

It is well established that stress, poor diet, and sedentary lifestyles have significant cumulative impacts on morbidity and mortality in the U.S. adult population.[4] To date, however, there is a notable lack of attention to how health care providers navigate their daily dietary choices and little longitudinal data on nutrition and the physical health of the American health care workforce.

Why Nutrition?

In their recommendations for improving clinician mental health in the postpandemic era, Schwartz and colleagues pointedly advocate for the provision of clinicians' basic needs, which include food, rest, shelter, transportation, and personal protective equipment (PPE).[5] However, the inclusion of nutrition into the daily professional life of clinicians has impacts beyond basic humanitarian considerations, such as clinician performance, quality of patient care, and physician well-being.

For example, mild dehydration can alter concentration, alertness, and short term memory, as evidenced by decreased performance on short term memory tests, perceptual discrimination, arithmetical ability, visuomotor tracking, and psychomotor skills.[6] This evidence has been established in athletes and airline pilots as well as physicians.[7,8] Humans require varying degrees of fluid intake between 2700 and 3700 mL a day, without the consideration of physical activity or other increased needs.[9] Mild to moderate dehydration can lead to dry mouth and skin, sleepiness, fatigue, headache, lightheadedness, and constipation. While adequate fluid intake seems to be an easy goal to maintain, it often goes ignored. Two separate studies have noted suboptimal fluid intake on physician call shifts with resultant body mass decreases and urine ketonuria.[10,11] There have also been studies using cognitive tests that demonstrated cognitive declines associated with dehydration during clinical shits.[12]

The quality and quantity of food intake also can affect performance and cognition, as evidenced by investigations in athletes, airline pilots, and physicians.[3] Caloric intake for humans varies between 1500 kilocalories and 3000 kilocalories per day independent of physical activity.[13] Health care workers can walk over 2 miles in an 8-hour shift, leading to more caloric requirement.[14] Symptoms of hypoglycemia include adrenergic responses such as sweating and tremor, glucagon responses such as hunger and nausea, and neuroglycopenic responses such as fatigue, dizziness, headache, lack of concentration, and confusion.[15] Of note, an investigation into nutrition and cognition during work hours of 20 staff physicians at a teaching hospital found 4 subjects to have hypoglycemic range serum glucose levels during work hours, and 40% describing symptoms of hypoglycemia.[16]

One caveat that could play into the perception of wellness on a daily basis is the timing of meals. In the chaotic and unpredictable realm of clinical medicine, it is often difficult to eat at regular intervals. Studied interventions in the health care setting include actions as simple as providing a healthy breakfast, nutrition logs, and intermittent snacking.[17–20] Additionally, as clinician sleep cycles may be regularly disturbed, it is important to know that eating near regular bedtimes can adversely affect circadian rhythms.[21]

From a food quality standpoint, high-fat diets and processed foods have been associated with anxiety and depressive disorders. Further exposure has been associated with a decline in cognitive function.[22–24] Research into the link between nutrition and mood has built an area of investigation called nutritional psychiatry. This discipline focuses both on diet quality as a modifiable risk factor for mental health disorders and the biological processes behind diet and mental health.[22] To date, proposed mechanisms of the interplay between diet and mental health include inflammation, oxidative stress, neuroplasticity, the microbiota–gut–brain axis, and mitochondrial dysfunction.[22,25]

Barriers to Physician Nutritional Wellness

It is easy to identify the main culprits of a physician's poor diet because they are ubiquitous in the hospital. Processed foods rife with preservatives, flavor enhancers, heavy salt, unsaturated fats, and refined sugars abound, especially in vending machines in a staff break room. While these foods provide quick, convenient satiation and can keep for ages, they are not compatible with a healthy lifestyle. The hospital cafeteria poses similar challenges to quickly finding a nutritionally balanced, convenient meal. From a business perspective, it is difficult to serve large quantities of food without reliance on industrial foodstuffs. However, the problem with ultraprocessed foods lies in their association with poor dietary quality; evidence suggests an association with an increased risk of adverse health outcomes spanning cardiovascular disease, diabetes, and mental health. [23,26,27] Thus, when these foods are presented as the only options in the workplace, are adequately tasty, and often supply the quick pick-me-up we all need, we may forget there are better alternatives.

When examining specific barriers to quality food choices in the health care environment, there is a small amount of investigation to date. In a 2008 cross-sectional survey of 328 British National Health Service doctors working in 2 NHS Trust Hospitals, limited cafeteria hours, lack of healthy food selections in the cafeteria, and limited time to eat were all noted as barriers to healthy eating.[28] Interestingly, this study correlated frequent hospital cafeteria reliance with less overall healthy lifestyle and younger age. When considering hospital cafeterias specifically, it is evident that healthy options are rare. This is accompanied by a high frequency of sweet "impulse buy" items at the register and "meal combo" deals that add unnecessary calories at reduced prices.[29]

Solutions

In an ideal world, there would be a personal chef doing all of the grocery shopping and showing up on cue to provide a preservative free, healthy, satiating meal. Sadly, our lives and careers do not allow this luxury. To break the cycle, we need to come up with practical, feasible solutions. Furthermore, these solutions need to be sustainable, affordable, and flexible for different health care systems, as one size rarely fits all.

The Mediterranean Diet

The Mediterranean diet is predicated on nutritional wellness and advocates for locally grown, seasonally fresh foods. First described by Keys, it is characterized by a high intake of fruits, vegetables, minimally refined breads and cereals, potatoes, beans, nuts, and seeds.[30] Artificially sweetened goods are replaced by the occasional use of honey or minimal sugar for interspersed desserts. Animal fats such as butter and lard are replaced by olive oil and other plant oils. Dairy and egg intake are minimized to a few times per week. Protein sources include fish and poultry in smaller amounts while red meat is minimized.[30,31] The health benefits of the Mediterranean diet have been amply described and are noted to include emotional well-being.[32]

The practical benefits of the Mediterranean diet can be derived by the average health care worker through thoughtful food choices. Seeking out unprocessed meals or snacks may equate to choosing fresh fruit rather than a graham cracker, resulting in an equal amount of satiation with added health benefits. Additionally, the prepacking of whole, unrefined foods in a lunch bag can offer an array of available food choices, rather than relying on the offerings of the hospital setting.

Mindful Eating

Mindfulness is a prevalent concept in the physician well-being armamentarium. Mindfulness is defined as an intentional focus on the present despite external distractions. Extending this concept to nourishment in the health care environment may be beneficial; for example, enacting a daily practice of mindful eating can provide a brief but effective respite. Practically, mindful eating can be used on a daily basis by sitting down purposefully, eating slowly with intent, and avoiding distractions such as cell phones, televisions, or magazines. Focusing on food texture, tastes, and smells can provide an excellent respite from stress as well as reduce the chances of overeating, poor satiety, and poor food choices.[33] Mindful eating also teaches the awareness of hunger and fullness cues as well as emotional responses to eating.[34] A multitude of guided exercises focused on mindful eating exist—this Sharkawy can allow for a more formal practice, which allows a novice to gain confidence with a new skill.

Food Journaling

Documenting daily food intake can add insight into calories consumed and behavioral eating patterns. Otherwise known as food journaling, this practice aims to offer feedback on caloric content, satiety, and hunger cues.[35,36] Traditionally, this is complicated by the time-intensive nature of the activity and user input inaccuracy. The advent of mobile-based food journaling platforms has revolutionized food journaling, specifically in the realm of smartphones. The specific strength of these mobile apps lies in the quick availability of nutritional information of commercially and commonly available products. This in combination with exercise inputs, step counting, and nutritional coaching offers exceptional flexibility for those interested in improving their diet and daily lifestyle within the confines of a high demand job such as clinical medicine.[37,38]

Water Dense Foods

In the past, focus was placed on the manipulation of fat, protein, and carbohydrate compositions of food. In turn, this has led to the introduction of heavily processed foods into the typical Western diet with ensuant deleterious health risks. An emerging concept is dietary energy density. People tend to eat a certain volume of food to obtain satiety. If a fixed volume of food contains more water, it has less dietary energy. Foods with lower dietary energy density lead to earlier satiety and fewer cravings.[39] A practical example is the choice between a box of raisins (130 calories) or eight ounces of fresh whole grapes (100 calories). The fresh grapes will lead to earlier and sustained satiety. Other healthy substitutions with high water content and low dietary energy include fruits, vegetables, soups, and stews. Consumption of high water content, low dietary energy foods could also lead to less cravings, snacking, and mood changes encountered on a busy clinical day.[40]

Home Cooking

Home meal preparation is one way to ensure the availability of sound food choices. While it may be perceived as a hindrance, home meal preparation provides optimal control over dietary intake and may have other potential benefits, including increased quality time spent between family members. Additionally, home meal preparation has been associated with the consumption of a healthy diet with the benefits passed on to other members of the household.[41] Strategies to increase the use of home meal preparation include recipe sharing among colleagues, designating one evening per week to cook based on call and family commitments, and using preassembled healthy meal kits from food services. A great option is a soup, which is easily made in advance in large batches, is not typically energy-dense, and is easily transported to work.

Building the Nutrition Environment

Practicing daily nutrition improvement and healthy eating habits does not have to be a lonely existence. Rather, there is a benefit to creating an environment that facilitates learning about nutrition. The hive mentality of exchanging tips, recipes, and resources can be synergistic and can strengthen the community in which you work. In the Department of Anesthesiology at the University of Colorado, we implemented f new formats to encourage physician well-being through food. Improved video conferencing software offers a fantastic platform for cooking events. The Anesthesiology Department at Children's Hospital Colorado invited a James Beard Award-winning chef to teach a cooking class on video conferencing software. Over 30 physicians, anesthetists, advanced practice nurses, and office staff joined online to prepare a vegetarian Mediterranean-inspired meal that was prepared in under an hour. We are now planning a series of cooking classes featuring healthy recipes from our group's diverse ethnic origins. These creative initiatives prove to be inexpensive, easily implemented, and well-received, all while fostering a sense of community. We are combining this effort with an online collection of healthy and easily prepared recipes from group members.

Nutritional education is another important tool that we further developed for trainee wellness retreats, as it is often not included in resident self-care education. Given that many trainees have moved from other cities and are new to the area, we focus on sharing local food resources, specialties, and seasonal offerings. This is combined with education on alcohol consumption, sleep hygiene, stress management, mindfulness training, and other resilience topics to foster a healthy lifestyle and coping habits throughout training. Promoting physician well-being through healthy food choices is an essential component of a wellness program and ultimately contributes to a well physician and a cohesive workforce.

Structural Changes

While personal choices are critical, the quality of food available in the health care environment plays an important role in day-to-day physician wellness. As described earlier in this article, most food available to clinicians in the hospital consists of ultraprocessed foods. Breaking this cycle has proved difficult, but there are many opportunities for improving access to healthy foods in the workplace.

An interesting case has been built for the establishment of the "Healthy Teaching Kitchen" (HTK) in the health care environment. This program was initially piloted at the Veterans Health Administration in 2007 for Veterans, a population with higher rates of poverty and obesity, and is currently active at 119 VAs across the United States due to its success. The Healthy Kitchen has been expanded to other health care systems. These are typically located in the hospital and aim to improve diets of both visitors to and employees of the hospital through novel, hands-on culinary education, and support of healthier dietary habits.[42] In these Teaching Kitchens, instruction occurs in the area of nutrition knowledge, hands-on healthy cooking skills, use of web-based sources and technologies, and mindfulness training in diet, portion control, and satiety. This has expanded to include multiple institutions and is even an elective for undergraduate medical students at Stanford to better both the students' nutritional awareness and their ability to educate patients. There is also a well-established online resource (https://teachingkitchens.org and www.healthykitchens.org)[43]

Finally, advocating for healthy eating in the workplace and raising awareness to hospital leadership are important starting points. Initiating dialogue with hospital food services may also be reasonable and in many cases, successful. Another technique may involve food labeling to help people make smarter and more informed decisions regarding meal choices. For example, Thorndike and colleagues conducted a 2-year-long study of hospital employee food purchasing in their cafeteria after instituting "traffic light label" changes to differentiate the healthiness of items. The results revealed a sustained decrease in the purchase of "red labels" or "unhealthy, more caloric" food choices by hospital employees during this time period which the authors felt could lead to weight loss and improved obesity over time.[44] Further, including calorie counts on menus, "choice" logos, "heart healthy" logos, product placement to encourage healthy choices and enhanced nutrition fact panels have also proven effective in steering people toward more healthier options including decreased calorie and fat intake and increased vegetable intake. Over time, these choices may lead to durational behavioral change and improved health.[42,44] Such changes could be instituted broadly throughout a hospital system and potentially yield substantive impact on the health of patients, families, and hospital employees.

Another behavioral method to encourage healthy choices is to incorporate subsidization. Studies have demonstrated the effects of subsidizing healthy food choices, given that nutrient-rich, energy-dense foods are often more costly, and have shown that if healthier food costs less, consumption increases. Subsidies could be created by way of discounts on the food itself, or the accumulation of rewards with repeated purchasing of healthy food items.[45] Conversely, consideration should be given to increased taxation of high-fat or high-sugar foods to further encourage healthy choices. The economic case for healthier hospital cafeteria choices has been difficult to establish. Fluctuating prices and supply chain problems can offset any potential benefits of employee wellness and reduction in absenteeism. According to some studies, modifying the cafeteria of a workplace to include healthier choices could lead to a savings to cost ratio of $5.81 to $1.[46] The Centers for Disease Control published Best Practices for the Financial Sustainability of Healthy Food Service Guideline in Hospital Cafeterias, in which sociologic interviews with hospital cafeteria directors identified common themes and challenges. They suggest regular taste tests for new dishes, analysis of sales of healthy dishes, new dish rollout plans, substitution suggestions, and discount realignment as ways to address financial concerns.[47]

Overall, medical provider well-being is multifactorial and should include nutritional wellness. Our goal was to emphasize the importance of nutrition with respect to physician self-care and to provide ideas of how to incorporate mindful and educated nutritional choices throughout the clinical day, as this can help lead to a longer and healthier career in medicine.

DISCLOSURE

Dr A. R. Bielsky has received speaking fees from Biogen relating to the administration of nusinersen in patients with Spinal Muscular Atrophy. Dr A. R. Bielsky has served as a paid reviewer for 2 legal cases in the past Dr C. B. Foley has no disclosures. University of Colorado Department of Anesthesiology has provided ongoing support for the development of a wellness program, and thus serves as a vital supporter for this literature.

REFERENCES

1. Hsu DP, Hansen SL, Roberts TA, et al. Predictors of Wellness Behaviors in U.S. Army Physicians. Mil Med 2018;183(11-12):e641–8.
2. Shanafelt T, Ripp J, Trockel M. Understanding and Addressing Sources of Anxiety Among Health Care Professionals During the COVID-19 Pandemic. JAMA 2020;323(21):2133–4.
3. Hamidi MS, Boggild MK, Cheung AM. Running on empty: a review of nutrition and physicians' well-being. Postgrad Med J 2016;92(1090):478–81.
4. Masters RK, Reither EN, Powers DA, et al. The impact of obesity on US mortality levels: the importance of age and cohort factors in population estimates. Am J Public Health 2013;103(10):1895–901 [Erratum in: Am J Public Health 2016;106(7):e15].
5. Schwartz R, Sinskey JL, Anand U, et al. Addressing Postpandemic Clinician Mental Health : A Narrative Review and Conceptual Framework. Ann Intern Med 2020;173(12):981–8.
6. Popkin BM, D'Anci KE, Rosenberg IH. Water, hydration, and health. Nutr Rev 2010;68(8):439–58.
7. Adan A. Cognitive performance and dehydration. J Am Coll Nutr 2012; 31(2):71–8.
8. Wilf-Miron R, Lewenhoff I, Benyamini Z, et al. From aviation to medicine: applying concepts of aviation safety to risk management in ambulatory care. Qual Saf Health Care 2003;12(1):35–9.
9. Kennedy E, Meyers L. Dietary Reference Intakes: development and uses for assessment of micronutrient status of women–a global perspective. Am J Clin Nutr 2005;81(5):1194S–7S.
10. Parshuram CS, Dhanani S, Kirsh JA, et al. Fellowship training, workload, fatigue and physical stress: a prospective observational study. CMAJ 2004;170(6): 965–70.
11. El-Sharkawy AM, Bragg D, Watson P, et al. Hydration amongst nurses and doctors on-call (the HANDS on prospective cohort study). Clin Nutr 2016;35(4): 935–42.
12. El-Sharkawy AM, Sahota O, Lobo DN. Acute and chronic effects of hydration status on health. Nutr Rev 2015;73(Suppl 2):S97–109.
13. McKinnon RA, Oladipo T, Ferguson MS, et al. Reported Knowledge of Typical Daily Calorie Requirements: Relationship to Demographic Characteristics in US Adults. J Acad Nutr Diet 2019;119(11):1831–1841 e6.
14. Peters GA, Wong ML, Sanchez LD. Pedometer-measured physical activity among emergency physicians during shifts. Am J Emerg Med 2020;38(1): 118–21.
15. Lemaire JB, Wallace JE, Dinsmore K, et al. Food for thought: an exploratory study of how physicians experience poor workplace nutrition. Nutr J 2011;10(1):18.
16. Lemaire JB, Wallace JE, Dinsmore K, et al. Physician nutrition and cognition during work hours: effect of a nutrition based intervention. BMC Health Serv Res 2010;10:241.
17. Tanaka M, Mizuno K, Fukuda S, et al. Relationships between dietary habits and the prevalence of fatigue in medical students. Nutrition 2008;24(10):985–9.

18. Chaplin K, Smith AP. Breakfast and snacks: associations with cognitive failures, minor injuries, accidents and stress. Nutrients 2011;3(5):515–28.
19. Kanarek R. Psychological effects of snacks and altered meal frequency. Br J Nutr 1997;77(Suppl 1):S105–18 ; discussion 118-20.
20. Kaplan RJ, Greenwood CE, Winocur G, et al. Dietary protein, carbohydrate, and fat enhance memory performance in the healthy elderly. Am J Clin Nutr 2001; 74(5):687–93.
21. Oosterman JE, Kalsbeek A, la Fleur SE, et al. Impact of nutrients on circadian rhythmicity. Am J Physiol Regul Integr Comp Physiol 2015;308(5):R337–50.
22. Marx W, Moseley G, Berk M, et al. Nutritional psychiatry: the present state of the evidence. Proc Nutr Soc 2017;76(4):427–36.
23. Adjibade M, Julia C, Alles B, et al. Prospective association between ultra-processed food consumption and incident depressive symptoms in the French NutriNet-Sante cohort. BMC Med 2019;17(1):78.
24. Tsan L, Decarie-Spain L, Noble EE, et al. Western Diet Consumption During Development: Setting the Stage for Neurocognitive Dysfunction. Front Neurosci 2021;15:632312.
25. Murciano-Brea J, Garcia-Montes M, Geuna S, et al. Gut Microbiota and Neuroplasticity. Cells 2021;(8):10. https://doi.org/10.3390/cells10082084.
26. Chen X, Zhang Z, Yang H, et al. Consumption of ultra-processed foods and health outcomes: a systematic review of epidemiological studies. Nutr J 2020; 19(1):86.
27. Gomez-Donoso C, Sanchez-Villegas A, Martinez-Gonzalez MA, et al. Ultra-processed food consumption and the incidence of depression in a Mediterranean cohort: the SUN Project. Eur J Nutr 2020;59(3):1093–103.
28. Winston J, Johnson C, Wilson S. Barriers to healthy eating by National Health Service (NHS) hospital doctors in the hospital setting: results of a cross-sectional survey. BMC Res Notes 2008;1:69.
29. Lesser LI, Hunnes DE, Reyes P, et al. Assessment of food offerings and marketing strategies in the food-service venues at California Children's Hospitals. Acad Pediatr 2012;12(1):62–7.
30. Keys A. Mediterranean diet and public health: personal reflections. Am J Clin Nutr 1995;61(6 Suppl):1321S–3S.
31. Guasch-Ferre M, Willett WC. The Mediterranean diet and health: a comprehensive overview. J Intern Med 2021. https://doi.org/10.1111/joim.13333.
32. Godoy-Izquierdo D, Ogallar A, Lara R, et al. Association of a Mediterranean Diet and Fruit and Vegetable Consumption with Subjective Well-Being among Adults with Overweight and Obesity. Nutrients 2021;(4):13. https://doi.org/10.3390/nu13041342.
33. Esquivel MK. Nutrition Strategies for Reducing Risk of Burnout Among Physicians and Health Care Professionals. Am J Lifestyle Med 2021;15(2):126–9.
34. Warren JM, Smith N, Ashwell M. A structured literature review on the role of mindfulness, mindful eating and intuitive eating in changing eating behaviours: effectiveness and associated potential mechanisms. Nutr Res Rev 2017;30(2):272–83.
35. Illner AK, Freisling H, Boeing H, et al. Review and evaluation of innovative technologies for measuring diet in nutritional epidemiology. Int J Epidemiol 2012; 41(4):1187–203.
36. Bruno V, Resende S, Juan C. A Survey on Automated Food Monitoring and Dietary Management Systems. J Health Med Inform 2017;8(3). https://doi.org/10.4172/2157-7420.1000272.

37. BVR ES, Rad MG, Cui J, et al. A Mobile-Based Diet Monitoring System for Obesity Management. J Health Med Inform 2018;9(2). https://doi.org/10.4172/2157-7420.1000307.
38. Yang Q, Mitchell ES, Ho AS, et al. Cross-National Outcomes of a Digital Weight Loss Intervention in the United States, Canada, United Kingdom and Ireland, and Australia and New Zealand: A Retrospective Analysis. Front Public Health 2021;9:604937. https://doi.org/10.3389/fpubh.2021.604937.
39. Rolls BJ. Dietary energy density: Applying behavioural science to weight management. Nutr Bull 2017;42(3):246–53.
40. Drewnowski A. Energy density, palatability, and satiety: implications for weight control. Nutr Rev 1998;56(12):347–53.
41. Wolfson JA, Bleich SN. Is cooking at home associated with better diet quality or weight-loss intention? Public Health Nutr 2015;18(8):1397–406.
42. Eisenberg DM, Righter AC, Matthews B, et al. Feasibility Pilot Study of a Teaching Kitchen and Self-Care Curriculum in a Workplace Setting. Am J Lifestyle Med 2019;13(3):319–30.
43. Chapman LS. Meta-evaluation of worksite health promotion economic return studies: 2012 update. Am J Health Promot 2012;26(4):TAHP1–12.
44. Jilcott Pitts S, Schwartz B, Graham J, et al. Best Practices for Financial Sustainability of Healthy Food Service Guidelines in Hospital Cafeterias. Prev Chronic Dis 2018;15:E58. https://doi.org/10.5888/pcd15.17047.
45. Shangguan S, Afshin A. A meta-analysis of food labeling effects on consumer diet behaviors and industry practices. Am J Prev Med 2019;56(2):300–14.
46. Black M, LaCroix R, Hoerster K, et al. Healthy Teaching Kitchen Programs: Experiential Nutrition Education Across Veterans Health Administration. Am J Public Health 2019;109(12):1718–21.
47. Thorndike A, Gelsomin E, McCurley J, et al. Calories purchased by hospital employees after implementation of a cafeteria traffic light-labeling and choice architecture program. JAMA Netw Open 2019;2(7):e196789.

Poetry and Medicine

Audrey Shafer, MD

KEYWORDS

• Poetry • Humanities • Health humanities • Medical humanities • Arts • Literature

KEY POINTS

- Poetry and medicine have multiple complex connections, because they both can address difficult human experiences.
- Anesthesiology, including the arc of patient care and attention to rhythms and precision, has much in common with the poem, including arcs of thought, rhythms, pauses, and resonances.
- Increasingly, access to reading and writing poetry has been found to decrease stress, enable reflection, and improve well-being.

INTRODUCTION

Poetry is in us, of us, and around us. Poetry is a way of meaning-making in a complicated, confusing world, which includes not only loss, terror, and hatred but also joy, gratitude, and love. The historical roots of poetry predate writing; intergenerational knowledge transfer included bards who memorized verse. For many centuries, poetry has imbued the writings and oral traditions of religions around the world. Our exposure to poetry starts when we are young: we are taught poems in nursery rhymes and children's songs. We ask in a slant rhyme at the end of the alphabet song: "Now I know my ABC's/Tell me what you think of me." However, we may lose our comfort with poetry as we progress through education. Poetry itself can feel confusing, and the effort to live with a poem, to mull it over, and accept its ambiguities can feel burdensome, as well as tangential to life. Poetry put to music, in the form of lyrics from musical theater to popular music to rap, may become the only poetry the public feels has worth.

Poetry is often put in opposition to prose as a form of literature, but in actuality, these 2 forms, which manifest in a diversity of ways, overlap. What is usually true of poetry, however, is that summarizing a poem so eviscerates the poem that a brief synopsis is meaningless. For example, parse Robert Frost's much quoted poem, "The

Anesthesiology, Perioperative and Pain Medicine, Stanford University School of Medicine, Veterans Affairs Palo Alto Health Care System, Anesthesia 112A VAPAHCS, 3801 Miranda Avenue, Palo Alto, CA 94304, USA
E-mail address: ashafer@stanford.edu

Anesthesiology Clin 40 (2022) 359–372
https://doi.org/10.1016/j.anclin.2022.01.009
1932-2275/22/Published by Elsevier Inc.

Road Not Taken," to "choices in life's journey matter," and we have not experienced the poem itself at all.[1] We have not walked in that "yellow wood," have not felt the rhythms of the words, the breaths, the spaces. In other words, a poem, whether a couplet, sonnet, free form, epic, or anything in-between, needs to be fully read, experienced, and hopefully heard, either aloud or in the mind's ear.

Poetry as incantation has a long history in healing, such as in shamanistic rituals. Such uses continue in tempered, more nuanced ways. Poetry is frequently invoked at gatherings to celebrate or mourn passages in life and death. Poetry creates community within such gatherings, and enables those present to access emotions—and, importantly, first gives permission to access such feelings. Think of the funeral scene in *Four Weddings and a Funeral*, where the bereaved Matthew recites the poem, "Funeral Blues" by W. H. Auden, as an elegy for his dead partner and lover, Gareth.[2,3] The poem creates a shared experience of grief and loss, and provides an avenue for collective and individual healing.

An outstanding way to start or continue an exploration of how to approach and live in a poem is through the podcast, *Poetry Unbound*, by poet, theologian, and educator, Pádraig Ó Tuama.[4] Each episode focuses on 1 poem, read twice within the space of 10 minutes, with an intervening dive into the poem, its poetics, the poet's life, and the ways in which the poem affects the host. The podcast, itself personal and universal, hence captures that which makes a poem both individual and revelatory of truths.

The value of poetry in medicine is demonstrated in the multiple medical journals that accept and publish poetry and the growing number of literary medicine contests that include poetry, or exclusively focus on poetry. For example, poems can be found in sections of the *Journal of the American Medical Association*, *The Lancet*, *Annals of Internal Medicine*, and *New England Journal of Medicine*. Medical specialty journals that include poetry include 2 major journals in anesthesiology: *Anesthesia and Analgesia* and *Anesthesiology*.[5,6]

Medical (or health) humanities, the academic discipline devoted to the intersections of the arts, humanities, and medicine, includes poetry readings at national conferences as well as the publication of poems in scholarly journals, for example, *Journal of Medical Humanities*. Medical literary journals, such as *The Pegasus Review*, *The Intima*, *Pulse: Voices from the Heart of Medicine*, *Literary AMWA* (American Medical Women's Association), and *Bellevue Literary Review* include poetry. Volumes or anthologies of literary writing can include poetry related to medicine, or can be exclusively composed of such poetry.[7] The extensive online resource chronicling literature, film, and arts related to medicine presented in the New York University Literature Arts Medicine Database includes 745 annotations of poetry.[8] Medical literary contests, such as the Paul Kalanithi Writing Award and the Irvin D. Yalom Literary Award (for students and trainees only) accept poetry entries.[9,10] Poetry contests on topics related to medicine and the human condition include those open to practitioners and the public, such as the Hippocrates Initiative for Poetry and Medicine, and those exclusively for medical students, such as the William Carlos Williams Poetry Competition for Medical Students.[11,12]

There are growing numbers of physician-poets publishing in the aforementioned venues or compiling chapbooks or poetry collections. Historically, the most famous physician-poets include William Carlos Williams and John Keats. Williams, a family doctor and pediatrician born in 1883, practiced in New Jersey. Part of both the modernist and the early imagist movements in poetry, Williams also wrote prose, including short stories and an autobiography. Although his stories tended to deal more directly with medicine and practice, occasional poems, such as "The Last Words of My English Grandmother," did as well.[13,14]

John Keats, born in 1795 in London, attended medical school, did surgery apprenticeships and received his apothecary license (for pharmacy, medicine, and surgery). However, he abandoned medicine and surgery to become a poet and died at age 25 years of tuberculosis. In his short career he wrote poems that have lasted in the Western poetry canon, which, like "Ode to a Nightingale," contain multiple references to the pharmaceutical and medical knowledge he had acquired in his studies.[15] There are also several physician-writers, such as Sir Arthur Conan Doyle, who wrote poetry but who remain far more known for their prose writing. Two contemporary physician-poets, Rafael Campo and Audrey Shafer, are featured in the documentary, *Why Doctors Write*, by filmmaker Ken Browne.[16]

This article explores some of the multiple relationships between poetry and medicine. The word "healing" is used in a broad, inclusive way, and no claim is made that poetry itself has direct curative powers. We will explore the following:

- How illness, health, and medicine are portrayed in poems, including how poetry enables us to understand the human condition in new or deeper ways.
- How poetry and anesthesiology, in particular, are related.
- How poetry and writing poetry can enhance our understanding of well-being.

This article will not provide an exhaustive overview of these topics, but rather will sample poems illustrative of such concepts and provide highlights for further contemplation.

PORTRAYAL OF ILLNESS, HEALTH, AND MEDICINE IN POETRY

Humans are embodied and mortal. For centuries, we have struggled to understand these truths through words. Philosopher Martha Nussbaum notes: "We have never lived enough. Our experience is, without fiction, too confined and too parochial. Literature extends it, making us reflect and feel about what might otherwise be too distant for feeling."[17] Poetry extends our understanding of the world, both across time and distance.

There are many poems that illustrate the powerful, subtle, lyrical, and heartbreaking ways in which poets explore what it means to be human, to be mortal, to be ill, to care for another that is ill, to mourn, to become and be a physician or health care worker, and to experience or witness suffering. Poems, in their crystalline, spare, allusive, and expansive ways, enable us to hold a moment in hand. To both stop and explode time. **Table 1** lists a sampling of poems currently online that can start the reader on this journey.

Table 1
Sample poems available online about the human condition and health[a]

Poet	Title	Online Source
bearheart, b: william	When I Was In Las Vegas And Saw A Warhol Painting of Geronimo	https://muse.jhu.edu/article/548715
Brooks, Gwendolyn	We Real Cool	https://www.poetryfoundation.org/poetrymagazine/poems/28112/we-real-cool
Campo, Rafael	The Chart	https://www.poetryfoundation.org/poetrymagazine/poems/57745/the-chart

(*continued on next page*)

Table 1
(continued)

Poet	Title	Online Source
Carver, Raymond	What the Doctor Said	https://utmedhumanities.wordpress.com/2014/10/12/what-the-doctor-said-raymond-carver/
Clifton, Lucille	Dialysis	https://utmedhumanities.wordpress.com/2014/10/12/dialysis-lucille-clifton-2/
Coulehan, Jack	On Reading Walt Whitman's "The Wound Dresser"	https://jackcoulehan.com/
Derricote, Toi	Pantoum for the Broken	https://wisepoets.com/2021/08/21/toi-derricotte-pantoum-for-the-broken/
Dove, Rita	Old Folks Home, Jerusalem	https://www.poetryfoundation.org/poetrymagazine/browse?contentId=36267
Hall, Donald	The Ship Pounding	https://www.ncbi.nlm.nih.gov/pmc/articles/PMC2839325/
Harper, Michael S.	Nightmare Begins Responsibility	https://www.poetryfoundation.org/poems/42829/nightmare-begins-responsibility
Hoagland, Tony	Emigration	https://journals.lww.com/academicmedicine/fulltext/2000/11000/emigration.19.aspx
Howe, Marie	What the Living Do	https://poets.org/poem/what-living-do
Kenyon, Jane	The Sick Wife	https://www.ncbi.nlm.nih.gov/pmc/articles/PMC2839325/
Lee, Li-Young	Persimmons	https://www.poetryfoundation.org/poems/43011/persimmons
Neruda, Pablo	The Dictators	https://www.poetryfoundation.org/poetrymagazine/browse?contentId=25873
Plath, Sylvia	Tulips	https://www.poetryfoundation.org/poems/49013/tulips-56d22ab68fdd0
Rilke, Ranier Maria	Washing the Corpse	https://poems.com/poem/washing-the-corpse/
Shafer, Audrey	Falling Fifth: The Neurosurgery Patient and the Anesthesiologist	https://pulsevoices.org/index.php/poems/falling-fifth-the-neurosurgery-patient-and-the-anesthesiologist
Vuong, Ocean	Seventh Circle of Earth	https://poetryschool.com/how-i-did-it/i-forward-first-collection-special-ocean-vuong-seventh-circle-earth/
Whitman, Walt	The Wound-Dresser	https://www.poetryfoundation.org/poems/53027/the-wound-dresser
Young, C. Dale	Corpus Medicum	https://www.poetryfoundation.org/poetrymagazine/browse?volume=187&issue=2&page=30

[a] Some of the poems contain strong imagery, and are on difficult topics, which can be triggering for some readers.

Three poems that explore these critical themes are provided here: a fragment by Sappho, a poem on pain by Emily Dickinson, and a modern poem on the pandemic by Adjoa Boateng. The poems cross time and oceans, and the reader is encouraged to read them aloud, to spend time with the words, the spacing, the rhythms. Sappho, born in Lesbos in 630 BCE, is known for her poetry on love and longing, much of which is only preserved as fragments on papyrus or pottery (**Fig. 1**). In poem 31, she explores the bodily manifestations of love and envy, including effects on the ribcage, tongue, skin, ears, vision, and the body as a whole. This is love sickness manifest.

FRAGMENT 31

By Sappho, translated by Chris Childers

[For the full version see reference 18 https://www.literarymatters.org/1-1-sappho-31/]

"He seems like the gods' equal…
sets the heart in my ribcage fluttering;…
and my tongue stiffens into silence…
flames underneath my skin prickle and spark…"

The poem fragment concludes:

"…my body shakes, suddenly sallower

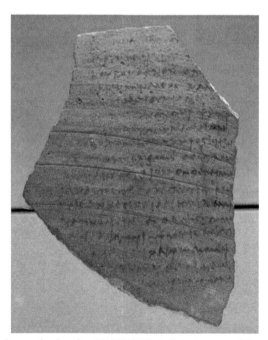

Fig. 1. Fragment of poem by Sappho. PSI XIII 1300: 3rd–2nd century BC ostrakon from Egypt, preserving four stanzas of Sappho fr. 2 (Voigt). Now in the collection of the Laurentian Library, Florence. (Photograph by Sailko. Used unchanged via license Creative Commons Attribution 3.0 Unported. Available at: https://commons.wikimedia.org/wiki/File:Ostrakon_PSI_XIII_1300,_II_sec._ac,_frammento_di_un%27ode_di_saffo_sul_culto_di_afrodite.JPG Accessed September 3, 2021.)

than summer grass, and death, I fear and feel,
is very near."[18]

Moving centuries forward, Emily Dickinson addresses the experience of pain, linking the experience to timelessness and the sway pain has over us.

PAIN HAS AN ELEMENT OF BLANK

By Emily Dickinson

Pain has an element of blank;
It cannot recollect
When it began, or if there were
A day when it was not.

It has no future but itself,
Its infinite realms contain
Its past, enlightened to perceive.
New periods of pain.[19]

(THE POEMS OF EMILY DICKINSON: VARIORUM EDITION, edited by Ralph W. Franklin, Cambridge, Mass.: The Belknap Press of Harvard University Press, Copyright © 1998 by the President and Fellows of Harvard College. Copyright © 1951, 1955, 1979, 1983 by the President and Fellows of Harvard College.)

Pain can make us speechless, preverbal, incoherent. The questions used to elicit clinical details of the type, onset, quality, and duration of pain can feel completely inadequate when one is in the throes of pain. The erasure that pain can cause, diminishing the rest of our lives, reducing social contact, narrowing our world, is contained in the poem—pain becomes the future itself, it swallows our past, it is a void that allows for nothing else, only its return.

Suffering has both universal and highly individualistic qualities. Poetry is particularly adept at enabling such qualities to be explored. Adjoa Boateng is an anesthesiologist-intensivist who worked in critical care during the coronavirus disease 2019 (COVID-19) pandemic. Her poem, "Grief, What Is Your Name," launched the new section, The Human Experience, in the journal, *Anesthesia and Analgesia*:

GRIEF, WHAT IS YOUR NAME?

By Adjoa Boateng

After encountering innumerable deaths in the ICU, ushering families through the dying process virtually, grieving a life once lived, simply, amidst so much death, this piece came to life.

Today, I write to those entities my mind cannot digest.

To the novel tastes that defy even umami, the ones chewed, looking upwards, with eyes closed, to give my tastebuds a bit more bandwidth.

Today I write to you, grief.

You arrive indiscriminately, luggage brimming with both overwhelming cacophony and also deafening silence.

You disrupt conversation, causing coffee to spill over freshly pressed linen.

I weep.

What was once the fluid and graceful nature of my tongue begins to stutter through poorly concocted words or use inappropriate comedy because life sometimes, is too much to bear.

Paradigm shift.

Grief is when the life preceding no longer mirrors life thereafter.

So I pause, stare toward the muted tones around me and whisper, "Grief, what is your name?"

When we are already in mourning and there is more death, what do we call it? From where does more pain emanate when numbness prevails? How do more tears spring from a dried well? Grief, who birthed you? From whose womb were you nourished and sung lullabies? What bosom fed you emotion-scattered, overwhelming, speechless pain? How did your mother come to be? Did she adorn with delicate, yet decadent lace that lingers long after death bringing reminders of what was, via song, scripture or sermon?

I ask you, again, grief, what is your name??

Do your eyes puff with sunrise's trickling red, yellow and orange embers as you awake from a night of tear-stained weeping; a reminder that the escape of dreaming is over.

Grief, do you also wish that same sleep would rescue you back to dream, because reality is too harsh, too stinging?

Acid to an open wound?

When the tone of my mother's voice becomes less rhythmic, more monotone, less laugh-filled, more littered with pause–I want to almost say the words with her as if to blunt the stab when she breathes deeply and whispers, "I have some bad news."

But grief, I don't know you.
Not like this.

You are to come with warning, preparation, a chance to reconcile replaying voice-mails when a voice is no longer.

A chance to find old pictures when flesh travels to morgue. You are to give us opportunity to go through ritual.

We need ritual…or so we thought.

Your son–tragedy, robs and steals from us. So we stand, rather, we crumble, shell-shocked.

Stranger, what is your name?

Until we meet again.

But oh! Shall I never you meet again. You make the taste of my own mortality too sweet.[20]

Boateng's poem, written and published during the COVID-19 pandemic, apostrophizes "grief." Grief is addressed, given attributes like lineage and the ability to carry "luggage," and yet remains a "stranger." Naming is one of the ways in life and in medicine that we categorize, and hence feel, we better understand, or even control, something. That something can be a diagnosis, which may hold unknowns within it, but it can also be far more elusive: a boundless, inchoate concept. This complex poem, in which we meet the narrator's mother bearing "bad news," conjures images of "flesh travel[ing] to morgue" *as* we witness the narrator repeatedly attempt to understand how and why grief came to be such a dominant part of the human condition, and contextualize the pandemic within the arc of human loss and suffering.

Some of the poems examined in this section relate directly to the practice of anesthesiology, particularly because such practice includes the witnessing and alleviation of pain and suffering. The following section deals even more directly with not only how anesthesiology is portrayed in poem but also how the act of providing an anesthetic holds poetic elements.

POETRY AND ANESTHESIOLOGY

For the purposes of the comparison of poetry and anesthesiology, "poetry" is used here to broadly include the genre of poetry, poetics, poetry making, and poems. Anesthesiology is also used broadly, to include providing anesthesia care (such as the practice of anesthesia, the delivery of anesthetics), the experience of general anesthesia, and the experience of the anesthesiologist or trainee.

Poetry and altered states are complex: they are both simultaneously specific and ambiguous, linear and defiant of boundaries, well-studied entities, and incompletely defined or partially known. The dynamics of poetry are applicable to the practice of anesthesiology, where both intimacy and detachment are experienced, at times, in intense and fraught ways. The reader of a poem brings their individual experience and history to the reading and thus forms a unique relationship with the poem and the poet. The patient and the anesthesiologist bring their own expectations and experiences to the discussion of an anesthetic, and this complicated, usually quite brief, interaction can have the feel of the creation of a new relationship, a new understanding of the other.

Although vastly different in purpose and outcome, anesthesiology training and classes on poetry are both replete with new and potentially uncomfortable, overwhelming experiences, as well as providing entrées to new language, specialty-specific jargon, and rituals. Such rituals are different in tone and embodiment, but each set, such as, for poetry: reading a poem aloud before class analysis, listening for rhythms, following themes for poetry courses, or, for anesthesiology: the donning of scrubs, entering a restricted area of the hospital, preparing equipment, anticipating the pace for preoperative, intraoperative, and postoperative care, has physical, intellectual, and emotional qualia.

Exploring the properties of poetry and anesthesia, such as allusion, boundedness, porosity, disruption, voice, breath, and surprise, can illuminate both poetics and anesthetics. **Fig. 2** compares poetry and anesthesia in 3 domains: form, rhythm, and purpose. For example, in the domain of form, the visual analysis of the poem as object — with its crisp hospital sheetlike border, the flush or ragged margins, the placement of title and poet's name, can be likened to a visual analysis of the anesthetizing location, with the patient center stage. Similarly, the anesthesiologist and the reader of poetry are both attuned to rhythms, disruptions in rhythms, and repetitions. However, the third domain, purpose, holds the widest divergence, because the purpose of poetry centers on interpretation and creativity, whereas the purpose of the anesthetic is caring for the individual patient.

Fig. 3, an image of the operating room with an imagined patient, and the following poem attempt to illustrate this comparison.

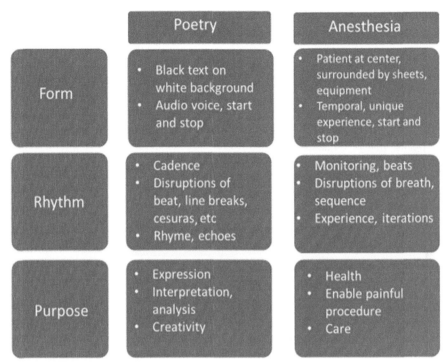

	Poetry	Anesthesia
Form	• Black text on white background • Audio voice, start and stop	• Patient at center, surrounded by sheets, equipment • Temporal, unique experience, start and stop
Rhythm	• Cadence • Disruptions of beat, line breaks, cesuras, etc • Rhyme, echoes	• Monitoring, beats • Disruptions of breath, sequence • Experience, iterations
Purpose	• Expression • Interpretation, analysis • Creativity	• Health • Enable painful procedure • Care

Fig. 2. A comparison of poetry and anesthesia along 3 domains: form, rhythm, and purpose.

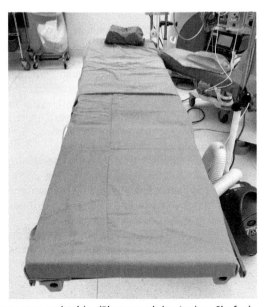

Fig. 3. An operating room and table. (Photograph by Audrey Shafer.)

ANESTHESIA IS A POEM

By Audrey Shafer

> Begin: an arc rises
> from pain, suffering, love
> tendrils flow to past and future
>
> but here, now, this matters
> demands: pay attention
>
> peaks, valleys, cadences
> pauses, surprises, turns, breaths
> echoes, comforts, but also
> a knowledge of the abyss
> a body exposed, raw
>
> intensely intimate
> layered mystery
>
> time expands, contracts
> and thus encapsulated, concludes
> the end opens our eyes
> light enters
> look: the arc sets
> just there, beyond the horizon.[21]

The caveat of depersonalization and hence dehumanization needs to be addressed, because the patient cannot be reduced, simplified to the text of a poem without loss and distortion. In anesthesia practice, the patient is frequently alluded to—transformed metonymically to lines on the monitor, for example, or metaphorically as in a vessel for disease—during the time that the patient's personhood is hidden by general anesthesia. The metaphoric resonances of the relatively innocuous phrase, "under anesthesia," wherein "anesthesia" becomes not only an entity but also something one is beneath in some way, with all the negative connotations of being down (such as death, misfortune, and poor status), are explored, along with metonyms for patients and their bodies, in the article, "Metaphor and Anesthesia."[22]

Although reification of the patient, particularly the incapacitated patient, is dehumanizing, to deny that patients are objectified during medical care is to forego critical analysis of the experience of illness. The risk of dehumanization increases when analogies of the nonhuman and the patient are too closely aligned, too tightly bound, leading to a distancing of the practitioner and the patient. For example, the main character of Margaret Edson's play Wit, Dr Vivian Bearing, whose life work was rigorous interpretation of John Donne's poetry, remarks on being ignored as a whole person while she is a patient with ovarian cancer. She attempts to confront the confusion of the physical and the metaphysical, the treatment of her as an individual versus as a vessel for anticancer therapies, while being in the disempowered position of being ill and hospitalized.[23]

The anesthesiologist frequently becomes the advocate, protector, and voice for the patient, both before and after rendering their patient incapacitated. The reliance on close attention paid to an individual under anesthesia is a hallmark of anesthesia care. The following points summarize this comparison of poetry and anesthesiology:

- The reading and writing of poetry, as well as the practice of anesthesia demand close attention
- Both a poem and the time frame of an anesthetic are bounded
- Poetry and anesthesia care depend on specialized language and norms
- Rhythms are critical to both poetry and anesthesia
- Altered states can be attributes of both poetry and anesthesia, but the cause, purpose, and nature of those states differ
- Critical differences between poetry and anesthesia include the life and health of an individual as the central focus in the practice of anesthesia, and the impetus to create new understanding through words in poetry
- Comparisons of the arts and medicine can illuminate both fields, but beware of dangers such as simplification, forced equivalence, and reification.

POETRY, WRITING POETRY, AND WELL-BEING

A growing interest in the beneficial effects of the arts on health and well-being for patients and health practitioners has led to research and subsequent literature reviews. In particular, access to a variety of art interventions, including poetry, with inclusion in care ("arts on prescription") or as part of health practitioners' opportunities, has demonstrated improvement in mental health, sense of well-being, and attitudes toward the work environment.[24]

The experience of reading poetry can frame and illuminate one's own experiences of illness and caregiving. Furthermore, the act of writing poetry can provide a much needed sense of perspective. Johanna Shapiro, the founder of the medical humanities program at University of California Irvine School of Medicine, writes, "Illness in my family and myself made me feel helpless and hopeless. Writing about illness for me restored a sense of control."[25]

Certain subspecialties may have particular interests in how poetry impacts health care and the experiences of those involved. For example, the range of powerful emotions, including the need for solace and feelings of anger, grief, and regret, in the multidisciplinary world of palliative care make this a particularly potent area to develop poetry and medicine workshops as opportunities for patients, families, and health care workers. Benefits ranging from breathing techniques by reciting short poems, to providing acknowledgment of difficult situations along with coping mechanisms, and community building and connection among staff have been postulated and are under study.[26]

Likewise, some illnesses can have particular symptoms or effects that benefit from the addition of poetry, and thus improve patient well-being. A preliminary study of patients with multiple sclerosis undergoing speech therapy for dysarthria found improved levels of confidence in communication when the speech pathologist was joined by a poet who included poetry in the exercises.[27] Cancer-related pain reduction through a poetry-based intervention may also improve coping skills and a sense of hope.[28] Poetry has been found to reduce a sense of isolation felt by some patients, such as those with depression or other mental health issues; this has led to ongoing studies of the potential impact on feelings of loneliness due to social isolation resulting from the COVID-19 pandemic. Poetry may thus impact public health. Poetry, by fostering "creative introspection," connects people to their surroundings, other people, and the world at large.[29]

Academic and independent centers offer ways for people to connect with and write poetry. The Medicine and the Muse Program at Stanford University School of Medicine, for example, hosts a variety of programs and collaborations. Pegasus Physician

Writers hold an annual poetry and music concert, featuring ekphrastic poetry written by physicians and students, with chamber music played by the St. Lawrence String Quartet.[30] The Stuck@Home concert series, started due to the isolation of pandemic, intermittently featured those in health care writing poetry.[31] Stanford medical students can apply for funding to complete a poetry project through the medical scholars program and the Biomedical Ethics and Medical Humanities Scholarly Concentration.[32] Led by writer Laurel Braitman, Director of Writing and Storytelling, students, trainees, physicians, and health professionals from around the world write and share their work through guided workshops such as retreats and the Writing Medicine program.[33] All the programs have generated comments on stress reduction and community building benefits.[34]

More research is needed on the health and well-being impacts of poetry reading and writing. In particular, studying the impact of illness, access to health care, systemic racism, and the rigors of medical training and practice through poetry analysis, reading, and writing by a variety of patients and health care workers could illuminate how issues of diversity, equity, inclusion, and justice influence health, health care, and well-being.

SUMMARY

Poetry and medicine interact in multiple ways, with educational and therapeutic possibilities. Because both poetry and medicine invest in understanding the human condition and forming connections, they overlap significantly in our attempts to understand life, health, mortality and our desire to create meaning. Reading poetry related to illness, debility, death, caregiving, and medical practice can enlarge our understanding of what health care workers do, and why they do it.

Anesthesiology is, in many ways, crystallized medicine—all the elements of patient interaction and care are there, but in a heightened timeframe and within highly stylized and specialized spaces. Similarly, poetry holds all the elements of literature, and even some nonverbal arts, yet compresses them, highlighting rhythms, individual word choices, and resonances. Both anesthesiology and poetry refer to past and future, while intensely focusing attention on the present, using creative and critical thinking.

Through poetry, whether reading, sharing, or writing, we give ourselves permission to think about our roles, our lives, our interactions with others, and our relationship with the world. Thus, poetry creates a space that enables us to pause, to reflect, to recharge. Ironically, poems about difficult subjects—loss, grief, regret, pain—can improve well-being by providing connection. Poetry shows us that our individual experiences and journeys are part of the larger human experience, and hence can improve understanding and well-being.

DISCLOSURE

The author has nothing to disclose.

REFERENCES

1. Frost R. The road not taken. Available at: https://www.poetryfoundation.org/poems/44272/the-road-not-taken. Accessed September 3, 2021.
2. Auden WH. Funeral blues. Available at: https://allpoetry.com/Funeral-Blues. Accessed September 3, 2021.
3. Excerpt from Four Weddings and a Funeral. Available at: https://www.youtube.com/watch?v=DDXWclpGhcg. Accessed September 3, 2021.

4. Tuama PÓ. Poetry unbound. On Being podcast platform. Available at: https://onbeing.org/series/poetry-unbound/. Accessed September 6, 2021.

5. Author guidelines, Anesthesia and Analgesia section: The Human Experience. Available at: https://edmgr.ovid.com/aa/accounts/ifauth.htm#thehumanexperience. Accessed September 4, 2021.

6. Author guidelines, Anesthesiology section: Mind to Mind. Available at: https://pubs.asahq.org/anesthesiology/pages/instructions-for-authors-paper-types#mindtomind. Accessed September 4, 2021.

7. Belli A, Coulehan J. Blood and Bone: Poems by Physicians. Iowa (USA): University of Iowa Press; 1998.

8. Litmed: literature, arts, medicine database, NYU Langone Health. Available at: https://medhum.med.nyu.edu/. Accessed September 4, 2021.

9. Paul Kalanithi Writing Award. Stanford Medicine and the Muse Program. Available at: https://med.stanford.edu/medicineandthemuse/events/paul-kalanithi-essay-contest.html. Accessed September 4, 2021.

10. Irvin D. Yalom Literary Award, Pegasus Physician Writers. Available at: http://www.pegasusphysicians.com/programs-awards. Accessed September 4, 2021.

11. Hippocrates Initiative for Poetry and Medicine. Available at: http://hippocrates-poetry.org/. Accessed September 4, 2021.

12. Williams WC. Annual Poetry Competition, Northeastern Ohio Medical University College of Medicine. Available at: https://www.neomed.edu/medicine/poetry-competition/. Accessed September 4, 2021.

13. For short stories, see Williams WC. The doctor stories, compiled by Robert Coles. New York: New Directions; 1984.

14. For sample poem, Williams WC. The Last Words of My English Grandmother. Available at: https://www.poeticous.com/william-carlos-williams/the-last-words-of-my-english-grandmother. Accessed September 6, 2021.

15. Keats J. Ode to a Nightingale. Available at: https://www.poetryfoundation.org/poems/44479/ode-to-a-nightingale. Accessed September 8, 2021.

16. Browne K. Documentary film, Why Doctors Write Trailer. available at: https://www.whydoctorswrite.org/. Accessed September 8, 2021.

17. Nussbaum M. Love's knowledge: essays on philosophy and literature. Oxford: Oxford University Press; 1990. p. 47.

18. Childers C. Translation of Sappho 31. In: Literary matters: The Association of Literary Scholars, Critics and Writers. Available at: https://www.literarymatters.org/1-1-sappho-31/. Accessed September 3, 2021.

19. Dickinson E. Pain has an element of blank. 1924. Available at: MedHumChat. https://www.medhumchat.com/discussionguides/2019/6/18/emily-dickinson-pain-has-an-element-of-blank. Accessed September 4, 2021. From Dickinson E. Complete Poems Part One: Life XIX. Boston: Little, Brown and Company.

20. Boateng A. Grief, what is your name? Anesthesia and Analgesia 2021; 133:289. Available at: https://journals.lww.com/anesthesia-analgesia/Fulltext/2021/07000/Grief,_What_Is_Your_Name_.36.aspx. Accessed September 6, 2021.

21. Shafer A. Anesthesia Is a Poem. Presented at the Aesthetics and anesthetics: Boundaries and crossings in poetry and anesthesia. International Health Humanities Consortium Conference. Chicago, poster, March 28, 2019.

22. Shafer A. Metaphor and anesthesia. Anesthesiology 1995;83:1331–42.

23. Edson M. Wit. New York: Farrar, Straus & Giroux; 1999.

24. Jensen A, Bonde O. The use of arts interventions for mental health and wellbeing in health settings. Perspect Public Health 2018;138(4):209–14.

25. Shapiro J. Healing words: My journey with poetry and medicine. Fam Syst Health 2020;38(3):334–7, 335.
26. Davies EA. Why we need more poetry in palliative care. BMJ Support Palliat Care 2018;8:266–70.
27. Balchin R, Hersh D, Grantis J, et al. "Ode to confidence": poetry groups for dysarthria in multiple sclerosis. Int J Speech Lang Pathol 2020;22(3):347–58.
28. Arruda MA, Garcia MA, Garcia JB. Evaluation of the effects of music and poetry in oncologic pain relief: A randomized clinical trial. J Palliat Med 2016;19(9): 943–8.
29. Xiang DH, Yi AM. A look back and a path forward: Poetry's healing power during the pandemic. J Med Humanit 2020;41:603–8, 605.
30. Pegasus Physician Writers. Available at: http://www.pegasusphysicians.com/. Accessed September 8, 2021.
31. Stanford Stuck@Home concert series. Available at: https://med.stanford.edu/medicineandthemuse/events/stuck-home-concert-.html. Accessed September 8, 2021.
32. Biomedical ethics and medical humanities medical scholars funded projects. Available at: https://med.stanford.edu/medicineandthemuse/Education/publications/projects.html. Accessed September 8, 2021.
33. Reflective writing session for healthcare workers and their loved ones. Available at: https://www.laurelbraitman.com/writingmedicine. Accessed September 8, 2021.
34. MacCormick H. How writing helps medical students and doctors handle stress. Scopeblog. 2020. Available at: https://scopeblog.stanford.edu/2020/05/20/how-writing-helps-medical-students-and-doctors-handle-stress/. Accessed September 8, 2021..

Well-being in the Intensive Care Unit
Looking Beyond COVID-19

Sheela Pai Cole, MD[a],*, Shahla Siddiqui, MD, DABA, MSc, FCCM[b]

KEYWORDS

- Compassion fatigue • Burnout syndrome • Compassion satisfaction
- Secondary traumatic stress • Moral injury • Psychological resilience

KEY POINTS

- Wellbeing in the intensive care unit (ICU) is affected by a combination of personal factors, organizational factors, quality of interpersonal relationships, and exposure to end-of-life issues.
- Moral injury occurs when an act is perpetrated, one bears witness to or fails to prevent an act that is against deeply held moral beliefs.
- Second victim syndrome is the guilt and other psychological onslaught faced by health care providers who hold themselves responsible following unexpected patient morbidity or mortality.
- Leadership held check-ins, active listening to feedback, and availability of wellness resources help mitigate health care worker (HCW) burnout.
- Training in communication, conflict resolution, and simulation of team-based care aid in creating collaborative scenarios and clarifying roles among multi-disciplinary teams.

INTRODUCTION

Critical care medicine is a subspecialty characterized by intense clinical situations balanced by immense reward in the care of critically ill patients in the intensive care unit (ICU).[1,2] Intensivists often work in multidisciplinary paradigms, frequently engaging with other physicians, advanced practice providers, nurses, and ancillary

[a] Department of Anesthesiology, Perioperative and Pain Medicine, Stanford University, 300 Pasteur Drive, H3580, Stanford, CA 94305, USA; [b] Department of Anesthesia, Critical Care and Pain Medicine, Beth Israel Deaconess Medical Center, Harvard Medical School, 330 Brookline Avenue, Boston, MA 02215, USA
* Corresponding author.
E-mail address: spaicole@stanford.edu
Twitter: @SheelaPaiCole (S.P.C.); @shahlasi (S.S.)

Anesthesiology Clin 40 (2022) 373–382
https://doi.org/10.1016/j.anclin.2022.01.010
anesthesiology.theclinics.com

staff.[3,4] The critical care team works in tandem to manage complicated, life-threatening illnesses, initiate end-of-life conversations, collaborate with consultants, among many other high-acuity tasks.[4] These cumulative demands may, over time, contribute to an intensivist's perceived lack of autonomy and poor work–life balance.[5,6] Coupled with frequent sleep deprivation, this may result in an increased incidence of depression, anxiety, and burnout syndrome (BOS) in ICU physicians compared with other physicians.[7] Burnout is more common among physicians compared with the general population. Global literature has shown a high rate of burnout within all specialties of medicine.[2] The 2020 National Physician Burnout and Suicide Report showed a 44% rate of burnout among ICU physicians compared with 41% of general anesthesiologists.[8,9] The above description has been amplified by the ongoing COVID-19 pandemic not only due to dying patients but also personal factors such as changes in workload and wages coupled with job insecurity.[10,11] There have been a multitude of metaphorical images depicting the "physician as hero" role, such as the submerged physician holding a patient bed afloat—in other words, saving the patient at the cost of drowning themselves.

Considering the existence of widespread incidence of BOS among all levels of ICU practitioners before the COVID-19 pandemic, in 2016 an official statement entitled "Burnout Syndrome in Critical Care Health care Professionals. A Call for Action," was jointly prepared and published by the American Thoracic Society (ATS), American College of Chest Physicians (CHEST), American Association of Critical-Care Nurses (AACN), and Society of Critical Care Medicine (SCCM) in their corresponding professional journals.[12] Although the statement predates the pandemic, many of the factors predisposing to BOS highlighted in the report are relevant and magnified in the current moment, such as at-risk personal characteristics, work–life balance, and organizational pressures. These factors may cumulatively lead to a high rate of turnover, poor quality of patient care, and reduced patient satisfaction. Another initiative in 2020 was the Critical Care Societies' collaborative National Summit and Survey on Prevention and Management of Burnout in the ICU. The summit identified that society is at risk of losing this essential workforce and it is imperative to investigate the root causes of ICU clinician BOS. Addressing physician and caregiver well-being is important for staff retention and is associated with improved patient outcomes, increased patient satisfaction, lower infection rates, and lower medication errors.[13]

Wellbeing Versus Burnout Syndrome

Well-being in the workplace is defined as "the presence of professional fulfillment and the absence of burnout."[14]Stamm and colleagues, coined the term Professional Quality-of-life (ProQOL) which consists of both positive and negative elements (ie, compassion satisfaction and compassion fatigue are important determinants of well-being in the workplace).[15,16] Maslach and colleagues, defined the term BOS by assessing 3 components: (1) emotional exhaustion, (2) depersonalization, and (3) lack of professional achievement or fulfillment.[17] The efficacy of validated instruments to assess burnout such as ProQOL and BOS increases when results are garnered from groups working in similar environments.[15]

Instruments for data collection such as Professional Quality of Life (ProQOL) have been used in various health care communities to demonstrate a direct association between the presence of compassion fatigue (ie, the negative feeling associated with constant self-giving leading to discomfort) and an increased incidence of BOS as well as an inverse relationship between compassion satisfaction (ie, the positive feeling associated with helping others and often the premise that leads health care workers (HCWs) to their careers) and BOS.[18] Compassion fatigue and BOS are more commonly seen among ICU nurses compared with ICU physicians, which might be attributed to the current crisis of nation-wide nursing shortages.

Concepts and Definitions Associated with Well-being Literature

Compassionate care is essential to health care delivery. Compassion satisfaction, compassion fatigue, burnout, and secondary traumatic stress are all frequently coined terms when discussing the correlates of total well-being. It is equally important to have the definitions imprinted as it is to have real-world examples to reflect on. Compassion satisfaction is the positive feeling associated with helping others. It is the passion that drives most physicians to start careers in medicine. It is the satisfaction an ICU physician experiences when a patient previously on life-support returns to the ICU for a visit after being discharged home. This is in direct contrast to compassion fatigue. Compassion fatigue was initially described by Figley in 1982 as "the cost of caring," which is amplified when health care workers are unable to refuel.[19,20] It describes the emotional toll that occurs with a continued outpouring of compassionate care. It is frequently seen among health care providers who seem unfazed by death and dying. BOS is the individual response to work-related events that occur in workers without baseline psychological disorders. A diagnosis of BOS requires all 3 components, as described by Christina Maslach: high depersonalization, high emotional exhaustion, and low personal fulfillment. Finally, secondary traumatic stress is the stress experienced by witnesses to trauma, usually as a "bystander."[21,22] This is especially true among ICU nurses who are frequently not decision makers but partake in the day-to-day care of the ailing patient.

Implications of the Coronavirus Pandemic

The COVID-19 pandemic has exacted enormous health care, economic, and psychological burdens globally.[23] Devastating effects of the pandemic include: high rates of infection and death, financial hardships faced by society and individuals, anxiety due to uncertainty of the future, personal health-related outcomes, and stress of childcare, to name a few.[24] HCWs are at the frontlines of the pandemic and face ongoing unprecedented challenges in treating unmanageable surges of patients with COVID-19, in working with public health officials to decrease the spread of infection, developing suitable short-term strategies, and formulating long-term plans.[25] The World Health Organization (WHO) estimates approximately 179,500 HCWs have died due to the COVID-19 pandemic worldwide.[26] The psychological burden and overall wellness of HCWs, and intensivists in particular, has received increased awareness, as the lay press and medical literature continue to report high rates of burnout, psychological stress, and suicide among clinicians including ICU providers.[27,28] Reports of increased COVID-19-related stress, anxiety, depression, burnout, suicide, and PTSD among frontline ICU staff including physicians are increasing.[28]

The high rate of COVID-19 mortality compounded by ongoing surges due to inconsistent vaccination in the US and globally and the politicization of COVID-19 therapies and inoculation has contributed to alarming rates of emotional exhaustion and burnout among HCWs, many of whom are now leaving the profession.[20] Additional challenges faced by intensivists include: fear of infecting family and loved ones, job insecurity due to potentially protracted personal illness, anxiety regarding the supply and quality of personal protective equipment (PPE), adapting to ever-changing hospital guidelines and operating procedures and policies, sustaining physically demanding and long work hours, particularly when faced with staffing shortages, and reconciling a professional commitment to helping others with the need to protect one's self.[18]

Risk Factors for Burnout among Intensive Care Unit Personnel

BOS risk factors can be grouped into 4 main categories.[12] Fessell and colleagues suggest a fifth category described later in discussion as a recent addition based on lessons learned from caring for patients during the pandemic.[25]

1. Personal characteristics: self-criticism, idealism, perfectionism, inadequate coping strategies, sleep deprivation, and overcommitment. These characteristics are often seen among highly productive workers.[21]
2. Organizational factors: unmanageable workload, lack of control over the work environment, insufficient rewards, and general breakdown in the work community. Specifically, for critical care physicians, night shifts and lack of time off between ICU weeks increased burnout, whereas for nurses, lack of ability in choosing days off and rapid patient turnover increased BOS.[23]
3. Quality of working relationships is an important modifiable risk factor for BOS. The conflicts between members of multidisciplinary teams caring for a complex patient as well as difficult HCW–patient relationships exact a toll on clinician well-being.
4. Exposure to end-of-life issues: Critical Care nurses cite increased burnout related to care of a dying patient—witnessing, and participating in transitions to comfort care Critical care physicians cite increased burnout due to: the constant exposure to inappropriate care (this can be related to delays in care and/or the wrong amount of care) (an example would include delivery of inaccurate information to a patient or family, disrespecting a patient's wishes, and advocating that another patient might benefit from an ICU bed as issues that compound).[24,29]
5. The pandemic has unearthed unprecedented anxiety and conflict among HCWs due to resource shortages and politicization of standard preventative measures such as wearing a mask, social distancing, avoiding super-spreader events, and vaccination to protect against severe disease. This is magnified among ICU personnel as they care for the most critically ill patients that often require resource-intensive advanced therapies including mechanical ventilation and extracorporeal membrane oxygenation.[25]

Moral Injury and Intensive Care Unit Practice

Moral injury occurs when an act is perpetrated, one bears witness to or fails to prevent an act that is against deeply held moral beliefs.[30] The term was first used in health care to describe the emotional turmoil suffered by nursing personnel after long hours of patient care that ultimately resulted in an unavoidable fatal outcome.[22] Among health care providers, any act that is in contradiction to the Hippocratic oath or serves as an impediment to deliver safe care to patients may be a source of moral injury. Intensivists may face several triggers for moral injury, such as observing undue patient suffering from delays in end-of-life discussions or poor clinical decision-making, communication challenges in brain death notifications, misunderstandings regarding do not resuscitate status, inappropriate or inaccessible care delivery, poor outcomes due to health delivery disparities, psychiatric issues and addiction leading to suboptimal outcomes, and engaging with grieving families.[31] Critical care physicians are often drawn to the field to care for the seriously ill; however, complex regulatory, insurance, and quality reporting requirements have led to increased documentation and other administrative activities, drawing away from time spent that would otherwise be spent at the bedside. This incongruence between clinician ideals and the reality of clinical medicine may further contribute to feelings of dissatisfaction. [31]

The COVID-19 pandemic has wrought additional moral injury, as intensivists continue to manage unprecedented volumes of high-acuity patients and navigate unknown and often futile treatment options.[28] The moral, psychological, and physical exhaustion and injury adds to compassion fatigue, medical errors, a lack of empathy in treating patients and caring for families, lower productivity, and higher staff turnover rates. The ability of HCWs to adequately cope with these stressors is important for their patients, their families, and for themselves. Left unchecked, long term, severe stressors can contribute to significant physical and mental health problems and low "psychological resilience" (the ability to positively adapt to adversity to protect themselves from stress). Another pandemic-induced burden to critical care personnel is the ethical constraints of shortages of ICU beds, ventilators, essential medicines, PPE, and staffing. Critical care personnel are tasked with enormously distressing difficult decisions around resource allocation, triaging patients, and assigning extremely limited resources that are essential to save a patient's life.[32] This further compounds moral burden and distress.[19]

Second Victim Syndrome

Second victim syndrome is defined as the guilt and psychological onslaught faced by health care providers who feel responsible following an unexpected patient morbidity or mortality event.[33] It may also refer to the struggle faced by HCWs from medical errors, unmanageably long working hours, under-supported medical practices, and lack of psychological support after a patient fatality or major adverse event.[34,35] In addition to the primary caregiver, second victims may include colleagues called in to help during an acute event, support personnel, students, and others who may have been involved in the event or the immediate aftermath.[36]

Second victims often experience fear, guilt, self-doubt, shame, anger, reliving of the event, sleep disturbance, and anxiety.[29,37] These emotions mirror symptoms of acute stress disorder and posttraumatic stress disorder and may affect HCWs both at work and at home. Such emotions may persist for weeks to years and lead to burnout, substance abuse, and even suicide. In a 2012 national survey of the impact of perioperative catastrophes on anesthesiologists, more than 60% of respondents experienced depression and 19% indicated that they never fully recovered from the experience and felt that their ability to provide care for the first 4 hours after an adverse event was impaired.[37] Although there is a dearth of literature among ICU physicians, the rate of second victim syndrome has been shown to be anywhere from 10% to 40% in this group.[35]

Solutions to Mitigate Burnout and Improve Intensivist Fulfillment

Later in discussion, we describe pandemic-specific measures to address well-being and discuss long-term solutions to mitigate BOS and improve overall well-being in the critical care community.

COVID-19-SPECIFIC MEASURES TO IMPROVE CRITICAL CARE CLINICIAN WELL-BEING
Community Building

The pandemic reified the importance of a workplace community in mitigating burnout and promoting well-being. Clinical leaders can build and reinforce resilience in their teams by displaying compassion. In the authors' collective experience, we have witnessed thoughtful leaders checking in frequently, listening to feedback, providing wellness resources and support, and demonstrating compassion to their team.[38] This sense of togetherness and care can significantly bolster team morale and sustain clinicians during highly stressful times. Guided conversations or town halls to foster communication can provide reassurance of future stability and help staff collectively envision a future beyond the pandemic.[39] "Work-from-home regime engagement activities" are useful for employees as well as for institutions. "Those organizations doing these kinds of engagement activities for their employees are learning new skills and developing themselves."[40] This hopeful outlook begins with leadership and serves as a sustaining source of team morale. Indeed, in times of extreme stress, teams need to trust and rely on one another and leadership for support.[41–43]

Long-term Measures to Mitigate Burnout

Communication training

Institutional commitment to mitigate intensivist BOS could include the incorporation of team building and community building programs that strengthen team dynamics and patient care. Incorporating daily multidisciplinary rounds (MDR) helps to clarify roles among various ICU providers including nursing, respiratory therapy, physical and occupational therapy, and social workers. MDRs also aid in the synthesis of comprehensive care plans for patients and facilitate ICU discharge.[44] In their postimplementation survey, O'Brien and colleagues, demonstrated the feasibility of incorporating MDR into the ICU workflow and improved overall communication between all members of the ICU team.[44] Debriefings after adverse events such as cardiac arrest are another example of fostering team building. Dedicated time for debriefing lauds effective team actions identifies opportunities for future growth and create collaborative scenarios between teams.[45,46] In a single-center postcode debriefing survey, code response satisfaction improved[47] and staff members described an increase in peer and institutional support after the implementation of a debriefing protocol.[48]

Further, dedicated training in communication and conflict resolution via team-based care simulation may be helpful. For example, *Vitaltalk,* a team-based simulation training program, is being adopted at many institutions to hone critical care trainees' communication skillsets to bridge patient values with treatment plans.[49] These programs intend to reduce BOS among ICU staff and hasten emotional healing after stressful events.

Post-intensive Care Unit Clinics and Longevity Programs

Post-ICU clinics help patients and their families re-acclimatize to normal life and allow ICU providers to experience post-ICU outcomes. Sharing details of patient survival constitutes continuity of care and serves as a form of evaluation and validation for the care provided during the ICU course and may boost clinician morale.[42] As an example, The Society of Critical Care Medicine's (SCCM) THRIVE program provides resources and education for ICU patient survivors and their families related to postintensive care syndrome and has had a significant impact on ICU physician morale and well-being.[42] Other benefits of post-ICU programs include identifying unforeseen outcomes of ICU therapies (eg, stop dates for certain medications), forming a network of ICU survivors as support for other critically ill patients and families, facilitating post-ICU follow-up education to ICU providers, and providing insight into the patient experience during an ICU stay. One challenge of sustaining a post-ICU program is that fiscal support typically falls outside traditional payment models and requires sustainable institutional investment.

Flexible Scheduling

Control of one's schedule is an important determinant of personal and professional satisfaction. With the advent of high acuity intensive care units (ICU) caring for patients on mechanical circulatory support, large-volume centers are attempting to move toward continuous in-house coverage by critical care faculty. Purported advantages of this model are improved patient care and patient satisfaction, especially when this care model is accompanied by a "system change." System change involves the institution of measures such as liberation from mechanical ventilation, goals of care conversations, and other interventions around the clock instead of deferring these "non-emergent" tasks to the day team caring for the patient.[41,43,50]

Traditional ICU coverage is allocated in 7-day assignments with integrated overnight coverage. This model can result in physicians spending more than 33 consecutive hours in the ICU. Proponents of the traditional model tout continuity of care and patient safety as the biggest advantages of this approach. Some institutions have mitigated long ICU shifts by creating a shift-based system (ie, separate day and night shifts). Concerns with shift-based models include discontinuity of care and patient safety as there are more frequent hand-offs between ICU personnel and greater coverage of nights and weekends throughout the year. Geva and colleagues, recently described a simulated model of shared service scheduling whereby 4 ICU attendings shared most of the day and nighttime service for 2 teams over a 2-week period with creative assignments to avoid 30 plus hour shifts.[51] This simulation study found more continuity of care and less handoffs, making it safer for patients while facilitating improved intensivist work–life balance with more weekends off throughout the year. Further, implementation data on this simulation paradigm are awaited.

SUMMARY

Advocating for personal well-being strategies such as self-care, self-forgiveness, and mindfulness may anecdotally help with reducing burnout and increasing professional well-being. However, institutional support in incorporating efficient practices and building a culture of wellness through systems-based changes may be more effective in recruiting and retaining a well workforce.[3,52,53] Appointing institutional or departmental well-being officers who are well versed in clinical workflow inefficiencies and have the skillset to advocate for their peers and colleagues are essential in supporting an institutional commitment to clinician well-being.[11] Finally, the COVID-19 pandemic has created a unique psychological quagmire among critical care professionals. Reducing intensivist burnout through proactive, multifaceted measures by institutions can help retain motivated and patient-centered clinicians that can continue providing the quality of care that we envision for our own loved ones.

DISCLOSURE

The authors have nothing to disclose.

CLINICS CARE POINTS

- Moral injury occurs when an act is perpetrated, one bears witness to or fails to prevent an act that is against deeply held moral beliefs, especially in the care of a patient at the end of their lives. Having multidisciplinary debriefings to discuss different viewpoints among the various caregivers may help the team to understand the varying opinions and basis of care being provided.
- Lack of control over one's control schedule can be addressed by incorporating flexible scheduling paradigms.
- Difficult relationships among members of different specialties caring for the same critically ill patient can be modified by providing communication and conflict resolution training, and simulation programs for team-based care

• Understanding a patient's progress after leaving the ICU by investing in post-ICU clinics helps HCWs realize the value of their efforts as well as gain perspective on the consequences of ICU therapies.

REFERENCES

1. Shanafelt T, Goh J, Sinsky C. The Business Case for Investing in Physician Well-being. Jama Intern Med 2017;177(12):1826.
2. Shanafelt TD. Enhancing Meaning in Work: A Prescription for Preventing Physician Burnout and Promoting Patient-Centered Care. Jama 2009;302(12): 1338–40.
3. Shanafelt T, Trockel M, Ripp J, et al. Building a Program on Well-Being: Key Design Considerations to Meet the Unique Needs of Each Organization. Acad Med J Assoc Am Med Coll 2019;94(2):156–61.
4. Cole SP. Burnout Prevention and Resilience Training for Critical Care Trainees. Int Anesthesiol Clin 2019;57(2):118–31.
5. Schäfer SK, Sopp MR, Staginnus M, et al. Correlates of mental health in occupations at risk for traumatization: a cross-sectional study. Bmc Psychiatry 2020; 20(1):335.
6. Geronazzo-Alman L, Eisenberg R, Shen S, et al. Cumulative exposure to work-related traumatic events and current post-traumatic stress disorder in New York City's first responders. Compr Psychiat 2017;74:134–43.
7. Mealer M. Burnout Syndrome in the Intensive Care Unit. Future Directions for Research. Ann Am Thorac Soc 2016;13(7):997–8.
8. Pines A, Maslach C. Characteristics of Staff Burnout in Mental Health Settings. Psychiatr Serv 1978;29(4):233–7.
9. Medscape National Physician Burnout & Suicide Report 2020: The Generational Divide.pdf. Available at: https://www.medscape.com/slideshow/2020-lifestyle-burnout-6012460. Accessed December 5, 2021.
10. Mitchell EP. Clinician Wellbeing during COVID-19. J Natl Med Assoc 2021; 113(5):481.
11. Dzau VJ, Kirsch D, Nasca T. Preventing a Parallel Pandemic — A National Strategy to Protect Clinicians' Well-Being. N Engl J Med 2020. https://doi.org/10.1056/nejmp2011027.
12. Moss M, Good VS, Gozal D, et al. A Critical Care Societies Collaborative Statement: Burnout Syndrome in Critical Care Health-care Professionals. A Call for Action. Am J Resp Crit Care 2016;194(1):106–13.
13. Kleinpell R, Moss M, Good VS, et al. The Critical Nature of Addressing Burnout Prevention: Results From the Critical Care Societies Collaborative's National Summit and Survey on Prevention and Management of Burnout in the ICU. Crit Care Med 2020;48(2):249–53.
14. Stobbs C. Maintaining personal resilience in this Covid-19 era. Practice 2021; 43(2):109–12.
15. Stamm Beth. ProQOL Manual.pdf. https://img1.wsimg.com/blobby/go/dfc1e1a0-a1db-4456-9391-18746725179b/downloads/ProQOL%20Manual.pdf?ver=1622839353725.
16. Xiong J, Lipsitz O, Nasri F, et al. Impact of COVID-19 Pandemic on Mental Health in the General Population: A Systematic Review. J Affect Disord 2020;277:55–64.
17. Lahav Y. Psychological distress related to COVID-19 – The contribution of continuous traumatic stress. J Affect Disord 2020;277:129–37.

18. Sterling MR, Tseng E, Poon A, et al. Experiences of Home Health Care Workers in New York City During the Coronavirus Disease 2019 Pandemic. Jama Intern Med 2020;180(11):1453–9.
19. Lai J, Ma S, Wang Y, et al. Factors Associated With Mental Health Outcomes Among Health Care Workers Exposed to Coronavirus Disease 2019. Jama Netw Open 2020;3(3):e203976.
20. Shen X, Zou X, Zhong X, et al. Psychological stress of ICU nurses in the time of COVID-19. Crit Care 2020;24(1):200.
21. Poncet MC, Toullic P, Papazian L, et al. Burnout Syndrome in Critical Care Nursing Staff. Am J Resp Crit Care 2012;175(7):698–704.
22. Jameton A. What Moral Distress in Nursing History Could Suggest about the Future of Health Care. Ama J Ethics 2017;19(6):617–28.
23. Embriaco N, Azoulay E, Barrau K, et al. High Level of Burnout in Intensivists. Am J Resp Crit Care 2007;175(7):686–92.
24. Piers RD, Azoulay E, Ricou B, et al. Perceptions of Appropriateness of Care Among European and Israeli Intensive Care Unit Nurses and Physicians. Jama 2011;306(24):2694–703.
25. Fessell D, Cherniss C. COVID-19 & Beyond: Micro-practices for Burnout Prevention and Emotional Wellness. J Am Coll Radiol 2020;17(6):746–8.
26. Organization WH, department H workforce. The Impact of COVID-19 on health and care workers: a closer look at deaths.
27. Chew NWS, Lee GKH, Tan BYQ, et al. A multinational, multicentre study on the psychological outcomes and associated physical symptoms amongst healthcare workers during COVID-19 outbreak. Brain Behav Immun 2020;88:559–65.
28. Restauri N, Sheridan AD. Burnout and Posttraumatic Stress Disorder in the Coronavirus Disease 2019 (COVID-19) Pandemic: Intersection, Impact, and Interventions. J Am Coll Radiol 2020;17(7):921–6.
29. Seys D, Wu AW, Gerven EV, et al. Health Care Professionals as Second Victims after Adverse Events. Eval Health Prof 2013;36(2):135–62.
30. Dean W, Talbot S, Dean A. Reframing Clinician Distress: Moral Injury Not Burnout. Fed Pract Heal Care Prof Va Dod Phs 2019;36(9):400–2.
31. Rosenthal MS, Clay M. Initiatives for Responding to Medical Trainees' Moral Distress about End-of-Life Cases. Ama J Ethics 2017;19(6):585–94.
32. Kenny N, Kotalik J, Herx L, et al. A Catholic Perspective: Triage Principles and Moral Distress in Pandemic Scarcity. Linacre Q 2021;88(2):214–23.
33. Wu AW. Medical error: the second victim. The doctor who makes the mistake needs help too. Bmj Clin Res Ed 2000;320(7237):726–7.
34. Busch IM, Scott SD, Connors C, et al. The Role of Institution-Based Peer Support for Health Care Workers Emotionally Affected by Workplace Violence. Jt Comm J Qual Patient Saf 2021;47(3):146–56.
35. Ozeke O, Ozeke V, Coskun O, et al. Second victims in health care: current perspectives</p&gt. Adv Med Educ Pract 2019;10:593–603.
36. Scott SD, Hirschinger LE, Cox KR, et al. The natural history of recovery for the healthcare provider "second victim" after adverse patient events. Qual Saf Heal Care 2009;18(5):325–30.
37. Gazoni FM, Amato PE, Malik ZM, et al. The Impact of Perioperative Catastrophes on Anesthesiologists. Anesth Analg 2012;114(3):596–603.
38. Giordano F, Cipolla A, Ungar M. Building resilience for healthcare professionals working in an Italian red zone during the COVID-19 outbreak: A pilot study. Stress Health 2021. https://doi.org/10.1002/smi.3085.

39. Mosanya M. Buffering Academic Stress during the COVID-19 Pandemic Related Social Isolation: Grit and Growth Mindset as Protective Factors against the Impact of Loneliness. Int J Appl Posit Psychol 2020;6(2):159–74.

40. Chanana N, Sangeeta. Employee engagement practices during COVID-19 lock-down. J Public Aff 2020;e2508.

41. Mikkelsen ME, Anderson BJ, Bellini L, et al. Burnout, and Fulfillment, in the Profession of Critical Care Medicine. Am J Resp Crit Care 2019;200(7):931–3.

42. Haines KJ, Sevin CM, Hibbert E, et al. Key mechanisms by which post-ICU activities can improve in-ICU care: results of the international THRIVE collaboratives. Intensive Care Med 2019;45(7):939–47.

43. Kerlin MP, McPeake J, Mikkelsen ME. Burnout and Joy in the Profession of Critical Care Medicine. Crit Care 2020;24(1):98.

44. O'Brien A, O'Reilly K, Dechen T, et al. Redesigning Rounds in the ICU: Standardizing Key Elements Improves Interdisciplinary Communication. Jt Comm J Qual Patient Saf 2018;44(10):590–8.

45. Couper K, Kimani PK, Davies RP, et al. An evaluation of three methods of in-hospital cardiac arrest educational debriefing: The cardiopulmonary resuscitation debriefing study. Resuscitation 2016;105:130–7.

46. Dine CJ, Gersh RE, Leary M, et al. Improving cardiopulmonary resuscitation quality and resuscitation training by combining audiovisual feedback and debriefing&ast. Crit Care Med 2008;36(10):2817–22.

47. Przednowek T, Stacey C, Baird K, et al. Implementation of a Rapid Post-Code Debrief Quality Improvement Project in a Community Emergency Department Setting. Spartan Med Res J 2021;6(1):21376.

48. Copeland D, Liska H. Implementation of a Post-Code Pause. J Trauma Nurs 2016;23(2):58–64.

49. Markin A, Cabrera-Fernandez DF, Bajoka RM, et al. Impact of a Simulation-Based Communication Workshop on Resident Preparedness for End-of-Life Communication in the Intensive Care Unit. Crit Care Res Pract 2015;2015:534879.

50. Nizamuddin J, Tung A. Intensivist staffing and outcome in the ICU. Curr Opin Anaesthesiol 2019;32(2):123–8.

51. Geva A, Landrigan CP, van der Velden MG, et al. Simulation of a Novel Schedule for Intensivist Staffing to Improve Continuity of Patient Care and Reduce Physician Burnout. Crit Care Med 2017;45(7):1138–44.

52. Shanafelt T, Swensen S. Leadership and Physician Burnout: Using the Annual Review to Reduce Burnout and Promote Engagement. Am J Med Qual 2017;32(5):563–5.

53. Shanafelt T, Ripp J, Trockel M. Understanding and Addressing Sources of Anxiety Among Health Care Professionals During the COVID-19 Pandemic. Jama 2020;323(21):2133.

Well-Being in Anesthesiology Graduate Medical Education
Reconciling the Ideal with Reality

Lauren Lisann-Goldman, MD[a], Christopher Cowart, MD[b], Hung-Mo Lin, ScD[c], Barbara Orlando, MD, PhD[d,*], Bryan Mahoney, MD[e]

KEYWORDS

- Graduate medical education • Resident well-being • Mindfulness
- Cognitive-behavioral therapy

KEY POINTS

- Burnout is an ongoing challenge in graduate medical education, especially in perioperative specialties.
- Mindfulness and cognitive-behavioral therapy (CBT) have shown promise in decreasing burnout; however, feasibility is likely context-dependent.
- Well-being interventions that address structural or systemic factors impacting well-being as opposed to interventions at the individual level may prove to be more effective in anesthesiology training programs.

INTRODUCTION

Burnout, "a state of mental and physical exhaustion related to work or caregiving activities," has been shown to impact 27% to 75% of graduate medical education (GME) trainees, with consequences including declining mental health, cardiovascular disease, poor sleep hygiene, chronically elevated stress levels, and malnutrition. Burnout rates in anesthesiology mirror those across medical specialties with rates between

[a] Department of Anesthesiology, Montefiore Medical Center, 111 E 210st, Bronx, NY 10467, USA; [b] Department of Anesthesiology and Perioperative Medicine, Penn State College of Medicine, 700 HMC Cres Road, Hershey, PA 17033, USA; [c] Department of Population Health Science and Policy, Icahn School of Medicine at Mount Sinai, 1 Gustave L. Levy Pl, NY 10029, USA; [d] Department of Anesthesiology, McGovern Medical School at the University of Texas Health Science Center- Houston, Memorial Hermann Hospital, 6431 Fannin Street, Houston, TX 77030, USA; [e] Department of Anesthesiology, Perioperative and Pain Medicine, Mount Sinai Morningside and West Hospitals, 1000 10th Avenue, NY 10019, USA
* Corresponding author.
E-mail address: barbara.orlando@uth.tmc.edu

Anesthesiology Clin 40 (2022) 383–397
https://doi.org/10.1016/j.anclin.2022.01.011
1932-2275/22/© 2022 Elsevier Inc. All rights reserved.

40% and 50%, with potential negative outcomes for patient care.[1–8] The negative consequences of burnout are particularly concerning among anesthesiology trainees given the high rate of substance abuse and suicide in this subspecialty.[9,10]

In response to this well-established causal relationship, the most recent core program requirements for the Accreditation Council for Graduate Medical Education (ACGME)-accredited programs, have included an emphasis on well-being guided by the rationale that "psychological, emotional, and physical well-being are critical in the development of the competent, caring, and resilient physician."[11] To this end, training programs are tasked with tracking resident well-being and implementing interventions when necessary. Anesthesiology training involves many relatively unmodifiable stressors such as production pressure, isolation from colleagues during the workday and a perceived lack of respect from surgical colleagues.[12] Programs confronted with evidence of burnout among trainees must, therefore, incorporate practical and effective interventions to mitigate the effects of the stressors inherent to anesthesiology residency training.

Interventions shown to reduce burnout include organizational initiatives targeting duty hours and workflow as well as individual-focused strategies.[13] Despite a growing call for structural or organizational approaches to address burnout, many programs continue to face economic or institutional barriers to such changes and are compelled to rely on individual-focused approaches.[14].

Our group thus attempted to develop and evaluate an individual-focused intervention to address anesthesiology resident burnout. The benefits of cognitive, behavioral, and mindfulness-based curricula have demonstrated benefit in burnout prevention.[13,15] MBSR has been implemented in anesthesiology training programs with mixed results based on validated survey tools assessing burnout and depression.[16] Acceptance of and attitudes toward these interventions among trainees in perioperative subspecialties significantly impact their efficacy and are poorly described in the literature.[17] Given the lack of evidence regarding the use and feasibility of in-person MBSR in conjunction with cognitive-behavioral therapy (CBT) in medical training programs, our group evaluated the effects of providing in-person MBSR and CBT on anesthesiology resident well-being and burnout.

We sought new strategies to address burnout among our trainees and developed a technique of directly querying residents in a safe space. "Confessions groups" have been demonstrated as an opportunity for residents to discuss and reflect on professional and personal challenges they face without fear of repercussion.[18] These sessions involve reading anonymous "confessions" aloud that have been previously submitted by group members. To develop specific interventions incorporating this feedback we used a structure inspired by the Delphi technique—an iterative process most often used to generate expert consensus—in which leadership responds to "confessions session" content with potential interventions that are then presented to the residents in subsequent sessions.[19,20]

Herein we chronicle a 2-part journey seeking effective interventions to address burnout among anesthesiology residents. Our initial intervention represented an individual-focused approach consisting of in-person MBSR and CBT. The impact on resident well-being and burnout was measured via hair cortisol levels, Maslach Burnout Inventory (MBI) scores, and sleep status level (SSL), all of which yielded insight into attitudinal and logistical barriers to wellness. To address these barriers, we pivoted to implement a "confessions session" model for generating ideas and program-level changes in work schedules and workflow. Efficacy was assessed through internal and external (eg, annual ACGME) anonymous surveys of resident burnout and well-being.

INDIVIDUAL-FOCUSED INTERVENTION: A MINDFULNESS-BASED STRESS REDUCTION (MBSR) PROGRAM FOR ANESTHESIOLOGY RESIDENTS EVALUATED WITH BIOPHYSICAL MARKERS OF STRESS AND VALIDATED BURNOUT ASSESSMENTS
Methods

Study Design: Approval from the Institutional Review Board (IRB) was obtained before this 2-year prospective cohort study. Participants included trainees in 2 urban anesthesiology training programs within a single health care system. The cohorts consisted of one training program which had in-person MBSR and CBT training made available while the second training program had a mobile app-based MBSR product made available to them. Inclusion criteria included Clinical Anesthesia CA-1 or CA-2 training level (ie, PGY-2 and 3). Exclusion criteria included PGY-1 and PGY-4 training levels given the limitations of the intern year schedule and the inability for PGY-4 residents to complete the 2-year study protocol.

After obtaining consent, study participants were followed over a 24-month period including a 3-month preintervention phase, an 18-month intervention phase and 3-month postintervention phase. Primary outcome variables included Maslach Burnout Inventory - Human Services Survey (MBI-HSS) scores, hair cortisol levels, and SSL collected through Fitbit Alta HR (Fitbit Inc., San Francisco, CA) wearable devices.

Intervention: The in-person training cohort was offered an MBSR and CBT course every other week during the 18-month intervention phase (36 sessions total) during regularly scheduled morning lecture time (6:30–7:00 AM) at a single training program. The instructors for these courses were certified in MSBR and CBT and were provided by the institutional office of Graduate Medical Education to all training programs in our system requesting this instruction. The MBSR course was based on the original MBSR curriculum developed by Jon Kabat-Zinn at the University of Massachusetts.[21] The resident curriculum consisted of 36-minute sessions, which deviated from the weekly 2.5 hour sessions over 8 weeks originally described for MSBR training due to scheduling restrictions imposed by operating room staffing requirements. Throughout these sessions, residents participated in sitting meditation, mindful movement, body scan, and walking meditation. The objective was to recognize stress and modify its effects through the incorporation of mindfulness and other de-stressing techniques into daily life. Session attendance was optional and available to all anesthesiology house staff in the program. The app-based cohort received access to moodgym (ehub Health Pty Ltd., Goulburn, AU), a mobile app-based CBT training product, and InsightTimer© (Insight Network Inc., San Francisco, CA) a mobile app-based MBSR product. The use of these products was voluntary and not recorded.

Data Collection: For all participants, MBI-HSS and hair cortisol levels were obtained on day one of the preintervention phases at which time SSL data collection with Fitbit Alta HR devices was initiated and continued through all study phases. The schedule for MBI-HSS and hair cortisol level collection included the end of the preintervention phase (day 90), three times during the intervention (days 180, 360, 540), and at the end of the postintervention phase (day 720). The data collection timeline is presented in **Table 1**.

The MBI-HSS is a validated 22-question survey to measure levels of burnout in clinicians on 3 scales: emotional exhaustion, depersonalization, and personal accomplishment.[22] Hair cortisol is an easily accessible means of testing when examining human cortisol levels over a period of several months. Samples were analyzed by the group that developed the method at the University of Massachusetts following the collection method originally described: hair was cut as close to the scalp as possible with clean scissors in an amount of hair roughly the width of a pencil from

Table 1 proposed study timeline with corresponding days for data collection						
	Preintervention			**Intervention Phase**		**Postintervention**
Study Day	1	90	180	360	540	720
MBI-HSS						
Hair Cortisol						
SSL						

Abbreviations: MBI-HSS, maslach burnout inventory human services survey; SSL, Sleep State Level collected from Fitbit Alta HR wearable devices.

the posterior vertex of the head.[23] Samples of 3 cm length, representing cortisol deposition over roughly the 3-month period before collection, were obtained using a ruler to measure the desired length (eg, 3 cm) from the cut end and cut again to yield the correct sample. Hair samples were wrapped in aluminum foil, clearly labeled with a permanent marker with each participant's unique identification number, stored at room temperature, and shipped overnight to an outside laboratory.

SSL was measured through a Fitbit Alta HR electronic fitness tracker which each participant was asked to wear 24 hours a day, except during charging times. This device is known to be safe in the operating room without interfering with operating room devices or monitors. Each participant was also asked to download Detalytics© (Detalytics Pte. Ltd, Singapore) onto their phone to allow for data from the Fitbit to be uploaded and eventually analyzed. This application was developed as a data collection hub and accessed for data analysis. Sleep cycles were analyzed to develop each participant's SSL. This was accomplished using the Detalytics© proprietary sleep analytics suite which analyzes the level and stability of sleep both during a single sleep cycle and across multiple episodes of sleep. The 3 data endpoints that comprise SSL include sleep quantity (eg, the duration of time the participant is asleep), sleep quality (eg, the time required to fall asleep and the number of awakenings experienced throughout a single sleep cycle), and sleep consistency (eg, the overall variability within multiple sleep cycle measurements).

Data Analysis: The primary objective of the analysis was to evaluate the impact of MSBR and CBT on MBI-HSS and hair cortisol levels at baseline, at 180 days, and at 360 days, and to determine variation changed over time. The secondary objective was to investigate the impact of the year of training. A mixed model was used with fixed effects including the intervention group, time point, clinical anesthesia year (CA1 and CA2), interaction between intervention group and time, and interaction between CA year and time. The random effects included the study subjects. The mixed model accounted for the within-subject correlation of the repeated assessments during the campaign periods.

Data are presented as median [interquartile range] and N (%). For comparisons of the Fitbit Alta HR and sleep data between the intervention group and control group, the Wilcoxon–Mann Whitney test was used for continuous data and Fisher's exact test was used for the categorical data, whereby appropriate. In general, a 2-sided P-value of less than 0.05 signifies statistical differences between the 2 groups. Although there are many items collected by the Fitbit device, the study sample size is also limited. Therefore, we chose to use 0.01 as the significance criterion instead of correcting the P-values for the multiple comparisons. The statistical analysis was performed using SAS Software (Version 9.4, SAS Institute, Cary, NC, USA).

Results

The control group was composed of 10 CA-1 and 8 CA-2 residents; the intervention group consisted of 10 CA-1 and 10 CA-2 residents ($P = .478$). Data collection was discontinued at the end of the first year of the study due to the low utilization of the MBSR and CBT in-person training.

The MBI for medical personnel consists of 3 domains: emotional exhaustion, depersonalization, and personal accomplishment. The results from each domain are scored on a 7-level scale from 0 to 6, with higher scores denoting worse burnout.

There was no significant difference between intervention and control groups on Maslach emotional exhaustion score at all-time points as seen in **Table 2**. However, we found a significant interaction between time and clinical training level ($P = .046$). The emotional exhaustion score (**Fig. 1**) was higher for CA2s at 180 days (Diff (SE): 0.87 (0.41); $P = .046$)) and 360 days (0.91 (0.53); $P = .095$) when compared with CA 1 s. This difference was not significant at baseline before the start of the mindfulness intervention (-0.02 (0.33); $P = .951$). Depersonalization score (**Fig. 2**) was consistently lower for the intervention group by -0.88 on average ((0.36); $P = .040$). Depersonalization score was higher for CA2s (1.08 (0.45), $P = .024$) at 180 days. This difference was not significant at baseline before the start of the mindfulness intervention (-0.40 (0.38); $P = .301$), nor at 360 days (0.17 (0.55); $P = .762$). At 180 days, depersonalization score declined for CA1s (-0.77 (0.26); $P = .007$) but increased for CA2s (0.72 (0.25); $P = .009$). This trend, however, was not observed at 360 days.

A significant difference in depersonalization scores existed when comparing depersonalization scores between CA1s and CA2s at day 180 and day 360 (respectively, -0.73 (0.28); $P = .0147$ at day 180 and -0.79 (0.36); $P = .037$ at day 360) (**Fig. 3**). There was also a significant difference in depersonalization scores over time between

Table 2
MBI-HSS between & within group comparisons

		Comparison	Ref.	Days	Difference	Standard Error	P-value	P-value for interaction
Group	EE	Intervention	Control	NA	0.29	0.31	.347	NA
	DEP				−0.78	0.36	.040	
	PA				0.04	0.21	.861	
	EETS				2.64	2.77	.347	
	DTS				−3.90	1.82	.040	
	PATS				0.26	1.66	.879	
Campaign by CA year	EE	CA2	CA1	0	−0.02	0.33	.951	0.046
				180	0.87	0.41	.046	
				360	0.91	0.53	.095	
	DEP	CA2	CA1	0	−0.40	0.38	.301	0.002
				180	1.08	0.45	.024	
				360	0.17	0.55	.762	
	PA	CA2	CA1	0	−0.11	0.22	.620	0.037
				180	−0.73	0.28	.015	
				360	−0.79	0.36	.037	
	EETS	CA2	CA1	0	−0.19	2.98	.950	0.048
				180	7.81	3.73	.047	
				360	8.08	4.75	.101	
	DTS	CA2	CA1	0	−2.01	1.90	.301	0.002
				180	5.40	2.25	.024	
				360	0.84	2.74	.762	
	PATS	CA2	CA1	0	−0.88	1.78	.626	0.033
				180	−5.85	2.23	.015	
				360	−6.35	2.84	.034	

Abbreviations: EE, emotional exhaustion; DEP, depersonalization; PA, personal accomplishment.

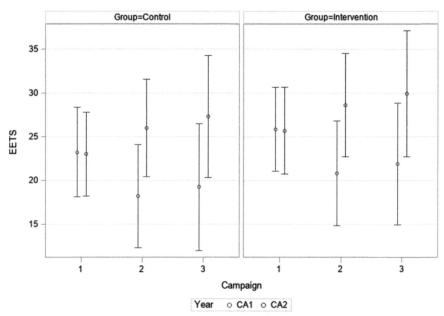

Fig. 1. Emotional Exhaustion Total Scores (with 95% CI) by Clinical Anesthesia Year over Campaign Time. Campaign 1 = day 0, Campaign 2 = day 180, Campaign 3 = day 360.

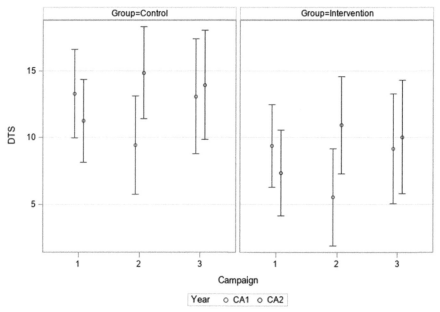

Fig. 2. Depersonalization Total Scores (with 95% CI) by Clinical Anesthesia Year over Campaign Time. Campaign 1 = day 0, Campaign 2 = day 180, Campaign 3 = day 360.

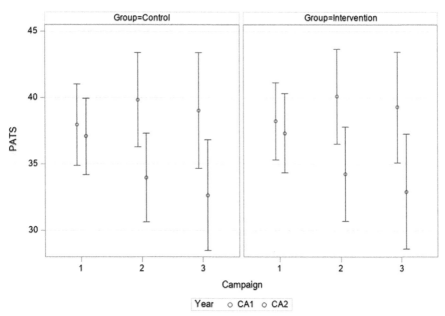

Fig. 3. Personal Accomplishment Total Scores (with 95% CI) by Clinical Anesthesia Year over Campaign Time. Campaign 1 = day 0, Campaign 2 = day 180, Campaign 3 = day 360.

baseline and day 180 in CA-2's (−0.38 (0.18); $P = .048$). No other meaningful comparisons over time or between groups for personal accomplishment scores were significant.

Fitbit Alta HR: Data from the Fitbit Alta HR showed no significant difference between the intervention group and the control group with the exception of minutes spent in Zone 2 heart rate (Intervention: median 285 minutes [IQR: 265–370] and control: 222 minutes [IQR: 183–498], Wilcoxon rank-sum test $P = .032$), and time spent performing vigorous exercise (Intervention: 4.01 minutes [3.52–5.76] vs control 16.46 [9.98–31.23], $P = .032$).

Hair Cortisol: There was no significant difference in hair cortisol levels between the control and intervention groups throughout the study.

DISCUSSION OF THE INDIVIDUAL-FOCUSED INTERVENTION AND TRANSITION TO AN ORGANIZATIONAL-FOCUS

Our experience conducting a 2-year study to assess the impact of in-person MBSR and CBT training for anesthesiology residents revealed many challenges in implementing an individual-focused intervention to combat burnout, while providing little benefit as measured by MBI-SSH scores and biometric data. The in-person and app-based resources were made available to our 2 cohorts while utilization was not mandated or tracked to maintain anonymity. The nature of residency training (ie, outside hospital rotations, vacation, and conference time) makes consistent attendance difficult. Of note, attendance was stymied by participants' willingness to attend, influenced by their personal time prioritization as well as lack of buy-in when introduced to MBSR and CBT. While the data collection of MBI-HSS and hair cortisol levels was discontinued after 1 year of the study, the in-person MBSR and CBT and app-based training continued throughout the duration of the original study design.

Our findings demonstrated a significant and consistent difference in depersonalization scores between the in-person MBSR and CBT training versus the app-based cohort may represent selection bias inherent in our study design given that this difference existed at the outset and persisted over time. Findings related to clinical training level may reflect the realities of anesthesiology training, unrelated to our study intervention. The CA1 year of training represents the steepest learning curve of residency, spent primarily in the practice of general anesthesiology. Most of the residents in their first year of training achieve a relative level of comfort by the second half of the year, with an accompanying sense of comfort and capability. The CA2 year of training, however, is a challenging year of new subspecialty rotations. Findings of decreased emotional exhaustion and increased personal accomplishment in CA1 residents are juxtaposed with the opposite pattern in CA2s, which may reflect this perceived difference between the 2 years of training.

This study design had multiple limitations. The inability to randomize trainees to study arms and therefore use a cohort design was necessitated by the logistics of delivering these interventions but led to inevitable selection bias. The lack of in-person training and the lack of tracking app usage limited our ability to determine the effect, or lack thereof, of the interventions. Inconsistent utilization of wearable sleep devices weakened the validity of our sleep state-level findings. Finally, the challenges of providing in-person MBSR and CBT training—and many of the factors we continue to face that likely influence resident burnout—may not be representative of other programs, in terms of productivity pressures present in a high-volume, tertiary urban training program. This initial study was motivated by a perceived need to address burnout, initially reported anecdotally and then tracked through both ACGME annual surveys and internal assessments by our health care system GME office. Perioperative subspecialty training programs (eg, anesthesiology, surgery, and surgical subspecialties) may face many barriers to both educational programming (ie, didactic, simulation, and small group sessions) and wellness offerings due to the demands of the operating room schedule and production pressure, which are also important drivers of burnout. The difficulties in this "have your cake and eat it too" approach (ie, reducing burnout without enacting structural change in address causes of burnout) came to light quickly during our investigation. While we did not conduct surveys to assess resident reception aside from those administered by the ACGME and our GME office, many comments were freely shared. A common theme involved resentment that our well-being intervention demanded additional time on the part of trainees in addition to their clinical demands despite each session replacing what would otherwise be a morning lecture. There was also a general lack of interest in both MBSR and CBT among our house staff. These factors led to poor attendance of our in-person sessions.

This experience of encountering multiple barriers and a lack of effectiveness in the use of MSBR and CBT motivated a shift to identifying new strategies to address ongoing evidence of burnout in annual surveys of well-being. To gather information from trainees and develop novel interventions, we used the confession sessions model as a vehicle, inspired by the iterative structure of the Delphi technique, for developing a more effective strategy for addressing resident burnout and well-being.

ORGANIZATIONAL-FOCUSED INTERVENTION: A CONFESSION SESSIONS MODEL INCORPORATING A MODIFIED DELPHI METHOD TO DEVELOP STRATEGIES FOR ADDRESSING ANESTHESIOLOGY RESIDENT WELL-BEING AND BURNOUT
Methods

Study Design: Exemption from the Institutional Review Board (IRB) was obtained before this 2-year prospective qualitative study. The study design involved confession sessions, or confidential meetings held every 3 months in place of regularly scheduled morning didactics. The goal was to identify and develop strategies to address themes resulting from the confessions sessions (**Table 3, Fig. 4**). Each session was used to elicit and incorporate resident feedback. The confessions sessions were initiated with the prompt: "What's on your mind?" We encouraged residents to include challenges or frustrations at work regarding schedule, work–life balance, adjusting to COVID-19, and so forth. Responses were collected anonymously through a secure web-based survey application (RedCap) then printed before each in-person session, or collected in a presentable format for virtual sessions during the COVID-19 pandemic. We then worked through the responses as a group to identify actionable changes in our residency program to improve well-being. All sessions were private and confidential, including only residents and facilitated by a chief resident. During discussion, the resident leader would record themes based on the presession responses and the conversations prompted by their presentation to the broader resident group. As these sessions were intended as a safe space for residents to openly discuss challenges they encountered in their residency training, recording, or transcription of these conversations was not used. This prevented the approach to theme identification through transcript analysis, a technique commonly used in qualitative research, but was considered essential to maintain confidentiality and spontaneous flow of conversation.[24]

Data analysis

Qualitative data: Following each confession session, themes were presented to residency program leadership to prompt concrete program and departmental change. The program director, while not present in the virtual discussions, also reviewed the initial anonymous responses to the presession prompts. Each session was structured to allow for new "confessions" while also collecting resident feedback on initiatives proposed by residency leadership in response to themes previously identified. This was facilitated by the addition of premeeting prompts specifically addressing departmental initiatives, in addition to the repetition of the open-ended prompt. All interventions proposed by program leadership were addressed by prompts preceding subsequent confession sessions to obtain resident feedback before and/or following implementation.

Quantitative data: Efficacy of the interventions developed through these iterative sessions was assessed through analysis of well-being and burnout surveys collected anonymously by the ACGME, which uses a 4-point Likert scale ranging from "strongly agree" to "strongly disagree." This aggregate outcome variable used by the ACGME as an assessment of program performance in addressing resident well-being and

Table 3		
Modified Delphi Structure incorporating confessions sessions		
Round	**Content/Structure**	
1	Open-ended prompt. Each "confession" is: • deidentified • submitted along with a corresponding severity score 1–10, with 10 being most problematic and 1 being least	
2	Each participant reviews & reacts to information provided in the first round	
3	Second iteration of reacting to information from prior round (in this setting with the goal of identifying targets for intervention)	

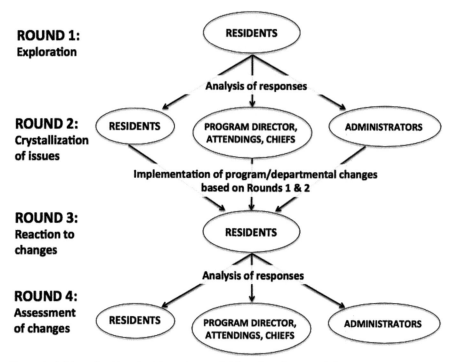

ROUND 1:
Exploration

RESIDENTS

Analysis of responses

ROUND 2:
Crystallization
of issues

RESIDENTS   PROGRAM DIRECTOR, ATTENDINGS, CHIEFS   ADMINISTRATORS

Implementation of program/departmental changes based on Rounds 1 & 2

ROUND 3:
Reaction to
changes

RESIDENTS

Analysis of responses

ROUND 4:
Assessment
of changes

RESIDENTS   PROGRAM DIRECTOR, ATTENDINGS, CHIEFS   ADMINISTRATORS

Fig. 4. Delphi-method inspired iterative model for identifying and developing strategies to address themes generated through confessions sessions.

burnout was identified as an appropriate means of assessing the effectiveness of the organization-focused interventions resulting from our qualitative study design. Well-being survey data collected anonymously through ACGME annual resident surveys of the training program from 2019 to 2021 was analyzed with the Benjamini–Hochberg Procedure or adjustment for false-discovery rate to detect changes in well-being survey items over the course of the intervention.

Results

Six confessions sessions were held over 2 academic years (2019–2021), and identified multiple themes that were then evaluated and addressed through meetings of residency program leadership (**Table 4**). Sessions were held in person before February 2020, and virtually from March 2020 onward. Content was presented to program administrators after each meeting, and several changes in the program were enacted. While certain themes were consistent over time (eg, feelings of burnout and difficulty finding time to study), some were context-dependent and impacted by the COVID-19 pandemic (eg, lack of auxiliary support, such as anesthesia technicians and perioperative nursing).

Several identified themes were clustered as stemming from our staffing model and its impact on work–life balance: difficulty finding time to study, need for personal days, need for predictable scheduling to allow for appointment scheduling, and feelings of burnout. To address these issues, the number of CRNAs covering evening shifts was increased, weekday 24-h calls were eliminated, and a novel shift was introduced that paired working late (ie, not overnight) with a postcall day free from clinical duties.

Table 4	
Themes identified through confessions sessions and leadership proposed responses	
Themes Identified	**Leadership Proposed Interventions**
Difficulty finding time to study	Elimination of weekday 24-h call assignments.
Need for personal days	• Pairing of free precall days with overnight
Need for predictable scheduling	call duties.
to allow for appointment	• Creation of a "Long" shift with the following
scheduling	day off.
Feelings of burnout	Expansion of evening CRNA staffing
Lack of transparency in	Selection of class representatives
departmental decision making	Funding for additional technician support
Need for anesthesia technician support	

This allowed for more predictability in relief times at day's end and provided relief from clinical duty both preceding and following weekday evening call responsibilities.

During the COVID-19 pandemic, with the shift to virtual sessions, it was apparent that frank discussion became less consistent, accompanying an expressed lack of insight into decision-making among departmental and residency leadership. This led to the creation of an elected class representative system allowing for a liaison between house staff and leadership who would participate in quarterly meetings with leadership, including program evaluation committee meetings.

One context-dependent theme resulted from nursing shortages caused by the COVID-19 pandemic, leading to anesthesiology residents being asked to help with recovering patients in the postoperative recovery unit. The residents' frustration with this development was identified through presession prompt responses and class representatives. The concern was addressed by the program director through a follow-up virtual meeting with the residents to explain the structural context leading to this development, along with a discussion with clinical coordinators to find alternative solutions that would not involve residents functioning outside of their expected roles. Additionally, workload increases caused by anesthesia technician shortages led to the expansion of hospital funding for additional hiring.

To address the consistent theme of burnout, our departmental "well-being champion," a role created by our institutional GME office, was included in all discussions and actively identified and shared institutional resources aimed at resident well-being. Analysis of aggregate annual anonymous well-being survey data conducted by the ACGME showed significant improvement in 7 out of 12 question items addressing both personal accomplishment and emotional exhaustion (**Table 5**). A greater than 70% ACGME-mandated response rate was achieved each of the 3 years surveys used for analysis were conducted.

DISCUSSION

GME leaders continue to seek effective means for improving widespread burnout across medicine.[13,14] The ACGME mandate to address resident well-being is motivated by a moral imperative, given the consequences of burnout and depression on both health care providers and patients.[8,9] However, like many aspects of residency training, implementation barriers exist based on economic, organizational, and historical factors that vary between region, context (ie, community vs. academic), and medical subspecialty. This may be due to the medical specialty, structure of the training program, departmental culture, or the economics dictating staffing models, region, context, and subspecialty specific. Our lack of success in implementing individual-

Table 5
Statistical analysis of change in annual aggregate anonymous well-being survey responses

Survey Item	Raw	BenjaminiHochberg	False Discovery Rate
		P-values	
I find my work to be meaningful.	0.0471	0.2355	0.0707
I work in a supportive environment.	0.0254	0.1524	0.0435
The amount of work I am expected to complete in a day is reasonable.	0.0168	0.1176	0.0336
I participate in decisions that affect my work.	0.1182	0.2476	0.1351
I have enough time to think and reflect.	0.1238	0.2476	0.1351
I am treated with respect at work.	0.0700	0.2476	0.0933
I feel more and more engaged in my work.	0.0006	0.0072	0.0072
I find my work to be a positive challenge.	0.0134	0.1072	0.0322
I find new and interesting aspects in my work.	0.0045	0.0470	0.0162
I often feel emotionally drained at work.	0.2910	0.2910	0.2910
After work, I need more time than in the past to relax.	0.0054	0.0486	0.0162
I feel worn out and weary after work.	0.0047	0.0470	0.0162

focused strategies such as MSBR versus success with organization-focused interventions, such as changes in staffing models and call duty structure, reveals the importance of identifying the appropriately tailored tool for each training program. Our use of a confession session model in conjunction with an iterative process of problem identification and strategy development based on a modified Delphi method can serve as a model for leaders in graduate medical education elsewhere.

Confessions sessions, regardless of the nature of the concerns, allow for effective identification and resolution of issues in an evolving health care training environment. They can provide a structured framework to address residents' concerns in real-time to improve resident well-being and the learning environment. While our experience proved an individual-focused intervention to be nonfeasible given resident attitudes and logistical barriers, other programs and specialties may find benefit with the provision of MSBR and CBT following the use of an iterative framework involving a confessions session approach such as the one described here. Given the heterogeneity across multiple domains in graduate medical education, the findings of the most well-designed study investigation strategies to address burnout may not apply to a large number of programs seeking to implement well-being initiatives.

While our experience yielded an improvement across many measures of resident well-being as evidenced by annual anonymous ACGME and internal surveys over the 2 years during which organizational-focused interventions were implemented following the use of an iterative confessions sessions approach, mustering the will to reach this goal required a great deal of support, both financial and institutional.

Our initial approach reflected the desire, likely shared by many leaders in graduate medical education, to achieve these gains without addressing structural issues requiring significant cost to our department and hospital. As with many goals worth achieving, results rarely come without great effort and cost. Asking trainees to develop effective coping skills to deal with the stressors of residency training, albeit with the departmental or institutional provision of this training, reflects a desire by leaders to "have their cake and eat it too;" in effect, outsourcing the work of dealing with what certainly represents an inherent externality of our industry, physician burnout. A responsible industry in a well-functioning society must be held accountable for the externalities resulting from that industry, and physician burnout should be regarded in this manner.

We found the ACGME to be a valuable resource in implementing organizational changes. Our existing call schedule and staffing models became insufficient to accommodate the rapidly expanding surgical volume of our health care system. As such, we determined an expansion of our residency program would be the best means of meeting that need while also providing flexibility to the current staffing model. Our submission to the ACGME to request a complement increase was predicated on the expansion of training opportunities and well-being and quality initiatives. Each year, as we saw an increase in our resident numbers with each new class, we implemented a change specifically designed to improve resident well-being. The first year, we eliminated 24-h calls for senior house staff and initiated our long call designation that provided a day free from clinical duties following a late shift. The second year, we effectively eliminated all 24-h calls, other than on weekends. Feedback from confessions sessions preceding and following these changes provided valuable insight into the strategy of our approach. Moving forward, we intend to develop a model to guarantee residents "on-demand wellness days," an additional theme identified in recent confessions sessions and a mandate of our GME office. This will facilitate a reliable and consistent backup model that will not disrupt our operating room staffing assignments or the rotation-based assignments of coresidents.

Our research journey has demonstrated the importance of tailoring well-being interventions to the individual training program. Implementing structural or organizational changes, while factoring in financial and logistical challenges, may yield the most benefit in confronting the epidemic of resident burnout. Departmental, institutional, and extra-institutional support is essential in meeting this goal.

DISCLOSURE

The authors have nothing to disclose.

REFERENCES

1. Freudenberger HJ. The staff burnout. J Soc Issues 1974.

2. IsHak WW, Lederer S, Mandili C, et al. Burnout During Residency Training: A Literature Review. J Grad Med Educ 2009. https://doi.org/10.4300/jgme-d-09-00054.1.

3. Grossi G, Perski A, Osika W, et al. Stress-related exhaustion disorder - clinical manifestation of burnout? A review of assessment methods, sleep impairments, cognitive disturbances, and neuro-biological and physiological changes in clinical burnout. Scand J Psychol 2015. https://doi.org/10.1111/sjop.12251.

4. Melamed S, Shirom A, Toker S, et al. Burnout and risk of cardiovascular disease: Evidence, possible causal paths, and promising research directions. Psychol Bull 2006. https://doi.org/10.1037/0033-2909.132.3.327.
5. Melo MCA, Das C, Medeiros F, De Bruin VMS, et al. Sleep quality among psychiatry residents. Can J Psychiatry 2016. https://doi.org/10.1177/0706743715620410.
6. Hamidi MS, Boggild MK, Cheung AM. Running on empty: A review of nutrition and physicians' well-being. Postgrad Med J 2016;92(1090):478–81.
7. Hyman SA, Michaels DR, Berry JM, et al. Risk of burnout in perioperative clinicians: A survey study and literature review. Anesthesiology 2011. https://doi.org/10.1097/ALN.0b013e318201ce9a.
8. De Oliveira GS, Chang R, Fitzgerald PC, et al. The prevalence of burnout and depression and their association with adherence to safety and practice standards: A survey of united states anesthesiology trainees. Anesth Analg 2013. https://doi.org/10.1213/ANE.0b013e3182917da9.
9. Bryson EO, Silverstein JH. Addiction and substance abuse in anesthesiology. Anesthesiology 2008. https://doi.org/10.1097/ALN.0b013e3181895bc1.
10. Alexander BH, Checkoway H, Nagahama SI, et al. Cause-specific mortality risks of anethesiologists. Anesthesiology 2000. https://doi.org/10.1097/00000542-200010000-00008.
11. Accreditation Council for Graduate Medical Education. 2020 ACGME Common Program Requirements (Residency). Available at: https://www.acgme.org/What-We-Do/Accreditation/Common-Program-Requirements.
12. Kuhn CM, Flanagan EM. Self-care as a professional imperative: physician burnout, depression, and suicide. Can J Anesth 2017. https://doi.org/10.1007/s12630-016-0781-0.
13. West CP, Dyrbye LN, Erwin PJ, et al. Interventions to prevent and reduce physician burnout: a systematic review and meta-analysis. Lancet 2016. https://doi.org/10.1016/S0140-6736(16)31279-X.
14. Wolpaw JT. It Is Time to Prioritize Education and Well-Being Over Workforce Needs in Residency Training. Acad Med 2019. https://doi.org/10.1097/ACM.0000000000002949.
15. Grensman A, Acharya BD, Wändell P, et al. Effect of traditional yoga, mindfulness-based cognitive therapy, and cognitive behavioral therapy, on health related quality of life: A randomized controlled trial on patients on sick leave because of burnout. BMC Complement Altern Med 2018. https://doi.org/10.1186/s12906-018-2141-9.
16. Goldhagen BE, Kingsolver K, Stinnett SS, et al. Stress and burnout in residents: Impact of mindfulness-based resilience training. Adv Med Educ Pract 2015. https://doi.org/10.2147/AMEP.S88580.
17. Wen L, Sweeney TE, Welton L, et al. Encouraging Mindfulness in Medical House Staff via Smartphone App: A Pilot Study. Acad Psychiatry 2017. https://doi.org/10.1007/s40596-017-0768-3.
18. Karan SB, Berger JS, Wajda M. Confessions of Physicians: What Systemic Reporting Does Not Uncover. J Grad Med Educ 2015;7(4):528–30.
19. Hsu CC, Sandford BA. The Delphi technique: Making sense of consensus. Pract Assessment, Res Eval 2007;12(10):1–8.
20. McMillan SS, King M, Tully MP. How to use the nominal group and Delphi techniques. Int J Clin Pharm 2016;38(3):655–62.
21. Santorelli SF, Kabat-Zinn J. Mindfulness-based stress reduction (MBSR): Standards of practice. Mindfulness-based Stress Reduct Stand Pract 2014.

22. Lim WY, Ong J, Ong S, et al. The Abbreviated Maslach Burnout Inventory Can Overestimate Burnout: A Study of Anesthesiology Residents. J Clin Med 2019. https://doi.org/10.3390/jcm9010061.

23. Meyer J, Novak M, Hamel A, et al. Extraction and analysis of cortisol from human and monkey hair. J Vis Exp 2014. https://doi.org/10.3791/50882.

24. Chun Tie Y, Birks M, Francis K. Grounded theory research: A design framework for novice researchers. SAGE Open Med 2019;7. https://doi.org/10.1177/2050312118822927. 205031211882292.

Moving Past Burnout, Looking Toward Engagement

Elizabeth W. Duggan, MD, MA[a],*, Malissa Clark, PhD[b]

KEYWORDS

- Engagement • Physician engagement • Burnout • Psychological safety
- Organizational justice • Job crafting • Job demands-resources (JD-R) model
- Physician well-being

KEY POINTS

- Engagement is a behavioral-affective workplace state defined by 3 dimensions: (1) vigor, (2) dedication, and (3) absorption. Engagement is negatively related to burnout and is a distinct construct with independent antecedents and outcomes.
- "Physician engagement" is a term frequently used in the medical literature; however, it lacks a cohesive and validated definition.
- Organizational psychology provides the opportunity to design and implement interventions demonstrated to augment engagement and combat burnout.
- Three key antecedents of engagement that offer opportunity to health care organizations include (1) psychological safety (2) organizational justice, and (3) job crafting
- Increasing employee engagement results in positive workplace outcomes at both individual (well-being, increased motivation, organizational commitment, job satisfaction, work initiative) and organizational levels (decreased turnover, higher performance levels, and increased customer [patient] satisfaction and loyalty).

INTRODUCTION

Over the previous decade, literature detailing physician burnout has vastly expanded, indicating that physicians continue to experience increasing symptoms of burnout, career dissatisfaction, and early career departure.[1] The rising symptoms were sufficiently heightened such that prior to the coronavirus disease 2019 pandemic, physician burnout was identified as a public health crisis.[2] This crisis has been further

---

[a] Industrial and Organizational Psychology, Department of Anesthesiology and Perioperative Medicine, University of Alabama Birmingham, 619 South 19th Street JT 804, Birmingham, AL 35249-6810, USA; [b] Department of Psychology, University of Georgia, 319 Psychology Building, Athens, GA 30602, USA
* Corresponding author.
E-mail address: eduggan@uabmc.edu

Anesthesiology Clin 40 (2022) 399–413
https://doi.org/10.1016/j.anclin.2022.01.012   **anesthesiology.theclinics.com**
1932-2275/22/© 2022 Elsevier Inc. All rights reserved.

exacerbated during the pandemic with mounting pressure placed on physicians to selflessly care for patients when exhausted, and at the potential risk of personal harm. As stated by Drs Dzau, Kirch, and Nasca in a *New England Journal of Medicine* perspective piece: "We are now facing a surge of physical and emotional harm that amounts to a parallel pandemic."[3]

A recent study by Afonso and colleagues[4] demonstrates that 59.2% of anesthesiologists are at risk of burnout, and 13.8% meet criteria for burnout syndrome. Burnout is associated with reduced work effort,[1] decreased professionalism, and increased medical errors.[5] At an organizational level, the annual economic cost associated with burnout related to turnover and reduced clinical hours is approximately $7600 per employed physician each year, an estimated system loss of $4.6 billion annually.[6] Academic departments experiencing a high incidence of burnout also suffer declining productivity, decreasing article authorship by approximately 15%.[7]

Burnout is a behavioral-affective work-related state classified by 3 dimensions. The 2 "core" dimensions—exhaustion and cynicism—are highly correlated.[8] In health care, cynicism often results in feelings of depersonalization, a negative and/or detached response toward patients. The third component, professional efficacy, is less often present in burnout but is supported by empirical evidence as being a critical component of the construct.[9] Discussions that exclusively focus on decreasing physician burnout overlook a critical construct that impacts physician careers: workplace engagement. Burnout and engagement are negatively related, and research reveals that efforts fostering engagement improve individual and organizational outcomes and mitigate the burnout state.[9–11]

WORKPLACE ENGAGEMENT

Work engagement was first defined in 1990 as a physical, cognitive, emotional, and mental expression during role performances.[12] This definition has transitioned over time with further academic study and is now generally accepted as a positive and fulfilling affective-motivational state of work-related well-being, composed of 3 dimensions: (1) vigor, (2) dedication, and (3) absorption.[13] Unlike employees who suffer from burnout, engaged employees have a sense of energetic and affective involvement with their work. These employees do not experience their work as stressful and demanding, but as challenging and connecting.[14]

Work engagement does not represent the same concept as job satisfaction; these constructs embody different behavioral-affective states. Job satisfaction is a positive or pleasurable state resulting from the "appraisal of one's job experience" and is marked by a sensation of contentment and positive feelings about or toward one's work.[15] The two constructs relate to workplace antecedents and outcomes in unique ways.[16] Antecedents of job satisfaction need to be present to prevent job dissatisfaction; however, these job components are unlikely to contribute to engagement. For instance, an acceptable salary and health insurance often increase job satisfaction however, they do not promote a state of employee engagement. A 2008 study surveying 750 academic physicians practicing in the United States (38% response rate) demonstrated that job security and incentives (eg, monetary and nonmonetary benefits) were the greatest contributors to job satisfaction.[17] However, when examining salary, fringe benefits, and bonuses in a hierarchical regression model predicting engagement, these factors neither increased model fit nor were they significant predictors of workplace engagement levels.[18]

Workplace engagement, unlike job satisfaction/dissatisfaction, is not represented by a state of contentment; it is characterized by energy (vigor), a motivational component to commit to tasks (dedication), and a willingness to invest personal resources (physical, cognitive and emotional) to accomplish the work (absorption). When individuals are engaged, they perform an action for its own sake, rather than the purpose of acquiring any material or social reward. According to Edward Deci and Richard Ryan's Self-Determination Theory, this type of motivation results in a "flow" state and is achieved under three experienced conditions: a sense of autonomy, competence, and relatedness.[19]

THE RELATIONSHIP BETWEEN BURNOUT AND ENGAGEMENT

Although solutions to burnout are needed and overdue, efforts must additionally move toward promoting physician engagement. A multifaceted approach to improving the workplace environment for physicians and health care providers will more quickly and assuredly address the burnout crisis in medicine. Although both burnout and work engagement are related to key job outcomes, burnout is more strongly related to personal health, whereas work engagement is tied to motivational outcomes.[14]

Organizational research has long debated the extent to which engagement is simply the opposite of burnout. If the two constructs are diametric sides of the same coin, work engagement would not explain variance over and above the effects of burnout. Early evidence suggested this relationship; the two constructs' dimensions appeared to be the others' opposite.[20,21] Emerging research, however, demonstrates that the antithetical relationship between constructs was misrepresented; burnout and engagement are independent constructs.[22] The most commonly used measure of work engagement (the Utrecht Job Engagement Scale) and the most frequently used assessment of burnout (the Maslach Burnout Inventory) have a great deal of overlap, creating an apparent relationship between emotional exhaustion with vigor and cynicism with dedication.[23,24] However, overlap of *measures* does not necessarily mean overlap of *constructs*.[22] At a conceptual level, burnout and engagement are distinguishable, and value is added by considering, measuring, and taking action to impact both.

JOB DEMANDS-RESOURCES MODEL

The Job Demands-Resources (JD-R) model provides a theoretic framework for understanding the unique predictors and outcomes of work engagement and burnout.[25] According to the JD-R model, the balance between job resources and job demands results in one of two psychological states: (1) engagement or (2) burnout.[26] Each state relates to important individual and organizational outcomes. Job and personal resources are key drivers of work engagement, which in turn, lead to improved individual and organizational outcomes through a motivational process.[14] Personal resources, including self-esteem, optimism, and self-efficacy, are considered distinct from resources built into the job itself. Job resources are situational and include autonomy, social support, supervisory coaching, relationship with one's leader, and professional development.[27,28] Engagement initiatives featuring these attributes help to outweigh negative experiences borne by employees on the job.[29]

Conversely, job demands are the key drivers of burnout.[9,30] Demands predict job strain, health impairment, and workplace burnout,[31,32] and include role ambiguity, role conflict, stressful events, excessive workload, and work pressure.[9] A sentinel meta-analysis on job demands and burnout argues that job demands are perceived by employees as "losses" that require effort, energy, and personal resources to overcome.[9] As a result, if these demands are not met with adequate personal and on-the-

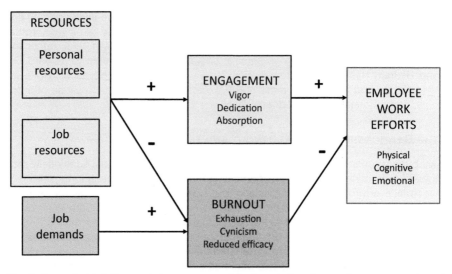

Fig. 1. Expanded Job Demands-Resources model of workplace burnout, engagement, and job satisfaction. The JD-R model was originally proposed by Demerouti et al. (2001)[33] and has been revised by the authors over time as research has progressed and expanded.

job resources, employees experience increasing burnout symptoms resulting in decreased work investment and effort (**Fig. 1**).

The JD-R model offers insight into operable and pragmatic antecedents that can be optimized to meet employee needs and improve work engagement. Higher levels of work engagement result when job and personal resources match or exceed demand levels.[26] Implementing these key job resources is critical for organizations seeking to offset job demands, empower and motivate employees to meet work challenges, and experience a positive and fulfilling work-related state.

ANTECEDENTS TO ENGAGEMENT

Organizational psychology research has examined engagement for more than 30 years, helping to define its components and validate its relationship with antecedents and outcomes. The medical community frequently uses the term "physician engagement" to describe a wide variety of work states, improvement efforts, and change initiatives. The citing literature has, however, neither rigorously used validated assessments nor scientifically explored its proven antecedents and outcomes. While efforts are underway to more accurately measure and assess engagement levels, health care studies must additionally include criterion validation before relationships are established between antecedents, constructs, and outcomes.

Health care institutions seeking to refine their strategy and build initiatives to enhance the work environment are best served by increasing their awareness and understanding of validated engagement research. The JD-R model was introduced to the scientific community in 2001 and has since been applied across a myriad of organizations to produce several empirical, peer-reviewed studies linking antecedents to outcomes.[14,16,25,33,34] In addition, these studies have demonstrated that job resources result in greater impact on employee engagement when job demands are high, critical to helping physicians meet the increasing demands of caring for patients in turbulent times.[35] Three antecedents that offer notable advantages to health care

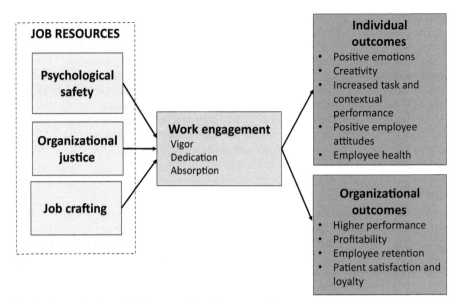

Fig. 2. Antecedents and outcomes of health care worker engagement

environments include (1) psychological safety, (2) job crafting, and (3) organizational justice (**Fig. 2**).

PSYCHOLOGICAL SAFETY

Psychological safety involves the ability to exercise one's authentic self without the fear (or actualization) of negative consequences.[12] Most often, the sense of safety is provided by an employee's direct supervisor but may also result from the workplace experience.[36] Companies characterized by open and supportive environments allow employees to experiment and innovate to solve problems, to express concerns and share obstacles, and to at times, falter or fail without consequence.[12]

May and colleagues[37] empirically tested dimensions of employee engagements and identified three key conditions present in psychologically safe work environments: (1) supervisory relationships, (2) coworker relationships, and (3) adherence to work group norms.

A supervisor demonstrating support and encouragement, as opposed to power or control, has an outsized impact on employee perception of the safety of their work environment.[38] In health care, perceptions of leadership correlate significantly with perceptions of psychological safety.[39] Reporting structures that intimidate and inhibit an employee's ability to express concerns or discuss unmet needs may increase employee vulnerability and/or decrease willingness to seek help when needed.[39] A workplace culture and organizational leader create learning space, and when they foster professional growth, limit shame and embarrassment and allow providers to disclose mistakes. These conditions build self-efficacy and encourage employees to engage in novel activities, take on new risks, and introduce innovative ideas.[38,39]

As relationships within work units demonstrate increasing affective trust, mutual respect, and value for each other's contributions, perceptions of psychological safety also increase.[37] A 2011 meta-analysis by Christian and colleagues[40] identified social support as a key predictor of employee work engagement. Edmondson and colleagues[39] confirmed that the variation in psychological safety is more heavily influenced by one's local workgroup cohesion than the medical center at large. Interactions between colleagues impact task and daily engagement, as well as engagement over time.[33,40]

Finally, work group norms govern behavior and attitudes of members.[41] Pressure can be placed among members to work within the boundaries of these norms.[12] Norms build safety for an "ingroup" (those working within group norms) while simultaneously cultivating deleterious effects on others. Group pressure can be coercive, forcing members to adhere to group "rules."[42] Norms that reinforce shame or fear limit psychological safety, prevent equitable participation and contribution, and fail to support employees in their efforts to be fully engaged at all levels of the organization.[43]

Recommendations

Supervisor/leader

- Create inclusive environments: Promote broad workplace membership.[44] Equitable mentoring, diverse leadership, and public celebration of employee differences foster workplace safety and are associated with inclusive and safe environments.[45]
- Set expectations and coach toward success: Provide clear and consistent directions for employees and model appropriate risk-taking initiatives and learning behaviors.[45–47]
- Build trust: The integrity, openness, and benevolence of the leader dictates perceptions of affective trust,[48] which is paramount to building psychological safety.[49,50]

Coworker groups

- Provide encouragement: Build systems that reinforce collegial support via formal exchange (eg, changing call or work schedules, second victim support groups, executive coaching, mentorship programs) and informal exchange (eg, providing advice and help, networking new members).
- Build peer groups: Create occasions for peer group interactions to discuss concerns and issues in their professional environment. This requires information sharing, resource exchange, peer feedback, and collective participation.

Group norms

- Power sharing: Consider formal facilitation training for groups to help members identify and promote opportunities to share ideas, concerns, and challenges.
- Ensure safe and private communication channels: Allow those who feel uncomfortable or intimidated to report (anonymously and/or via group ombudsman) behaviors and/or norms that limit their expression of authentic self.
- Team accountability: Groups who win (and lose) together are more likely to express concerns, work together, and admit failure.[51] Shared team rewards are associated with positive psychological safety.

ORGANIZATIONAL JUSTICE

Organizational justice involves an employee's subjective perception of fairness in the workplace and is impacted by three key factors: (1) organizational decisions, (2) processes and actions, and (3) employee treatment. Employee perceptions of organizational justice are linked to a wide range of outcomes such as engagement, job satisfaction, organizational commitment, task performance, and trust in management.[52]

Initial research on organizational justice focused primarily on the fairness of decision outcomes, referred to as distributive justice.[53] For example, John Stacey Adams' Equity Theory posits that individuals' perceptions of fairness were determined by an evaluation of their own input/output ratio when compared with the input/output ratio of others.[54] If the ratios match, the employee considers the distribution to be equitable. Researchers have since expanded these theories to include the processes that determine outcome allocation (procedural justice). Justice perceptions are also influenced by the extent to which individuals in positions of power fairly communicate procedural details (informational justice), and the degree to which employees feel that they are treated with respect and dignity (interpersonal justice).[55] Perceptions of justice are often assessed in relation to a supervisor or organization, in regard to a particular event (eg, a specific decision about pay, rewards, or promotions) or a collection of workplace decisions over time.[56]

Justice issues surface in work environments for a variety of reasons, but the most common theme emerging during these deliberations is uncertainty. Uncertainty Management Theory posits that under a state of uncertainty (lacking direct information regarding an aspect of one's workplace), employees react more strongly to fairness variations (perceived injustice).[57] In search of renewed predictability and to offset the anxiety of uncertainty, an individual seeks fairness in the social environment.[57] For instance, when organizational outcomes are negative (eg, layoffs, pay cuts), procedural, informational, and interpersonal justice perceptions become paramount in an employee's willingness to understand and accept the outcome.[58]

Health care is constantly introducing uncertainty into the work environment. Providers are regularly adjusting medical care pathways, shifting to meet the needs of patients, adapting to novel research, working with new technology, and acclimatizing to novel payment and service models. Being expected to manage frequent change, within an ongoing pandemic, has elevated provider uncertainty to previously unexperienced levels. Employee perceptions of justice feed into their overall global perceptions of fairness, which in turn impact workforce engagement.[56] When treatment by a work authority is considered unfair, the employee suffers an emotional reaction deemed "moral outrage," resulting in anger and resentment.[59,60] When employee uncertainty is managed through fair treatment, individuals are more likely to feel fully invested and engaged in their work.[16]

Recommendations

- Reduce uncertainty: Foster justice when key changes are made in the workplace.[56] Provide timely communication providing transparent explanations. Be candid as to the challenges faced, information known and unknown, and anticipated next steps.
- Manage communication: Formal and informal sources of communication message information about the organization and its decisions, risking uncertainty if messages are mixed.[56] Augment electronic communication with in-person discussions, question and answer sessions, and open-door policies to facilitate interpersonal justice.
- Respect: Model a considerate, respectful, and trustworthy voice when providing information about organization, when speaking with coworkers, and when conversing with individuals external to one's immediate work group.[56]
- Be consistent: Inconsistent justice evokes negative emotions and creates uncertainty. Communicate and adhere to guidelines for recruitment, selection, opportunity, performance evaluations, and promotion. In addition, offer a correctional process for outcomes deemed "unfair."[55]

- Model "just" cultures, including 3 key culture components.[61]
  - *Basic assumptions* are the foundation of an organization. When leaders and employees embrace justice and equity as a premise of the organization, behaviors reflect and enact the assumption.
  - Declare justice as an *espoused value* and build formal expectations accordingly.
  - *Artifacts* are those items easily visible to the work community that reflect culture messages. Feature justice themes in language, discussions, and celebrations.

JOB CRAFTING AND PERSONALIZED DEVELOPMENT

Amy Wrzesniewski and Jane Dutton (2001) coined the term *job crafting* to describe the proactive changes employees make in their work patterns and tasks to redefine their environment and further work meaning.[62] This term has further been refined to include the self-directed job changes workers make to offset demands and augment resources.[63] Organizations that encourage employees to job craft, offset work demands by increasing job resources (eg, mentorship, social support, mastering a new skill). Job crafting also includes seeking new opportunities and assignments to expand the scope of one's jobs to meet professional capabilities and interests. Through these activities, employees optimize their work environment to best suit their intrinsic motivators and thereby increase their workplace engagement. Employees who seek both resources and challenges are more engaged with their job and experience less burnout.[64]

Early job crafting literature in the 1970s examined the concept of job crafting from a "top-down" approach.[63,65] The organization was expected to design the job, set forth its tasks, and align resources to meet demands. When the job required new tasks, the organization designed change programs to resource these novel demands. However, as the knowledge and service economy began to expand, organizations became more reliant on employee ideas and innovation. Labeled "bottom-up" job crafting, workers identified and created resources to better meet the dynamic conditions of their work environment.[65] Organizations excelled as employees innovated against competitors, adeptly responded to customer needs, and flexed to rising challenges.[66]

During this same time, however, medical practices experienced an opposite shift. Historically, physician practices were small and independent, and work-design decisions were predominantly driven by the doctors who concomitantly owned the practice and cared for its patients. Today, hospitals and health systems increasingly acquire physician practices critical to their core operations and/or hire physicians directly. These health care conglomerates, facing the demands of private and public insurers, patient service needs, pay-for-performance models, and growing investment costs (eg, technology, electronic medical record, required reporting) often use a "top-down" job crafting approach. To increase efficiency, optimize safety, and minimize cost, employers increasingly outline physician roles and prescribe accompanying resources. This approach fails to consider the employee's motivations and underrecognizes unique work environment demands.

Attributes within a job (eg, autonomy, skill variety, task significance) are "core" characteristics that increase job meaning.[67] Doctors who can actively craft their roles to include these attributes as resources are more likely to experience personal meaning in their work and meet job demands critical for organization success.[68]

Recommendations

- Schedule autonomy: As possible, allow individuals to choose work hours/shifts to better meet both organization and personal needs. Flex call schedules to

manage off-hour assignments (eg, nights, weekends, holidays) to balance unique home-work needs.
- Task variety: Encourage employees to outline their professional interests and proactively write ideal job descriptions. Incorporate skill variety into the current job or find stretch assignments to increase access to those tasks/assignments that are most exciting.
- Significant work: Ensure that physicians can see, and are reminded of, the positive outcomes and significance of their work. The degree to which an employee appreciates the impact of their work influences their sense of fulfillment and meaning.
- Job challenges: Individuals seeking tasks/roles to pursue cognitive interests are exercising personal motivators; this empowers personal learning and development, improves capability and performance, and consequently enhances work engagement.[69]
- Personalized development: Offer development conferences separate from performance discussions; this provides a forum for open discourse and structured feedback. When tied to performance, employees may be less likely to ask for support, accept candid feedback, or admit weaknesses and training needs.
- Method autonomy: Jointly create work goals to align personal interest with organization goals. Encourage physicians to design and innovate the needed processes and methods to achieve the expected outcomes.

Currently, job crafting opportunities within health care organizations are inadequate and if available, may be limited to senior level physicians. Job crafting should be promoted at all physician levels. Unrelieved job demands cause employee strain, which leads to increasingly negative job perceptions over time.[70] Employees who are unable to receive and/or procure resources to manage work demands increasingly experience burnout. Early work intervention—allowing physicians to craft their roles, tasks, and time—not only serves to manage stressful role requirements but also additionally offsets the strain of future work pressures by matching resources to job demands.[25,72]

OUTCOMES

As health care leaders expand their understanding of workplace psychology, they are better equipped to combat physician burnout and promote workplace engagement, as well as impact organizational outcomes.[14,16] Validated assessments measuring employee engagement and perceptions of job resources offer organizations the opportunity to study the impact of interventions. A suggested list of validated assessments is provided in **Table 1**.

Table 1
Recommended assessments for burnout, engagement, and reviewed antecedents

Construct A	Assessment
Burnout	Maslach Burnout Scale, General Inventory[25]
Engagement	Job Engagement Scxale[16]
Psychological safety	Edmondson's Survey Scale (Appendix, pp. 382–383)[38]
Organizational justice	Colquitt's Justice Measure (Table 1, p. 389)[52]
Job crafting scale	The Job Crafting Scale (Table 1, p. 177)[63]

Individual Outcomes

Evidence demonstrates that engaged employees experience better health, less frequent work absences, and more positive work morale.[25,71,73] Engaged employees express more positive emotions regarding their work role; highly engaged supervisors report feeling more "inspired, energetic, cheerful and enthusiastic" than those with lower levels of engagement.[74]

The resulting positive emotional state has been shown to increase an employee's organizational attachment resulting in decreased turnover intention, and increased commitment.[16]

Engaged employees also demonstrate a greater receptivity to novel lines of thinking and willingness to learn, including both the daily pursuit of learning and learning over time.[75,76] There is a positive relationship between engagement and proactive behaviors including taking initiative, openness to new experience, and exhibiting higher levels of creativity, as rated by colleagues.[75,77–79] A 2011 meta-analysis by Christian and colleagues[40] confirmed that engagement positively predicts both required (in-role) and contextual (extra-role) performance. The extra-role "above and beyond" attitude is also associated with improved workplace safety.[16,31,34]

Organizational Outcomes

Engaged employees tend to be higher performers, furthering the organization's goals and mission.[16,80] Examining 587 employees, Halbesleben and Wheeler[81] (2008) confirmed that engagement levels predict later performance as rated by both one's coworkers and supervisor. Organizations with higher levels of employee engagement are also more likely to report higher levels of job satisfaction, yielding an upturn in productivity. Engaged employees are more likely to engender organizational citizenship behaviors, taking on tasks that are not part of formal job requirements, and cannot be required in advance, but can be performed by employees to foster organizational functioning.[27] A positive relationship exists between overall employee engagement levels and customer satisfaction and service climate, and as a result customer loyalty.[82] A meta-analysis by Harter and colleagues[83] (2002) confirmed that an engaged workforce results in higher organization profitability, customer satisfaction, and loyalty. Engagement is also thought to provide a competitive advantage by increasing employees' affective commitment to their organization.[77,84]

SUMMARY

Although multiple articles have been published outlining the prevalence and outcomes of physician burnout, there is limited knowledge and appreciation for the mitigating role of workplace engagement. Engaged employees experience better health, are more present, and demonstrate higher levels of motivation in their work environment.[25,71] An engaged workforce provides organizations with a competitive advantage resulting in numerous positive outcomes including optimized employee potential, an upturn in job satisfaction, increased productivity and creativity, enhanced organizational citizenship behaviors, and decreased employee burnout and turnover intentions.[14] Applying organizational psychology principles and evidence offers physicians the opportunity to strategically design workplace changes to combat burnout, enhance patient care, and reengage doctors in the clinical mission.

DISCLOSURE

The authors have nothing to disclose.

REFERENCES

1. Shanafelt TD, Dyrbye LN, West CP, et al. Potential impact of burnout on the U.S. physician workforce. Mayo Clin Proc 2016;91(11):1667–8.
2. Jha AK, Iliff AR, Chaoui AA, et al. A crisis in health care: a call to action on physician burnout. Waltham, MA: Massachusetts Medical Society; 2019. https://cdn1.sph.harvard.edu/wp-content/uploads/sites/21/2019/01/PhysicianBurnoutReport2018FINAL.pdf.
3. Dzau VJ, Kirch D, Nasca T. Preventing a parallel pandemic - a national strategy to protect clinicians' well-being. N Engl J Med 2020;383(6):513–5.
4. Afonso AM, Cadwell JB, Staffa SJ, et al. Burnout rate and risk factors among anesthesiologists in the United States. Anesthesiology 2021;134(5):683–96.
5. Panagioti M, Geraghty K, Johnson J, et al. Association between physician burnout and patient safety, professionalism, and patient satisfaction: a systematic review and meta-analysis. JAMA Intern Med 2018;178(10):1317–31.
6. Han S, Shanafelt TD, Sinsky CA, et al. Estimating the attributable cost of physician burnout in the United States. Ann Intern Med 2019;170(11):784–90.
7. Turner TB, Dilley SE, Smith HJ, et al. The impact of physician burnout on clinical and academic productivity of gynecologic oncologists: a decision analysis. Gynecol Oncol 2017;146(3):642–6.
8. Lee RT, Ashforth BE. On the meaning of Maslach's three dimensions of burnout. J Appl Psychol 1990;75(6):743–7.
9. Lee RT, Ashforth BE. A meta-analytic examination of the correlates of the three dimensions of burnout. J Appl Psychol 1996;81:123–33.
10. Halbesleben JR, Buckley MR. Burnout in organizational life. J Management 2004;30:859–79.
11. Bakker AB, Hakanen J, Demerouti E, et al. Job resources boost work engagement, particularly when demands are high. J Educ Psychol 2007;99:274–84.
12. Kahn WA. Psychological conditions of personal engagement and disengagement at work. Acad Manage J 1990;33:692–724.
13. Schaufeli WB, Salanova M, Gonzalez-Roma V, et al. The measurement of engagement and burnout: a two-factor confirmatory analytic approach. J Happiness Stud 2002;3:71–92.
14. Bakker AB, Demerouti E, Sanz-Vergel AI. Burnout and Work Engagement: The JD-R Approach. Annual Review of Organizational Psychology and Organizational Behavior. P 389-411.
15. Locke EA. The nature and causes of job satisfaction. In: M.D., editor. Handbook of industrial and organizational psychology. Chicago: Rand-McNally; 1976. p. 1297–349.
16. Rich BL, Lepine JA, Crawford ER. Job engagement: antecedents and effects on job performance. The Academy of Management Journal; 2010. p. 617–35.
17. Janus K, Amelung VE, Baker LC, et al. Job satisfaction and motivation among physicians in academic medical centers: insights from a cross-national study. J Health Polit Policy Law 2008;1133–67.
18. Kulikowski K, Sedlak P. Can you buy work engagement? The relationship between pay, fringe benefits, financial bonuses and work engagement. Current Psychology; 2020. p. 343–53.
19. Deci EL, Ryan RM. Self-determination theory. In: Van Lange PAM, Kruglanski AW, Higgins ET, editors. Handbook of theories of social psychology. Newbury Park, CA: Sage Publications Ltd.; 2012. p. 416–36.

20. Cole MS, Walter F, Bedeian AG, et al. Job burnout and employee engagement: a meta-analytic examination of construct proliferation. J Management 2012;38(5): 1550–81.
21. Gonzalez-Roma V, Schaufeli WB, Bakker AB, et al. Burnout and work engagement: independent factors or opposite poles? J Vocational Behav 2006;62: 165–74.
22. Byrne ZS, Peters JM, Weston JW. The struggle with employee engagement: Measures and construct clarification using five samples 2016;101(9):1201–27.
23. Schaufeli WB, Bakker AB. Utrecht Work Engagement Scale: Preliminary Manual. Utrecht: Utrecht University; 2003.
24. Maslach C, Jackson SE, Leiter MP. Maslach Burnout Inventory Manual. Palo Alto, CA: Consulting Psychologists Press; 1996.
25. Demerouti E, Bakker A, Nachreiner F, et al. The job demands-resources model of burnout 2001;86(3):499–512.
26. Bakker AB, Demerouti E. The Job-Demands-Resources model; State of the art. J Managerial Psychol 2007;22:309–28.
27. Bakker AB, Demerouti E, Verbeke W. Using the job demands-resources model to predict burnout and performance. Hum Resour Manag 2004;43:83–104.
28. Xanthopoulou D, Bakker AB, Demerouti E, et al. The role of personal resources in the job demands-resources model. Int J Stress Management 2007;14(2).
29. Demerouti E, Bakker AB, de Jonge J, et al. Burnout and engagement at work as a function of demands and control. Scand J Work Environ Health 2001;27(4):279–86.
30. Alarcon G. A meta-analysis of burnout with job demands, resources, and attitudes. J Vocat Behav 2011;79:549–62.
31. Bakker A, Demerouti E, Schaufeli W. The Socially Induced Burnout Model. In: Shohov S, editor. Advances in Psychology Research. Hauppauge, NY: Nova Science Publishers; 2003. p. 13–30.
32. Hakanen J, Bakker AB, Schaufeli WB. Burnout and work engagement among teachers. J Sch Psychol 2006;43:495–513.
33. Halbesleben JR. A meta-analysis of work engagement: relationships with burnout, demands, resources, and consequences. In: Bakker AB, Leiter MP, editors. Work Engagement: A Handbook of Essential Theory and Research. East Sussex, United Kingdom: Psychology Press; 2010. p. 102–17.
34. Nahrgang J, Moregeson F, DA H. Safety at work: a meta-analytic investigation of the link between job demands, job resources, burnout, engagement and safety outcomes. J Appl Psychol 2011;96(1):71–94.
35. Bakker A, Van Veldhoven M, Xanthopoulou D. Beyond the demand-control model: thriving on high job demands and resources. J Personnel Psychol 2010;3–16.
36. Saks A. Antecedents and consequence of employee engagement. J Managerial Psychol 2006;21(7):600–19.
37. May D, Gilson R, Harter L. The psychological conditions of meaningfulness, safety and availability and the engagement of the human spirit at work. J Occup Organizational Psychol 2004;77:11–37.
38. Edmondson A. Psychological safety and learning behavior in work teams. Administrative Sci Q 1999;350–83.
39. Edmondson A, Higgins M, Singer S, et al. Understanding psychological safety in health care and education organizations: A Comparative Perspective. Research in Human Development 2016;13(1):65–83.
40. Christian M, Garza A, Slaughter J. Work engagement: a quantitative review and test of its relations with task and contextual performance. Personnel Psychol 2011;64(1):89–136.

41. Hochschild A. Emotion work, feeling rules and social structure. Am J Sociol 1979; 85(3):551–75.
42. Barker J. Tightening the iron cage: concertive control in self-managing teams. Administrative Sci Q 1993;408–37.
43. Shore L, Cleveland J, Sanchez D. Inclusive workplaces: a review and model. Hum Resource Management 2018;28:176–89.
44. Newman A, Donohue R, Eva N. Psychological safety: a systematic review of the literature. Human Management Resource Review 2017;3:521–35.
45. Singh B, Winkel D, Selvarajan T. Managing diversity at work: does psychological safety hold the key to racial differences in employee performance? Journal of Occupational and Organizational Psychology 2013;86:242–63.
46. Hirak R, Pang A, Carmeli A, et al. Linking leader inclusiveness to work unit performance: The importance of psychological safety and learning from failures, The Leadership Quarterly, 23, 2012,107-117.
47. Walumbwa F, Schaubroeck J. Leader personality traits and employee voice behavior: mediating roles of ethical leadership and work group psychological safety. J Appl Psychol 2009;1275–86.
48. Leroy H, Dierynck B, Anseel F, et al. Behavioral integrity for safety, priority of safety, psychological safety, and patient safety: a team-level study. J Appl Psychol 2012;97:1273–81.
49. Li A, Tan H. What happens when you trust your supervisor? Mediators of individual performance in trust relationships. J Organizational Behav 2012;407–25.
50. Schaubroeck J, Lam S, Peng A. Cognition-based and affect-based trust as mediators of leader behavior influences on team performance. J Appl Psychol 2011; 96:863–71.
51. O'Neill O. Workplace expression of emotions and escalation of commitment. J Appl Soc Psychol 2009;39:2396–424.
52. Colquitt J. On the dimensionality of organizational justice: A construct validation of a measure. J Appl Psychol 2001;86:386–400.
53. Colquitt J, Conlon D, Wesson M, et al. Justice at the millennium: A meta-analytic review of 25 years of organizational justice research. J Appl Psychol 2001;86(3):425–45.
54. Adams J. Inequity in Social Exchange. In: Berkowitz L, editor. Advances in Experimental Social Psychology2. Cambridge, MA: Academic Press; 1965. p. 267–99.
55. Colquitt J. Organizational Justice. In: Kozlowski S, editor. The Oxford Handbook of Organizational Psychology. Oxford, England: Oxford University Press; 2012. p. 526–47.
56. Colquitt J, Zipay K. Justice, Fairness and employee reactions. Annu Rev Organ Psychol Organ Behav 2014;2:11.1–11.25.
57. Lind E, Van den Bos K. When fairness works: toward a general theory of uncertainty management. Res Organ Behav 2002;24:181–223.
58. Greenberg J. Employee theft as a reaction to underpayment inequity: the hidden cost of pay cuts. J Appl Psychol 1990;75(5):561–8.
59. Bies R. The predicament of injustice: the management of moral outrage. Res Organ Behav 1987;9:289–319.
60. Folger R, Martin C. Relative deprivation and reference cognitions: distributive and procedural justice effects. J Exp Soc Psychol 1986;22:531–46.
61. Schein E. Organizational Culture and Leadership. 16th. San Francisco, CA: Jossey-Bass Publishers; 2010.
62. Wrzesniewski A, Dutton J. Crafting a job: revisioning employees as active crafters of their work. Acad Manag Rev 2001;26:179–201.

63. Tims M, Bakker A. Job crafting: towards a new model of individual job redesign. South Afr J Ind Psychol 2010;36:1–9.
64. Petrou P, Demerouti E, Peeters MCW, et al. Crafting a job on a daily basis: Contextual antecedents and the effect on work engagement. J Organizational Behav 2012;33:1120–41.
65. Hackman JR, Oldham GR. Work Redesign. Boston, MA: Addison Wesley; 1980.
66. Lee J, Lee Y. Job crafting and performance: literature review and implications for human resource development. Hum Resource Development Rev 2018;17(3): 277–313.
67. Hackman J, Oldham G. Motivation through the design of work: test of a theory. Organ Behav Hum Perform 1976;16:250–79.
68. Grant A, Parker S. Redesigning work design theories: the rise of relational and proactive perspectives. Acad Manag Ann 2009;3:317–75.
69. Petrou P, Demerouti E, Schaufeli W. Job crafting in changing organizations: Antecedents and implications for exhaustion and performance. J Occup Health Psychol 2015;20(4):470–80.
70. Zapf D, Dormann C, Frese M. Longitudinal studies in organization stress research: A review of the literature with reference to methodological issues. J Occup Health Psychol 1996;1(2):145–69.
71. Xanthopoulou D, Bakker A, Dollard M, et al. When do job demands particularly predict burnout? The moderating role of job resources. J Managerial Psychol 2007;22(8):766–86.
72. Schaufeli WB, Leiter MP, Maslach C. Burnout: 35 years of research and practice. Career Development International 2009;14(3):204–20.
73. Bailey C, Madden A, Alfes K, et al. The meaning, antecedents and outcomes of employee engagement: a narrative synthesis. Int J Management Rev 2017;19: 31–53.
74. Schaufeli W, Van Rhenen W. About the role of positive and negative emotions in managers' well-being: a study using the Job-related Affective Wellbeing Scale (JAWS). Gedrag Organ 2006;19:323–44.
75. Bakker A, Demerouti E, Ten Brummelhuis L. Work engagement, performance, and active learning: The role of conscientiousness. J Vocat Behav 2012;80: 555–64.
76. Sonnentag S. Recovery, work engagement and proactive behavior: a new look at the interface between nonword and work. J Appl Psychol 2003;88:518–28.
77. Hakanen JJ, Schaufeli WB, Ahola K. The job-demands resources model: a three-year cross-lagged study of burnout, depression, commitment and work engagement. J Appl Psychol 2008;22:224–41.
78. Frederickson B. The role of positive emotions in positive psychology: the broaden-and-build theory of positive emotions. Am Psychol 2001;56:218–26.
79. Bakker A, Xanthopoulou D. Creativity and charisma among female leaders: The role of resources and work engagement. Int J Hum Resour Manag 2013;24: 2760–79.
80. Bakker A. Building Engagement in the Workplace. In: Burke R, Cooper C, editors. The Peak Performing Organization. Oxon, United Kingdom: Routledge; 2009. p. 50–72.
81. Halbesleben J, Wheeler A. The relative role of engagement and embeddedness in predicting job performance and turnover intention. Work Stress 2008;22: 242–56.

82. Salanova M, Agut S, Peiro J. Linking organizational resources and work engagement to employee performance and customer loyalty: The mediation of service climate. J Appl Psychol 2005;90:1217–27.

83. Harter J, Schmidt F, Hayes T. Business-unit-level relationship between employee satisfaction, employee engagement, and business outcomes: a meta-analysis. J Appl Psychol 2002;87:268–79.

84. Schaufeli WB, Bakker AB. Job demands, job resources and their relationship with burnout and job engagement: A multi-sample study. J Organizational Behav 2004;25:293–315.

Quality of Life Improvement
A Novel Framework and Approach to Well-Being

Jina L. Sinskey, MD, FASA*, Joyce M. Chang, MD[1],
Dorre Nicholau, MD, PhD[2], Michael A. Gropper, MD, PhD[1]

KEYWORDS

- Physician well-being • Wellness • Burnout • Human-centered design
- Quality improvement • Implementation science • Change management

KEY POINTS

- Physician burnout is a complex problem that requires creative solutions and an iterative approach.
- Successful physician well-being efforts incorporate both individual-level and systems-level interventions.
- Two frameworks, the areas of worklife model and modified Maslow's hierarchy of physician burnout and wellness needs can promote a consistent approach to thinking about clinician well-being.
- As each health care organization faces different challenges to clinician well-being, tools to help design customized well-being interventions are more practical than a blanket list of well-being initiatives.
- We introduce the quality of life improvement (QOLI) approach, a novel approach that incorporates principles of human-centered design (HCD), quality improvement (QI), and implementation science (IS).

INTRODUCTION

Physician burnout is a complex problem, and it requires creative solutions that are adaptable to the ever-changing health care environment. While there is increasing awareness of the importance of systems approaches to combat burnout and foster physician well-being, few tools exist for organizations to operationalize the concept of well-being in the clinical setting. Abstract discussions of well-being without

Department of Anesthesia and Perioperative Care, University of California, 550 16th Street, San Francisco, CA 94158, USA
[1] Present address: 521 Parnassus Avenue, 4th Floor, San Francisco, CA 94143-0648.
[2] Present address: 505 Parnassus Avenue, San Francisco CA 94117.
* Corresponding author. 550 16th Street, San Francisco, CA 94158.
E-mail address: Jina.Sinskey@ucsf.edu
Twitter: @JinaSinskeyMD (J.L.S.); @DrJoyceChang (J.M.C.); @gropperUCSF (M.A.G.)

Anesthesiology Clin 40 (2022) 415–432
https://doi.org/10.1016/j.anclin.2022.01.013
1932-2275/22/© 2022 Elsevier Inc. All rights reserved.
anesthesiology.theclinics.com

concrete action can paradoxically contribute to burnout by eroding physicians' trust in leadership and the institution.

Nearly 60% of practicing anesthesiologists report symptoms of burnout with negative consequences for patient safety, physician health, physician retention, and health care system costs.[1,2] The National Academy of Medicine (NAM) released a report in 2019 emphasizing the need for a systems approach to clinician well-being.[3] This represents a shift from traditional well-being efforts, which had disproportionately focused on the individual rather than the organization.

Organizational efforts to enhance well-being require a strategic plan and system-wide initiatives.[4,5] NAM recommends the use of human-centered design (HCD) processes to co-design, implement, and continually improve solutions and interventions that address clinician burnout.[3] Quality improvement (QI) is a well-established process in medicine that functions to continuously improve the delivery of patient care and enhance patient safety. Implementation science (IS) is the scientific study of methods used to promote the uptake of evidence-based interventions into clinical practice. We propose that clinician well-being efforts should be reframed as clinician quality of life improvement (QOLI) to build on existing QI processes that are familiar to clinicians and health care organizations. At the same time, success with this approach will very likely improve patient safety. Here we outline an operational framework and approach that incorporates principles of HCD, QI, and IS to address clinician well-being. Additionally, we share our experience using this approach in a large academic anesthesiology department.

WELL-BEING FRAMEWORKS

Well-being is not simply the absence of burnout, but rather a multidimensional concept that refers to a state of happiness and contentment, fulfillment, engagement, and satisfaction with life. Well-being and quality of life (QOL) are closely related, and the dimensions of well-being closely mirror the domains of QOL (**Fig. 1**).[6,7] The World Health Organization (WHO) defines QOL as "individuals' perception of their position in

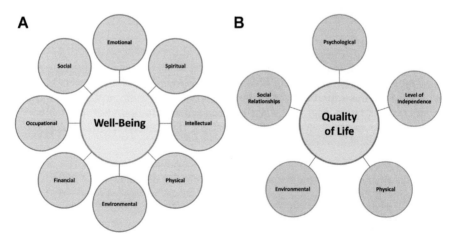

Fig. 1. (*A*) The 8 dimensions of well-being. (*B*) The 5 domains of quality of life. (*[A] Adapted from* Substance Abuse and Mental Health Services Administration (SAMHSA): Creating a Healthier Life: A Step-by-Step Guide to Wellness, 2016; with permission; and [B] Data from World Health Organization. Programme on Mental Health: WHOQOL User Manual. 2012 revision. World Health Organization; 1998).

life in the context of the culture and value systems in which they live and in relation to their goals, expectations, standards, and concerns."[7] It has already been demonstrated that efforts to enhance QOL for patients require a multidisciplinary approach with consistency among the administration, clinical management, and frontline caregivers.[8] Given the overlap between well-being and QOL, reframing clinician well-being as clinician QOL can shift the focus away from a strategy that relies solely on individual-level interventions to one that incorporates both individual-level and systems-level interventions. A recent study found that both individual (eg, family income, personality traits) and organizational factors (eg, workplace atmosphere, relations with hospital management) are associated with increased work-related QOL in anesthesiologists.[9]

A clear structural framework can promote a consistent approach to thinking about clinician well-being. Two such frameworks are (1) the 6 areas of worklife model proposed by Leiter and Maslach and (2) a modified Maslow's hierarchy of physician burnout and wellness needs (**Fig. 2**).[10,11] The areas of worklife model provides an organizational context of burnout by identifying areas of worklife whereby the degree of mismatch between a person and their work is predictive of burnout.[10] These areas are workload, control, reward, community, fairness, and values. This framework allows institutions to develop tailored initiatives to improve matches in these 6 areas. An assessment of clinicians' satisfaction within the 6 areas can provide valuable information to design a well-being strategy that builds on existing strengths while targeting key stressors in the work environment.

The modified Maslow's hierarchy of physician burnout and wellness provides a mechanism to prioritize clinician well-being needs.[11] This practical model states that well-being efforts should start by addressing the basics (eg, physical and mental health), followed by safety (eg, threats to personal safety from time pressure or inadequate staffing) and job security. Once these needs are met, well-being efforts can gradually move up the hierarchy to address clinician needs for respect, appreciation, and the ability to practice medicine fully.

Each health care institution and clinical work unit has its own distinct work culture and environment, and therefore a single cookie-cutter solution will not suffice. These

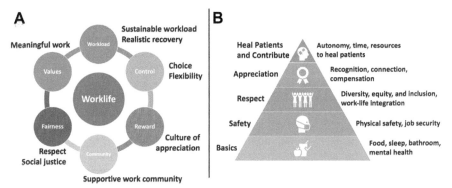

Fig. 2. Well-being frameworks. (*A*) Six areas of worklife. (*B*) Health professional wellness hierarchy. ([A] *Data from* Leiter MP, Maslach C. Six areas of worklife: a model of the organizational context of burnout. J Health Hum Serv Adm. 1999 Spring;21(4):472-89 and Maslach C, Leiter MP. New insights into burnout and health care: Strategies for improving civility and alleviating burnout. Med Teach.2017 Feb;39(2):160-163; and [B] *Adapted from* Shapiro DE, et al. Beyond Burnout: A Physician Wellness Hierarchy Designed to Prioritize Interventions at the Systems Level. Am J Med. 2019 May;(132);556-563;with permission.)

2 frameworks, when used in tandem, can form a dynamic tool to help identify target areas and guide well-being efforts across a variety of clinical settings to build customized solutions.

APPLYING CHANGE MANAGEMENT TO WELL-BEING

Change management is a structured approach to ensure sustainable changes are thoroughly and seamlessly implemented. Kotter developed an 8-step change model for understanding and managing change.[12] Kotter's framework emphasizes that the first steps of change may be invisible. One must lay the groundwork by creating an organizational climate conducive to change and empowering the entire organization to move toward a new way of doing things, before attempting to implement change.

In business, the goal of change management is to make fundamental changes in how business is conducted to help cope with a new, more challenging market environment. This can be applied to addressing physician well-being; we must change how we practice medicine to achieve physician well-being in an evolving health care environment. A core tenet of Kotter's change model is that change requires time, should not be rushed, and must go through a series of steps to achieve success and lasting results.[12] Critical mistakes in any step can have a devastating effect, slowing momentum and negating hard-fought wins. Until now, well-being efforts have been exceedingly reactive, with a focus on treating the symptom of burnout (eg, yoga and meditation) and not the underlying disease itself. A systematic, organizational approach to clinician well-being that addresses the disease, and not just the symptom, is a relatively newer concept. This approach takes time and can invite skepticism as progress may not be readily visible. Incorporating change management principles can help mitigate the risks of introducing this new paradigm for clinician well-being.

LESSONS FROM HUMAN-CENTERED DESIGN, QUALITY IMPROVEMENT, AND IMPLEMENTATION SCIENCE
Human-centered design

Design thinking is an HCD approach used in business and design, with increasing applications in medicine including medical education and learner well-being.[13] Design thinking differentiates itself from other problem-solving methods through (1) early stakeholder engagement to identify the correct problem, (2) a collaborative approach, and (3) continuous and rapid prototyping.[14] HCD has been adopted by numerous health care organizations as a powerful tool to drive innovation in medicine. HCD aims to create solutions that are feasible, viable, and desirable.[14] Feasibility explores what can reasonably be achieved within the foreseeable future, while viability refers to clinical and financial sustainability. Desirability asks whether the problem, and the solution, meet the needs of the target group. For the purposes of clinician well-being efforts, clinicians are the target group. The emphasis on desirability differentiates HCD from traditional problem-solving approaches; the question here is not *how* we solve a given problem, but *what* problem we should solve and *why*. Innovation must occur at the intersection of these 3 criteria to propel sustainable, achievable, and meaningful change. Design thinking involves 5 steps: empathize, define, ideate, prototype, and test.[15] The HCD process is not linear; testing may spawn more ideas and, in some cases, prompt designers to redefine the problem itself.

Quality Improvement

QI is a systematic, formal approach to analyzing and developing interventions to improve practice performance and processes. QI embodies the idea that the system and infrastructure, and not the individual, should be the focus of efforts to improve the quality of care and prevent future harm. Therefore, QI efforts emphasize system issues rather than individual shortcomings in an ongoing process of reassessment, readjustment, and continuous improvement.[16] QI is characterized by a rigorous feedback process which includes systematically defining and evaluating metrics to determine whether improvement efforts lead to intended changes and ensure that there are no unintended negative consequences. Due to the complexity and variability of health care, QI does not equate to blindly implementing a simple solution across all health care organizations. Thoughtful QI efforts require a framework and a toolkit of strategies and processes rather than a list of QI interventions.

Implementation Science

Implementation science is the systematic study of how to design and evaluate a set of activities to facilitate the successful uptake of an evidence-based health intervention.[17] In health care, there is a long history of failure to translate evidence into routine clinical practice due to a lack of systematic assessments of crucial barriers, enablers, and target factors that are critical for successful implementation. The fundamental principles of IS aim to bridge this gap. A key IS principle is behavior change theory, which attempts to explain why human behaviors change and apply this insight to design implementation strategies. A second important principle is engaging the right individuals and stakeholders upfront. Successful implementation requires insights from members of the target group as well as key decision makers and stakeholders with funding and resources. IS benefits from flexibility and nonlinear approaches to fit within real-world situations.[17] Similar to QI, a cyclical rather than linear approach is more effective.

THE QUALITY OF LIFE IMPROVEMENT APPROACH TO WELL-BEING

We believe that framing clinician well-being efforts as clinician QOLI will help organizations adopt a systems approach by (1) viewing well-being as a multidimensional concept akin to QOL and (2) using QI techniques and strategies that are already integrated into many health care institutions' organizational culture. We have developed a novel approach to designing clinician well-being interventions, the QOLI approach, which integrates principles of HCD, QI, and IS (**Fig. 3**, **Table 1**). The 3 methods of HCD, QI, and IS are powerful tools for designing and implementing health care solutions on their own. Hybrid approaches that incorporate one or more of these methods can yield synergistic results.[18,19] The QOLI approach consists of three phases presented as 3 questions: (I) why is this problem important, (II) what are we going to do about it, and (III) how do we keep improving? Detailed strategies and techniques for each step of the QOLI approach as well as relevant concepts from HCD, QI, and IS are presented in **Table 1**. The QOLI approach is an iterative process, and steps should be repeated as necessary.

Phase I: Why is this Problem Important?

For complex issues such as the ongoing threat to physician well-being, the defining parameters of the problem will determine how it is addressed. As Albert Einstein stated, "If I had an hour to solve a problem, I'd spend 55 minutes thinking about the problem and 5 minutes thinking about solutions." The first phase of the QOLI approach focuses on establishing the problem by building a team, assessing the landscape, and defining the problem.

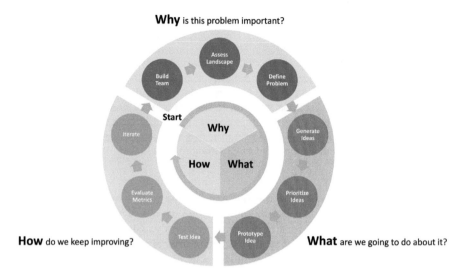

Fig. 3. The quality of life improvement (QOLI) approach.

Step 1: build the team

Well-being efforts require a core team consisting of members with different areas of expertise and diverse backgrounds (**Fig. 4**). As in QI, well-being teams should include members with 3 kinds of expertise: system leadership, technical expertise, and day-to-day leadership.[20] Sponsors provide system leadership and support for well-being efforts by committing necessary resources and lowering barriers. Front-line clinician well-being champions bring technical expertise as they are familiar with specific workplace stressors and drivers of engagement. They also provide day-to-day leadership to drive well-being initiatives forward. Per IS principles, well-being teams should include individuals in the target group (ie, front-line clinicians). A formal appointed role combined with protected time can increase the efficacy of front-line clinician well-being champions.[4] Depending on the specific well-being initiative and target clinical setting, the core team may include satellite members with additional technical expertise and day-to-day leadership.

Physician well-being efforts hinge on creating psychological safety to empower clinicians to share issues without fear of retribution. A team structure with designated front-line clinician well-being champions lowers the barrier for clinician input by alleviating concerns of stigmatization. Psychological safety is difficult to create and easy to destroy. Hence, all well-being core team members must actively engage in behaviors that nurture a safe atmosphere. Sponsors set the tone for well-being efforts, as well as for overarching workplace culture and work environment. A recent model of Wellness-Centered Leadership outlines specific skills and behaviors for leaders and sponsors to promote clinician well-being.[21] Ideal, effective front-line clinician well-being champions are individuals who are receptive to feedback, respected by their peers, approachable, and readily accessible in the clinical setting. Furthermore, they should be comfortable sharing well-being concerns directly and openly with leadership. Such qualities, combined with a strong commitment to enhancing well-being, are more important than specific expertise in well-being improvement science.[4]

Our department's well-being core team consisted of the department chair and department vice-chair of professionalism and well-being as sponsors, and front-line

Table 1
Strategies for each step of the quality of life improvement (QOLI) approach with relevant principles and tools from human-centered design, quality improvement, and implementation science

	Human-Centered Design[15]	Quality Improvement[23]	Implementation Science[17]	QOLI Strategies and Techniques
Build Team	• Engage stakeholders early	• Team needs 3 types of expertise: System leadership, technical expertise, day-to-day leadership	• Three categories of stakeholders to consider: Individuals, delivery systems, government agencies • Team should include members of the target group	• Sponsors: Provide resources and public support for well-being initiatives, lower barriers, drive culture • Clinician well-being champions: Frontline clinicians have insight into key stressors and technical expertise
Assess Landscape	• Empathize: Start by focusing on people, not the problem	• Use objective data • Identify whereby there is an opportunity for improvement • Go to the genba	• Identify evidence-based practice that should translated into clinical practice	• Internal assessment: Visit the clinical setting, surveys, focus groups/interviews • External assessment: Literature search, knowledge sharing with other institutions/departments • Maximize psychological safety during the internal assessment
Define Problem	• Define a problem statement	• Write a problem statement with the audience in mind • Lean A3 template	• Determine the evidence-practice gap to address	• Frame problem statements as "How might we…" questions • Do not include potential solutions in the problem statement • Create problem statements of appropriate scope • Write a problem statement with stakeholders in mind

(continued on next page)

Table 1
(continued)

	Human-Centered Design[15]	Quality Improvement[23]	Implementation Science[17]	QOLI Strategies and Techniques
Generate Ideas	• Ideate: Go broad ("flare") Tools: The 5 whys	• Tools: Cause and effect ("fishbone") diagram, process mapping, the 5 whys	• Behavior change theory: COM-B Model, Behavior Change Wheel	• Do not limit potential solutions too early • Can use QI tools to encourage brainstorming of ideas • Consider behavior change theory in developing ideas • Categorize ideas before moving on to the prioritization step
Prioritize Ideas	• Ideate: Select ideas ("focus") • Four categories, post-it voting • Three criteria of design thinking: feasibility, viability, desirability	• PICK chart: Possible, Implement, Challenge, Kill	• Consultation with local stakeholders for feasible, appropriate, and acceptable ideas	• Ideas must be feasible, viable/appropriate, and desirable/acceptable • Start with ideas that are easy to implement with a high payoff • Consider ideas that are easy to implement with a low payoff to generate early wins • Create a plan for ideas that are difficult to implement with a high payoff
Prototype Idea	• Prototype: Rapid prototyping • Contextual prototyping • User-driven prototyping			• Design each prototype to test a particular aspect of a given idea • Have a plan to test prototypes in the clinical setting with clinicians • Invite clinicians to engage in prototyping
Test Idea	• Test	• Plan-Do-Study-Act (PDSA) cycle: Plan, Do • Plan to test change: Who? What? When? Where? Why?	• Select key evaluation questions for process evaluation (was intervention implemented as intended) and summative evaluation (did the change occur because of the intervention)	• Create a plan for collecting data before running the test • Establish metrics before running the test

Evaluate Metrics	• Test	• PDSA cycle: Study • Measures: Outcome, process, balancing (unintended consequences)	• Perform process evaluation and summative evaluation • Assess for unintended consequences	• Use a systematic approach • Gather feedback and data after each test cycle
Iterate	• Rapid prototype-test cycles	• PDSA cycle: Act • Iteratively reassess	• Use a cyclical approach to fit within real-world situations • Keep in mind that the environment and context may change over time	• Several mini pilots are better than a single large pilot • Have a plan to regularly reassess

(*Data from* Stanford d.school. Design Thinking Bootleg.; 2018.; Quality Improvement Essentials Toolkit. Institute for Healthcare Improvement. Boston, MA. Accessed September 21, 2021. http://www.ihi.org/resources/Pages/Tools/Quality-Improvement-Essentials-Toolkit.aspx.; Handley MA, Gorukanti A, Cattamanchi A. Strategies for implementing implementation science: a methodological overview. Emerg Med J EMJ. 2016;33(9):660–664. https://doi.org/10.1136/emermed-2015-205461.

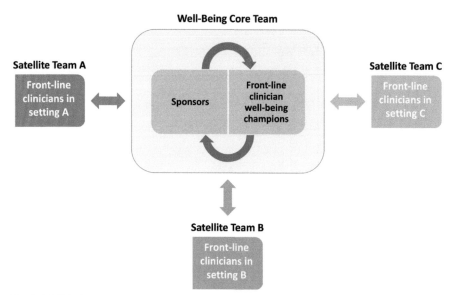

Fig. 4. Well-being team structure.

clinician well-being champions representing faculty members at various career stages including junior faculty. This team structure promoted early stakeholder engagement while ensuring buy-in and public support from departmental leadership. Subsequently, an associate chair of well-being and director positions for faculty and learner well-being was established to provide formal roles and dedicated time. The associate chair position uniquely represents a hybrid of both sponsor and front-line clinician well-being champion roles. We believe the most effective type of leader to tackle the complex issue of clinician well-being is one that can combine the strengths of a sponsor with the strengths of a front-line clinician well-being champion. This will enable the well-being team to identify new threats to well-being on an ongoing basis and address them expeditiously.

Step 2: assess the landscape
The next step is to perform an internal and external assessment of the well-being landscape. A core tenet of HCD is to start by focusing on the people instead of the problem. For clinician well-being efforts, an internal assessment is required to better understand clinician needs. The internal assessment must include visits to the clinical setting for all core team members, especially sponsors. In Lean Six Sigma, a QI methodology, this is called "going to the genba," with genba literally translated as "the real place," or whereby the real work happens. According to Toyota chairman Fujio Cho (Lean grew out of the Toyota Production System), going to the genba allows leaders to "go see, ask why, show respect." Clinician well-being efforts, at their core, are about supporting people and building engagement. Showing respect for clinicians translates to designing interventions that help, and at minimum, do not hinder daily clinical practice. Focus groups, one-on-one interviews, and surveys can provide additional information about the internal landscape. The internal assessment should be planned and performed with an emphasis on maximizing psychological safety by ensuring confidentiality and anonymity as desired by clinicians sharing their concerns.

An external assessment can create a foundation for well-being efforts and avoid "reinventing the wheel." As in IS, which focuses heavily on evidence-based frameworks and interventions, the external assessment may take shape as a literature review of evidence-based approaches to well-being in anesthesiology, other medical specialties, and those outside of the medical field. As evidence remains limited for systems-level well-being interventions, another approach to the external assessment is through knowledge sharing with other departments and health care institutions.[3]

The first step of our internal assessment was to solicit faculty member input through a department-wide e-mail asking faculty to share concerns and constructive ideas to improve their workload, work environment, and scheduling. To ensure psychological safety, responses were sent to the well-being core team, excluding the department chair, and compiled to maintain anonymity. Responses were then discussed at fireside chats moderated by the vice-chair of professionalism and well-being and a front-line clinician well-being champion. Attendees included the department chair and all faculty who wished to participate. Fireside chats improved transparency by fostering open dialogue.

Our external assessment involved a review of well-being literature as well as virtual and in-person discussions with well-being thought leaders and champions. To gain a broader perspective, our well-being core team connected with individuals from other departments in our institution (eg, hospital medicine) as well as anesthesiology departments across the country.

Step 3: define the problem

The next step is to define a problem statement based on insights gained from internal and external assessments. In HCD, a problem statement begins with the phrase, "How might we...?". Problem statements should have a scope that is narrow enough to be actionable, yet broad enough to encourage creativity. In addition, the problem statement should remain fact-based and not include a potential solution. Incorporating a potential solution will introduce bias and can misdirect efforts to solve problem. A problem statement should be written with the audience (eg, leadership, clinicians) in mind to provide clear communication and a unified vision, which in turn will encourage buy-in from stakeholders.

We defined several problem statements based on themes that emerged during the fireside chats (**Table 2**). One common theme was the lack of control and predictability related to scheduling. For example, faculty members were concerned about reliably attending to personal matters (eg, medical appointments, picking up children from daycare after work) on noncall days given the prevalence of noncall faculty leaving late in the evening due to unpredictability in the operating room (OR) schedule. For this theme we defined our problem statement as, "How might we increase scheduling predictability?" and mapped it to the "Workload" and "Control" areas of worklife.

Phase II: What are we going to do about it?

Once the problem has been defined, the focus shifts to finding potential solutions. In phase two of the QOLI approach, the well-being core team should brainstorm and prioritize potential solutions, then develop prototypes for testing.

Step 4: generate ideas

When generating ideas, it is important to consider all possibilities with the mindset that no idea is off-limits. Brainstorming is, by definition, a team effort. Psychological safety must be established and maintained within the team to encourage the participation and sharing of ideas. Four rules of brainstorming are (1) emphasize quantity over

Table 2
Faculty well-being problem statements mapped to the areas of worklife

Problem Statement	Area(s) of Worklife
How might we build a sense of community?	Community
How might we decrease nonphysician work?	Workload
How might we find more meaning in work?	Values
How might we increase scheduling predictability?	Workload Control
How might we improve lactation support for women faculty?	Fairness
How might we enhance transparency and fairness?	Fairness

quality of ideas, (2) withhold criticism, (3) welcome unusual or wild ideas, and (4) combine and improve ideas.[22] This can create fluency (ie, volume) and flexibility (ie, variety) in potential solutions.[15] QI tools such as process maps, cause-and-effect diagrams (eg, fishbone diagrams) and the Five Whys (ie, tool to identify root cause) can be useful to help brainstorm ideas.[23] These tools provide a systematic way of generating ideas when the team slows or gets stuck. Brainstormed ideas can be grouped into categories or themes to facilitate prioritization.

For the problem statement "How might we increase scheduling predictability?", ideas ranged from creating early leave shifts to not performing elective surgeries after a certain time (**Fig. 5**). These ideas were categorized into 2 groups: individual scheduling predictability and OR scheduling predictability.

Step 5: prioritize ideas

An essential step to operationalizing well-being is to identify which interventions have the highest yield for the level of investment. The answer to this question, like most questions in medicine, is that it depends. Every health care organization has a different culture and work environment, and therefore key stressors vary by clinical setting.

Generate

- Decrease PACU holds
- Create early leave shift
- Increase late shift staffing
- No elective cases after a certain time
- Shorten turnovers between cases
- Enforce on-time starts for first cases

Categorize

Increase individual scheduling predictability:
- Create early leave shift
- Increase late shift staffing

Increase operating room scheduling predictability:
- Decrease PACU holds
- No elective cases after a certain time
- Shorten turnovers between cases
- Enforce on-time starts for first cases

Fig. 5. Example of generating and categorizing ideas for increasing scheduling predictability. Note: this is note an exhaustive list of generated ideas.

Thus, tools to help prioritize ideas are more practical than a universal list of recommended well-being initiatives.

Two methods from HCD, IS and QI can help with prioritization. The first method builds on 3 criteria aligned between HCD and IS. The 3 criteria of HCD solutions are feasibility, viability, and desirability. In IS, these criteria translate to feasibility, appropriateness, and acceptability. Feasibility is defined as the extent to which an intervention can be successfully implemented.[24] Appropriateness refers to the perceived relevance or usefulness of the intervention, while acceptability refers to whether a proposed solution is agreeable, palatable, or satisfactory. When assessing ideas, those that have been successfully implemented in other departments and health care organizations may receive higher marks for feasibility and viability. Ideas must meet all 3 criteria to be implemented. Well-being initiatives that are viable and feasible, but not desirable, will detract from clinician well-being.

The second method is to determine the perceived payoff and level of difficulty of each idea. The PICK (Possible, Implement, Challenge, and Kill) chart is a Lean Six Sigma tool commonly used to prioritize QI efforts in health care by assessing ease of implementation and level of payoff.[25] Well-being initiatives that fall in the "Implement" category should be prioritized first, followed by "Possible," which represent quick wins. Creating a plan for "Challenge" initiatives can help build a long-term strategy. Initiatives in the "Kill" category should not be pursued further.

Ideas to increase scheduling predictability were prioritized using the 2 methods (Table 3). One idea was to create an early leave position for faculty. Faculty members could request to be scheduled as "early leave" on certain days and would be prioritized to be relieved of their clinical duties that day. Using our 2 methods, an early leave shift met the 3 HCD/IS criteria and fell into the "Implement" category on the PICK chart. Another idea was to create late stay positions for faculty. In this new position, faculty would start their shift later in the day and be responsible for relieving noncall faculty. This would increase flexibility for faculty wanting to fulfill nonclinical commitments and personal appointments in the morning while facilitating earlier leave times for noncall faculty. The late stay position also met all 3 HCD/IS criteria and fell into the "Implement" category. Therefore, ideas for both early leave shifts and late stay positions advanced to the prototype step. Not performing elective surgeries after a certain time, on the other hand, was not feasible or viable and fell into the "Kill" category. As a result, this idea was not moved forward.

One major stressor that was identified during the internal assessment was the prevalence of postanesthesia care unit (PACU) holds. PACU holds refer to a bottleneck

Table 3
Example of prioritizing ideas for increasing scheduling predictability

Idea	Three Criteria			PICK Chart Category
	Feasible	Viable	Desirable	
Create early leave shift	Yes	Yes	Yes	Implement
Increase late shift staffing	Yes	Yes	Yes	Implement
Decrease PACU holds	Unsure	Yes	Yes	Challenge
No elective cases after 5 PM	No	No	No	Kill
Shorten turnovers between cases	Unsure	Yes	Yes	Challenge
Enforce on-time starts for first cases	Unsure	Yes	Yes	Challenge

Note: this is not an exhaustive list of generated ideas. OR: operating room.

between the OR and PACU when the PACU reaches capacity and patients must remain in the OR. As a result, the workday becomes longer, and subsequent surgeries may be delayed or canceled. This is detrimental to patient care and resource utilization as well as the well-being of perioperative team members. Reducing PACU holds was desirable and viable, but there were questions about feasibility. This idea fell into the "Challenge" category and was tabled with plans to gather more information.

Step 6: prototype idea

The next step after ideation is prototyping. Prototypes provide opportunities to determine whether further investment in the idea is warranted and if so, what specific improvements should be made. Strategies for rapid prototyping in HCD are integrated into the QOLI approach.[15] Prototypes should be designed to test a particular aspect of the idea as opposed to testing a full-scale solution. Prototypes for well-being interventions should be tested in the clinical setting with clinicians (contextual prototyping) and clinicians should be invited to actively engage in the prototyping process (user-driven prototyping) with the goal of revealing undetected needs and insights. We have found it best to prototype and test a maximum of 3 to 5 well-being interventions at any given time. Details regarding how to test a prototyped idea will be discussed in the next step.

For the early leave shift, an initial prototype was created to determine (1) whether the concept of an early leave position was feasible at a busy clinical site and (2) whether the position facilitated early leave faculty members being able to make their commitments.

For the late stay positions, a prototype was created to determine (1) whether the concept of a late stay position was feasible at a busy clinical site, (2) whether the positions facilitated noncall faculty leaving earlier in the day, and (3) whether the position facilitated late stay faculty members being able to make their commitments.

Phase III: How do we Keep Improving?

The final phase of the QOLI approach is to create a plan for continuous improvement. This phase closely resembles a Plan-Do-Study-Act (PDSA) cycle, which is a systematic process used to design health care QI initiatives and provides a structure to promote iterative testing.[26] The goal of each PDSA cycle is to test a change. Steps are to plan the test (Plan), run the test (Do), analyze and learn (Study), and determine what modifications, if any, to make for the next cycle (Act).[23]

Step 7: test idea

As in HCD, rapid prototyping should occur with multiple prototype-test cycles. However, this should not happen at the expense of careful planning to maximize learning from each cycle. The testing plan should include the purpose of the test, the "5 Ws" (Who, What, When, Where, Why) of the testing process, and indicators of success to be measured.[27] Tests should occur on a small scale to refine the idea before implementation on a broader scale.[26]

For both the early leave shift and late stay position, the first prototype was rolled out at one clinical site and tested over several months. With the prototype goals in mind, a testing plan for the early leave shift was made to (1) ask a group of charge anesthesiologists who "run the board" (ie, coordinate OR assignments and scheduling) whether they could reliably relieve the "early leave" faculty, (2) ascertain leave times for faculty who were assigned to this shift, and (3) ask faculty assigned to the early leave shift whether they were able to make their commitments. For the late stay position, a testing plan was created to (1) ask a group of charge anesthesiologists whether they could reliably staff all ORs at the beginning of the day, (2) ascertain leave times for noncall faculty, and (3) ask faculty assigned to the late stay position whether they were able to make their commitments.

Step 8: evaluate metrics

Although evaluating metrics falls under testing, we have intentionally labeled it as its own step to underscore the importance of collecting feedback and data related to predetermined measures after each test, as posttest feedback informs the rest of the process. There are 3 outcomes of a PDSA cycle: adapt (refine and run another test), adopt (test on a larger scale), or abandon (do not perform more testing on this idea).[23]

Testing of the first early leave shift prototype revealed that the shift was feasible to implement from an overall scheduling standpoint, based on feedback from charge anesthesiologists. However, faculty leave times demonstrated that the shift was consistently longer on certain days; for example, faculty members scheduled as "early leave" during July (ie, when new anesthesiology residents and faculty were paired one-on-one) and on resident education days (ie, protected time for resident didactics) stayed much later. Feedback from faculty indicated that the shift successfully enabled faculty members to make their commitments outside of clinical work. Based on this information, the decision was made to "adapt" by maintaining the early leave shift but avoiding scheduling early leave shifts during July and on resident education days.

Testing of the late stay position showed that the position was feasible based on feedback from charge anesthesiologists, facilitated earlier leave times for noncall faculty, and allowed late stay position faculty to meet their morning commitments. Therefore, the decision was made to "adopt" by keeping these new positions with minimal change.

Step 9: iterate

The QOLI approach is iterative by design, which is a unifying feature of HCD, QI, and IS. Each step of the QOLI approach informs all other steps, whether they precede or follow the step. For example, testing an idea "may reveal that, not only did you get the solution wrong, but you also framed the problem incorrectly."[15] If this is the case, the team needs to revisit step 3 to redefine the problem. The team should regularly revisit ideas in the "Challenge" category as well as potential solutions that were not implemented to determine whether they should be moved forward. Even when a solution is deemed to improve clinician well-being, it should be revisited regularly, as new threats to well-being can appear at any time that may render an implemented solution irrelevant. Regular internal assessments through surveys and visits to the clinical setting will help identify additional opportunities to improve well-being.

Once we completed the prototype-test cycle for the early leave shift and late stay positions, we decided to revisit the PACU hold idea, which had been deferred due to questions about feasibility with a plan to collect more information. While testing the other 2 ideas, our vice-chair worked with perioperative and medical center leadership to identify potential solutions to decompress the PACU. One prototype was the creation of additional recovery beds to improve PACU throughput. This prototype was tested, and it was determined that despite requiring considerable resources, creating additional recovery beds would be worth the investment due to its high payoff. Additional recovery beds were created for postoperative short-stay patients and patients receiving anesthesia outside of the OR (ie, non-OR anesthesia), which resulted in a marked decrease in PACU holds.

Our department's efforts to increase scheduling predictability predated the coronavirus disease 2019 (COVID-19) pandemic. Early in the pandemic, elective surgeries were canceled, which resulted in a complete overhaul of faculty scheduling and new stressors due to faculty being under-scheduled with financial ramifications. Following the first wave of the pandemic, surgical volume ballooned, which then led to gross over-scheduling of faculty. These abrupt changes in the surgical volume demonstrate the ever-changing nature of the perioperative environment and underscore the necessity of an iterative approach to well-being.

NEXT STEPS

Anesthesiologists do not practice in a vacuum and well-being initiatives will have limited success without the participation of all stakeholders. Efforts to address the perioperative culture and work environment require buy-in from anesthesiologists, surgeons, and perioperative nurses. We have assembled a team of stakeholders from these 3 groups and will apply the QOLI approach to design and implement broader perioperative well-being initiatives. We hope these efforts will facilitate a comprehensive and systematic approach to improve perioperative clinician well-being.

SUMMARY

Physician well-being efforts must include systems-level interventions to address the work culture and environment. Each health care organization faces different challenges to clinician well-being, and tools to help design customized well-being interventions are more practical than a blanket list of well-being initiatives. Operationalizing well-being at the organizational level requires a consistent framework and approach. As demonstrated during the COVID-19 pandemic, new threats to well-being can arise at any time, and well-being teams must adopt an iterative approach to enhance clinician well-being. The QOLI approach incorporates principles of HCD, QI, and IS and serves as a pragmatic tool to bridge the gap between well-being theory and practice.

FINANCIAL DISCLOSURE

J. L. Sinskey, J. M. Chang, and D. Nicholau have nothing to disclose. M. A. Gropper has received royalties from Elsevier and his spouse is an officer and shareholder for Kindbody, Inc. (no conflict related to this work).

CONFLICTS OF INTEREST

J. L. Sinskey is the Vice-Chair of the American Society of Anesthesiologists' Committee on Physician Well-being. J. M. Chang, D. Nicholau, and M. A. Gropper have nothing to disclose.

REFERENCES

1. Afonso AM, Cadwell JB, Staffa SJ, et al. Burnout rate and risk factors among anesthesiologists in the United States. Anesthesiology 2021;134(5):683–96.
2. West CP, Dyrbye LN, Shanafelt TD. Physician burnout: contributors, consequences and solutions. J Intern Med 2018;283(6):516–29.
3. National Academies of Sciences, Engineering, and Medicine. Taking Action Against Clinician Burnout: A Systems Approach to Professional Well-Being. Washington, DC: The National Academies Press; 2019.

4. Tait S, Sherilyn S, Jill S, et al. A blueprint for organizational strategies to promote the well-being of health care professionals. NEJM Catal 2020;1(6). https://doi.org/10.1056/CAT.20.0266.
5. Shanafelt TD, Noseworthy JH. Executive leadership and physician well-being: nine organizational strategies to promote engagement and reduce burnout. Mayo Clin Proc 2017;92(1):129–46.
6. Rockville MD. Substance Abuse and Mental Health Services Administration (SAMHSA): Creating a healthier life: a step-by-step guide to wellness. US Dept of Health and Human Services 2016.
7. World Health Organization. Programme on Mental Health: WHOQOL User Manual, 2012 revision. Geneva (Switzerland): World Health Organization; 1998. https://apps.who.int/iris/handle/10665/77932.
8. Sagha Zadeh R, Eshelman P, Setla J, et al. Strategies to improve quality of life at the end of life: interdisciplinary team perspectives. Am J Hosp Palliat Care 2018;35(3):411–6.
9. Gafsou B, Becq MC, Michelet D, et al. Determinants of work-related quality of life in French anesthesiologists. Anesth Analg 2021;133(4):863–72.
10. Maslach C, Leiter MP. New insights into burnout and health care: strategies for improving civility and alleviating burnout. Med Teach 2017;39(2):160–3.
11. Shapiro DE, Duquette C, Abbott LM, et al. Beyond burnout: a physician wellness hierarchy designed to prioritize interventions at the systems level. Am J Med 2019;132(5):556–63.
12. Kotter JP. Leading Change. Boston (MA): Harvard Business Review Press; 2012.
13. Thomas LR, Nguyen R, Teherani A, et al. Designing well-being: using design thinking to engage residents in developing well-being interventions. Acad Med 2020;95(7):1038–42.
14. IDEO (Firm). The field guide to human-centered design : design kit.; 2015.
15. Stanford d.school. Design Thinking Bootleg. Stanford, California; 2018.
16. Varkey P, Reller MK, Resar RK. Basics of quality improvement in health care. Mayo Clin Proc 2007;82(6):735–9.
17. Handley MA, Gorukanti A, Cattamanchi A. Strategies for implementing implementation science: a methodological overview. Emerg Med J 2016;33(9):660–4.
18. Beres LK, Simbeza S, Holmes CB, et al. Human-centered design lessons for implementation science: improving the implementation of a patient-centered care intervention. J Acquir Immune Defic Syndr 2019;82(Suppl 3):S230–43.
19. Fischer M, Safaeinili N, Haverfield MC, et al. Approach to human-centered, evidence-driven adaptive design (AHEAD) for health care interventions: a proposed framework. J Gen Intern Med 2021;36(4):1041–8.
20. Institute for Healthcare Improvement. Science of improvement: forming the team. Available at: http://www.ihi.org/resources/Pages/HowtoImprove/ScienceofImprovementFormingtheTeam.aspx. Accessed August 8, 2021.
21. Shanafelt T, Trockel M, Rodriguez A, et al. Wellness-centered leadership: equipping health care leaders to cultivate physician well-being and professional fulfillment. Acad Med J Assoc Am Med Coll 2020. https://doi.org/10.1097/ACM.0000000000003907.
22. Osborn AF. Applied Imagination; Principles and Procedures of Creative Thinking. New York: Scribner; 1953.
23. Quality improvement essentials toolkit. Institute for Healthcare Improvement. Boston, MA. Available at: http://www.ihi.org/resources/Pages/Tools/Quality-Improvement-Essentials-Toolkit.aspx. Accessed September 21, 2021.

24. Proctor E, Silmere H, Raghavan R, et al. Outcomes for implementation research: conceptual distinctions, measurement challenges, and research agenda. Adm Policy Ment Health 2011;38(2):65–76. https://doi.org/10.1007/s10488-010-0319-7.
25. PICK chart. Wikipedia; 2021. Available at: https://en.wikipedia.org/w/index.php?title=Pick_chart&oldid=1033045071. Accessed August 25, 2021.
26. How to Improve | IHI - Institute for Healthcare Improvement. Available at: http://www.ihi.org/resources/Pages/HowtoImprove/default.aspx. Accessed December 16, 2020.
27. Health Quality Ontario. Measurement for Quality Improvement. Toronto (ON): Health Quality Ontario; 2013.

Moving?

Make sure your subscription moves with you!

To notify us of your new address, find your **Clinics Account Number** (located on your mailing label above your name), and contact customer service at:

Email: journalscustomerservice-usa@elsevier.com

800-654-2452 (subscribers in the U.S. & Canada)
314-447-8871 (subscribers outside of the U.S. & Canada)

Fax number: 314-447-8029

Elsevier Health Sciences Division
Subscription Customer Service
3251 Riverport Lane
Maryland Heights, MO 63043

*To ensure uninterrupted delivery of your subscription, please notify us at least 4 weeks in advance of move.

9780323987813